Male Lower Urinary Tract Symptoms
and Benign Prostatic Hyperplasia

Male Lower Urinary Tract Symptoms and Benign Prostatic Hyperplasia

EDITED BY

Steven A. Kaplan, MD

E. Darracott Vaughan Jr. Professor of Urology
Weill Cornell Medical College
Director, Iris Cantor Men's Health Center
New York Presbyterian Hospital
New York, NY, USA

Kevin T. McVary, MD, FACS

Professor and Chair
Division of Urology
Southern Illinois University School of Medicine
Springfield, IL, USA

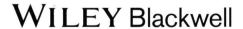

This edition first published 2014 © 2014 by John Wiley & Sons, Ltd

Registered Office

John Wiley & Sons, Ltd, The Atrium, Southern Gate, Chichester, West Sussex, PO19 8SQ, UK

Editorial Offices

9600 Garsington Road, Oxford, OX4 2DQ, UK

The Atrium, Southern Gate, Chichester, West Sussex, PO19 8SQ, UK

111 River Street, Hoboken, NJ 07030-5774, USA

For details of our global editorial offices, for customer services and for information about how to apply for permission to reuse the copyright material in this book please see our website at www.wiley.com/wiley-blackwell

Library of Congress Cataloging-in-Publication Data

Male lower urinary tract symptoms and benign prostatic hyperplasia / edited by Steven A. Kaplan, Kevin T. McVary.
    p. ; cm.
  Includes bibliographical references and index.
  ISBN 978-1-118-43799-5 (cloth)
  I. Kaplan, Steven A., editor. II. McVary, Kevin T., editor.
  [DNLM: 1. Lower Urinary Tract Symptoms. 2. Prostatic Hyperplasia. WJ 752]
  RC877
  616.6′5–dc23
                        2014013140

A catalogue record for this book is available from the British Library.

Wiley also publishes its books in a variety of electronic formats. Some content that appears in print may not be available in electronic books.

Cover image: ©iStockphoto/Artopat
Cover design by Andy Meaden

Set in 9.5/13pt Meridien by SPi Publisher Services, Pondicherry, India
Printed and bound in Malaysia by Vivar Printing Sdn Bhd

1   2014

Contents

Contributors

Aaron M. Bernie, MD, MPH
Department of Urology
Weill Cornell Medical College
New York-Presbyterian Hospital
New York, NY, USA

Benjamin N. Breyer, MD, MAS
University of California San Francisco
Department of Urology
San Francisco, CA, USA

Reginald Bruskewitz, MD
University of Wisconsin
Madison, WI, USA

Christopher R. Chapple, BSc, MD, FRCS(Urol)
Department of Urology
Royal Hallamshire Hospital
Sheffield, UK

Bilal Chughtai, MD
Department of Urology
Weill Cornell Medical College
New York-Presbyterian Hospital
New York, NY, USA

Anne Darves-Bornoz, MD
Garden City
New York, NY, USA

Jean J. M. C. H. de la Rosette, MD, PhD
Department of Urology
Academic Medical Center
University of Amsterdam
Amsterdam, The Netherlands

Christopher P. Filson, MD, MS
University of Michigan
Department of Urology
Division of Health Services Research
Ann Arbor, MI, USA

Nathaly François, MD
Division of Urology
Southern Illinois University School
of Medicine
Springfield, IL, USA

Claudius Füllhase, MD
Department of Urology
Großhadern Hospital
Ludwig-Maximilians-University
Munich, Germany

Mauro Gacci, MD
Department of Urology
University of Florence
Careggi Hospital
Florence, Italy

Robert H. Getzenberg, PhD
GTx Inc.
Memphis, TN, USA

Peter J. Gilling, MBChB, MD, FRACS
University of Auckland
Urology BOP Limited
Tauranga, New Zealand

Christian Gratzke, MD
Department of Urology
LMU Munich
Munich, Germany

Stavros Gravas, MD
Department of Urology
University of Thessalia
Larissa, Greece

Annika Herlemann, MD
Department of Urology
LMU Munich
Munich, Germany

Aaron E. Katz, MD
Garden City
New York, NY, USA

Prakash Kulkarni, PhD
James Buchanan Brady Urological Institute
Johns Hopkins University School of Medicine
Baltimore, MD, USA

Richard Lee, MD MBA
Departments of Urology
Weill Cornell Medical College
New York-Presbyterian Hospital
New York, NY, USA

Casey Lythgoe, MD
Division of Urology
Southern Illinois University School of Medicine
Springfield, IL, USA

Marty M. Miner, MD
Warren Alpert School of Medicine
Brown University, Providence, RI, USA

Matthias Oelke, MD, FEBU
Department of Urology
Hannover Medical School
Hannover, Germany

Nadir I. Osman, MBChB, MRCS
Department of Urology
Royal Hallamshire Hospital
Sheffield, UK

Raunak D. Patel, MS
Division of Urology
Southern Illinois University School of Medicine
Springfield, IL, USA

John B. Riley
Mid Michigan Health Centers
Jackson, MI, USA

Claus G. Roehrborn, MD
Department of Urology
UT Southwestern Medical Center
Dallas, TX, USA

Raymond C. Rosen, PhD
New England Research Institutes
Watertown, MA, USA

Matt T. Rosenberg, MD
Mid Michigan Health Centers
Jackson, MI, USA

Matteo Salvi, MD
Department of Urology
University of Florence
Careggi Hospital
Florence, Italy

Arcangelo Sebastianelli, MD
Department of Urology
University of Florence
Careggi Hospital
Florence, Italy

Roberto Soler, MD, PhD
Division of Urology
Federal University of São Paulo
São Paulo, Brazil

Alexis E. Te, MD
Department of Urology
Weill Cornell Medical College
New York-Presbyterian Hospital
New York, NY, USA

Simon van Rij, MBChB, FRACS
Tauranga Hospital
Tauranga, New Zealand

John T. Wei, MD, MS
University of Michigan
Department of Urology
Division of Health Services Research
Ann Arbor, MI, USA

CHAPTER 1

Etiology and Pathogenesis

Robert H. Getzenberg[1] & Prakash Kulkarni[2]

[1]GTx Inc., Memphis, TN, USA
[2]James Buchanan Brady Urological Institute, Johns Hopkins University School of Medicine, Baltimore, MD, USA

Key points

- Lower urinary tract symptoms (LUTS) corresponding to benign prostatic hyperplasia (BPH) are a complex disease that may represent distinct etiologies.
- By deciphering the molecular underpinnings, we can begin to delineate the distinct causes and identify different readouts, and therefore formulate and individualize therapies.
- BPH/LUTS involves the cellular components of the prostate including the epithelial and stromal cells.
- A number of steroid hormones including androgens, estrogens, and progesterone, along with various growth factors and chemokines have been demonstrated to contribute to the abnormal regulation of prostatic growth.
- Although inflammation has been demonstrated to be associated with BPH/LUTS, anti-inflammatory treatment approaches have, in general, not been shown to be effective.
- Cancer/testis antigens have been shown to be associated with BPH with more severe symptoms and therefore may serve as novel biomarkers thereof.

Introduction

Diseases of the prostate are some of the most common and devastating diseases in men, especially as they age. Indeed, the prevalence of BPH is estimated to begin its increase in the third decade of life from 5–10% to greater than 90% for men above 85 years of age [1]. One in four males will undergo surgery at some time in their life to relieve symptoms of BPH, which compresses the urethra and produces urinary-outflow obstruction. Although the use of pharmacologic agents has increased in the treatment of this disease, transurethral resection of the prostate (TURP) is still a leading surgical procedure in the United States, second only to cataract extraction, with an annual cost to the health-care system in excess of $5 billion [2].

Although we currently have a great deal of knowledge regarding the prostate, there are still many questions that need to be answered. Several of these questions, relating to clinically relevant prostatic diseases, such as prostatitis, BPH, and so on, involve normal prostate growth, differentiation, and aging, or aberrations in these processes, or both. Indeed, the earliest manifestation of BPH is the appearance of

Male Lower Urinary Tract Symptoms and Benign Prostatic Hyperplasia, First Edition.
Edited by Steven A. Kaplan and Kevin T. McVary.
© 2014 John Wiley & Sons, Ltd. Published 2014 by John Wiley & Sons, Ltd.

the mesenchyme in periurethral nodules, which has a similar morphology to the prostatic mesenchyme during embryogenesis [3]. In later stages of BPH development, glandular budding and branching toward a central focus lead to further nodule growth [3]. Such morphological evidence suggests that BPH is intrinsically a mesenchymal disease that results from a reawakening of embryonic inductive interactions between the prostatic stroma and epithelium [3]. Therefore, it is critical to understand the elements of prostatic regulation that play a role in the normal growth and differentiation of the prostate that can then be applied to the diseased gland.

What is BPH/LUTS? The biology

In this chapter, we will focus on the disease known historically as BPH but perhaps more appropriately termed LUTS. BPH or LUTS is one of the most common diseases occurring in aging men in the United States. Pathologically diagnosed BPH is characterized by the nonmalignant proliferation of the epithelial and stromal components of the prostate. Such histological BPH may or may not be associated with clinical BPH, which is characterized by the progressive development of LUTS. LUTS primarily results from constriction of the urethra and resulting resistance to urinary flow, and may take the form of urgency, frequency, nocturia, and a weak urine stream with incomplete emptying. If left untreated, LUTS can result in acute urinary retention, urinary incontinence, recurrent urinary-tract infections, and or obstructed uropathy [4]. Interestingly, some men with significantly enlarged prostates do not present with LUTS, while some men with normally sized prostates experience severe LUTS.

BPH is a chronic condition that increases in its prevalence and severity with age. The presence of histological BPH in men is estimated to be 8%, 50%, 70%, and 90% in their fourth, sixth, seventh, and eighth (and older) decades of life, respectively. The presence of moderate to severe LUTS (i.e. clinical BPH) is estimated to be 26%, 33%, 41%, and nearly 50% for the same respective age groups [5]. The extremely high prevalence of BPH and its associated symptoms can lead to a severe impact on quality of life, making it one of the nation's major health expenditures. In 2006, the management of BPH/LUTS was estimated to cost $4 billion/year in the United States alone [6]. Inclusion of prescription and nonprescription medication costs, and in-direct costs associated with morbidity (e.g. work limitations), increases this estimate significantly.

Medical treatment for clinical BPH has evolved over the last decade with a growing focus on pharmacological management of LUTS over more invasive therapies. A steady decline in surgical treatments for clinical BPH has been reported since the 1990s and is concomitant with an increase in nonsurgical interventions designed to manage symptoms [7,8]. This is likely due, at least in part, to the increased use of two largely effective drug categories in the treatment of LUTS, 5α-reductase inhibitors, which in effect shrink the prostate by inducing prostatic epithelial apoptosis and atrophy, and α_1-adrenergic receptor antagonists, which reduce prostatic urethral smooth muscle tone [9]. A number of short-duration clinical trials have compared the relative efficacy of these drug modalities individually and in combination. In these trials, 5α-reductase inhibitors and α_1-adrenergic receptor antagonists proved effective in treating clinical BPH symptoms but in combination showed no increased effect in alleviating symptoms or improving flow rate [7].

A relatively recent trial was performed to fully determine the efficacy of these approaches. To further investigate the effectiveness of individual and combination drug therapy for the medical management of clinical BPH, the National Institute of Diabetes and Digestive and Kidney Diseases conducted a long-term, randomized trial known as the Medical Therapy of Prostatic Symptoms (MTOPS) study. The MTOPS trial investigated whether finasteride, a 5α-reductase inhibitor, and doxazosin, an $α_1$-adrenergic receptor blocker, alone or in combination would specifically delay or prevent clinical progression of BPH. The results demonstrate that dual-drug therapy significantly reduced the risk of overall BPH clinical progression more than either drug monotherapy alone or placebo with a mean follow-up of 4.5 years [8]. Importantly as a component of the study protocol, serum samples were collected from MTOPS patients prior to randomization and at yearly intervals during the trial as well as at the end of the study. Prostate biopsy samples were also collected at baseline at year 1 and at the end of the study from a patient subgroup. These bio-samples were collected and banked in anticipation of analyses of potential molecular changes associated with patient responses to the MTOPS clinical protocol.

A number of theories have been proposed to explain the biology of the prostatic changes associated with BPH/LUTS. These include embryonic awakening, as described above [3], hormonal changes, and inflammation. Although there are significant data to support each of these that are summarized in this chapter, today, we still do not understand the full etiology of the prostatic changes and their associated symptoms. In all likelihood, it appears to be a combination of these changes that contribute to BPH/LUTS.

Regulation of the normal prostate

The human prostate is a walnut-sized gland, located at the base of the bladder and surrounding the urethra. The prostatic epithelial cells contribute secretions that empty through ducts into the urethra to form a major component of seminal plasma. There are 15–30 excretory ducts from the prostate that enter the urethra as it passes through the prostate, and each of these is surrounded by four to six prostatic lobules that contain acini lined by tall columnar epithelial cells. The endocrine system has been extensively documented to affect the prostate via testosterone, which is the major serum androgen that stimulates prostatic growth. During development, androgens and the androgen receptor regulate several key events that include development and differentiation of major target tissues such as the prostate, seminal vesicles, and epididymis [10]. Furthermore, it is generally held that androgens are not only required for normal function of the prostate gland but also implicated in prostate disease. Thus, identifying novel target genes, particularly those that are androgen regulated, may help to better understand the molecular basis of prostate physiology during health and disease.

Androgen regulation of the prostate

The prostate is composed principally of stromal and epithelial cells that are in close proximity to one another. BPH is a disease that is thought to involve stromally induced hyperplastic changes in the epithelium [1] and clearly demonstrates the interrelationships between stromal and epithelial cells.

Interactions between the stroma and the epithelium have been shown by a number of investigators to be critical in the regulation of prostatic growth and differentiation, and many of these stromal–epithelial interactions have been shown to work through soluble and structural signaling systems [11]. BPH has been compared with the fetal prostate, at which time the gland is also highly proliferative, and upon histological examination of BPH sections of the prostate gland, the morphology is similar to the fetal prostate. In the developing prostate, the effects of androgens have been demonstrated to be primarily on the underlying stromal cells, which, in the developing prostate, are the only cell type found to contain androgen receptors [12,13]. As the prostate matures, androgen receptors are found in both epithelial and stromal cells, suggesting that androgen action at this time may occur directly in both cell types [14]. However, 5α-reductase, the enzyme that is responsible for the conversion of testosterone to dihydrotestosterone (DHT), is localized only in the stromal cells, again demonstrating the importance of stromal cells in the hormonal regulation of prostatic growth. Androgen-receptor complexes affect prostatic function by interacting with androgen-response elements, specific DNA sequences located in the regulatory regions of a number of androgen-responsive genes. In addition, DHT has been demonstrated also to influence the expression of other prostatic growth factors.

Estrogens, progesterone, prostatic regulation, and BPH

While estrogens have been shown to diminish prostatic growth therapeutically, the classical thinking is that this is believed to be an indirect effect, mediated by blocking pituitary function and decreasing LH, which subsequently inhibits testicular testosterone production [15]. More recent studies have demonstrated more direct effects of estrogens on prostatic regulation and diseases. The impact of estrogens on the prostate and on BPH has recently been reviewed [16]. In classic studies, administration of androgens and estrogens to male beagles resulted in more highly symptomatic BPH in these animals as they aged [17]. In humans, while testosterone levels have been shown to decrease with age, estrogens do not follow this pattern. Therefore, correlations between serum estrogen levels and prostatic volume have been observed [18]. While estrogens have been shown to be direct contributors to the regulation of both stromal and epithelial cells within the prostate, the specific impact on the development of the prostatic changes associated with BPH is less clear. The principal estrogen receptors, ERα and ERβ, have both been shown to have roles in the differential regulation of the prostate, which is even more complex based upon the contextual and temporal nature of these interactions [16].

Growth factors and chemokines in BPH/LUTS

Over the past three decades, several lines of evidence have emerged that strongly suggest that prostatic growth is under the immediate control of specific autocrine and paracrine growth factors and their receptors, and is indirectly modulated by steroids. Thus, the complex milieu includes members of the fibroblast (FGF), insulin and insulin-like growth factor (IGF), transforming growth factor (TGF) families, and several other growth-regulatory proteins. Several studies have observed that these proteins and their downstream effector molecules are overexpressed in BPH and create a landscape of increased stromal and epithelial growth, and mesenchymal transdifferentiation that leads to disease progression [19]. Interestingly, in contrast to the prevailing notion that BPH is due to a pathological proliferation of prostatic fibroblasts/myofibroblasts and epithelial cells, Gustafsson and coworkers [20] have suggested that BPH is due to an epithelial-to-mesenchymal transition (EMT) that results in the accumulation of mesenchymal-like cells derived from the prostatic epithelium and endothelium. Since TGF-β is thought to play a key role in EMT, the authors suggest that TGF-β/Smad should be considered as targets for treatment of BPH [20].

In addition to growth factors, a variety of chemokines are actively secreted by the prostatic microenvironment. The primary driving forces behind the chemokine secretion appears to be the accumulation of senescent stromal fibroblasts, and possibly epithelial cells in the aging and enlarged prostate. Furthermore, chronic prostatitis/chronic pelvic pain syndrome (CP/CPPS) and histological inflammation could also serve as rich sources of chemokine secretion in the prostate. By binding to their cognate receptors, chemokines can stimulate powerful proproliferation signal transduction pathways and thus function as potent growth factors in the development and progression of BPH/LUTS [21]. A few reports in the literature also suggest that chemokine-mediated angiogenesis may be a contributing factor to BPH/LUTS development and progression. Thus, low-level secretion of multiple chemokines within the aging prostatic microenvironment may promote a concomitant and cumulative overproliferation of both stromal fibroblastic and epithelial cell types associated with increased prostatic volume. Though the accumulated evidence is rudimentary and fragmented, it argues favorably for the conclusion that chemokines can, and most likely do, promote BPH/LUTS, and justifies further investigations examining chemokines as potential therapeutic targets to delay or ablate disease initiation and progression [21].

Diabetes is another significant risk factor for BPH/LUTS due to the resulting hyperinsulinemia. Hyperinsulinemia stimulates the liver to produce more IGF, another mitogen and an anti-apoptotic agent that binds insulin receptor/IGF receptor and stimulates prostate growth. The levels of IGFs and IGF-binding proteins in prostate tissue and in blood are associated with BPH risk, with the regulation of circulating androgen and growth hormone [22].

Two other growth-regulatory molecules that have been implicated in prostatic growth and enlargement are sonic hedgehog and Cyr61. Hedgehog (Hh) signaling has long been recognized for its role in axial patterning, mesenchymal–epithelial inductive signaling, and growth regulation during fetal development. In many embryonic tissues, Hh functions as a proliferative stimulus. Robust Hh signaling is commonly found in the adult human prostate, and sonic hedgehog and Indian hedgehog are both expressed by the urothelium of the fetal prostate anlage where they regulate cell proliferation and differentiation, and play a role in prostate ductal budding [23]. Cyr61, a member of the CNN family of secreted regulatory proteins that is upregulated in BPH, has also been shown to be induced by lysophosphatidic acid and act as a secreted autocrine and/or paracrine mediator in stromal and epithelial hyperplasia [24]. As we begin to unravel the precise mechanisms involved, new treatments for BPH aimed at these interacting pathways involving various growth factors may emerge. Therefore, targeting growth factors potentially represents an attractive therapeutic approach to the regulation of abnormal enlargement of the prostate and the amelioration of other symptoms associated with BPH.

Inflammatory changes associated with BPH

Among the biomarkers that have been evaluated, those associated with inflammation appear to have taken center stage [1]. It seems that a form of inflammation may be activated in more highly symptomatic BPH [25]. As discussed above, these chemokines that are released by the prostatic environment in response to inflammation have been shown to be associated with increased prostatic cellular growth and have been proposed perhaps to play a role in the enlargement of the prostate as well as LUTS [21].

Inflammatory infiltrates were identified in more than 80% of men with complicated and/or symptomatic BPH, and both International Prostate Symptom Score and prostatic volume were higher in men with these inflammatory cells [26]. The prognostic significance of utilizing inflammation and tissue necrosis scores has been investigated, and while they seem promising, they require further study [27].

In the prostate cancer prevention trial, while there were modest associations between the use of nonsteroidal anti-inflammatory agents (NSAIDs) and the risk of BPH, NSAID use was not directly correlated with it [28]. Similar findings resulted from the Prostate, Lung, Colorectal, and Ovarian Screening Trial [29]. Several studies have now evaluated the utilization of anti-inflammatories as modulators of the symptoms associated with BPH.

Macrophages have been proposed to be a target for some of the inflammation that has been associated with BPH development. CD68(+) macrophages have been found in both the stromal and epithelial compartments in men with BPH/LUTS [30]. Monocyte chemotactic protein-1 (MCP-1/CCL2) has been associated with BPH as well, suggesting at least one mechanism through which macrophages are attracted to the prostate [31].

The stress response involves not only the epithelial components of the prostate but also the stromal elements. In fact, it may be the stromal components that are the key regulators of the prostatic changes associated with BPH, regardless of whether the disease presents as more epithelial or stromal predominant. The stress response may be either a driver or a passenger in the process that results in the prostatic changes corresponding to the observed symptoms, but regardless, it seems to be an important contributor.

Prostate-associated Gene 4 as a stress modulator within the prostate

Since most BPH is diagnosed not pathologically but as part of a spectrum of symptoms, there is an obvious need for a relatively noninvasive tool that can aid in the personalization of BPH treatment. In an effort to characterize molecular changes associated with symptomatic BPH, we performed an analysis of patterns of gene expression associated with highly symptomatic disease as defined by their American Urological Association symptom score [32]. From this analysis, we identified a series of proteins encoded by the differentially expressed genes that were associated with severe symptoms. Among these proteins was a Cancer/Testis Antigen, Prostate-associated Gene 4 (PAGE4), alternatively termed JM-27. PAGE4 was demonstrated to be relatively specific to the prostate and was approximately

18-fold higher in expression in BPH associated with significant symptoms [32]. When PAGE4 protein levels were examined, they were found to be associated not with the prostatic epithelium, like most prostatic biomarkers, but with the prostatic stroma. The relatively high level of expression within the stromal cells of the prostate associated with symptomatic BPH makes PAGE4 a unique protein. In preliminary studies, PAGE4 expression appears to be expressed within the fetal prostate but then turned off in the normal adult prostate and is reactivated in the stroma of the men with symptomatic but not asymptomatic BPH. When we artificially overexpressed the protein, we found that the PAGE4-overexpressing cells were able to protect themselves from stresses including glucose deprivation, tumor necrosis factor-α, and adriamycin challenge [33]. Thus, it appears that PAGE4 may represent a marker of the stress-associated changes that appear to accompany symptomatic BPH. This stress reaction may include inflammation, which, as described above, has been associated with more highly symptomatic disease.

In an effort to identify noninvasive biomarkers of BPH, we have been measuring PAGE4 in the blood as a potential indicator of disease type. These studies should reveal whether PAGE4 has the potential to serve as a serum-based biomarker of symptomatic BPH.

The need for biomarkers of BPH

BPH is a term used to describe an enlargement of the prostate that is associated with symptoms that have been described as LUTS. Although the term BPH refers to the prostate, it is known that other organs, including the bladder, are centrally involved in many of the symptoms that are associated with the disease. Despite the fact that BPH is among the most common urologic conditions affecting aging men, we still know very little about its etiology, and the frequently utilized medical therapies are focused on symptom improvement rather than on the biology of the disease(s). It is clear that not all BPHs are created the same. Some men present with large prostates, and others present with prostates within the normal size range. Furthermore, BPH is currently treated differently than most diseases as a result of its symptomatic description. As opposed to diseases like cancer, BPH is not diagnosed pathologically and is described by the reported symptoms and their severity. Typically a disease presents, and earlier treatment is better than later. In opposition to the approach of catching and treating a disease early, in BPH, treatments are usually reserved for those with some of the most severe symptoms, as opposed to those with histologic disease. Therefore, there is an urgent need to improve our molecular understanding of BPH so that we can discern novel biomarkers that could identify early on in their disease course men with severe disease that could have or may go into urinary retention. No such biomarkers exist or are currently being used. Furthermore, biomarkers are needed that can stratify patients into categories of potential response to therapies, that is, which patients may respond better to a particular therapy. This type of approach would allow us to focus potentially efficacious therapies on those with the disease type known to be most responsive rather than our current strategy of treating and seeing if symptoms improve.

Conclusions

We need to move beyond the currently used model where we treat BPH as merely a collection of symptoms rather than focusing on the

Dos and Don'ts

- There are currently no available serum or tissue biomarkers with clinical utility in stratifying patients with BPH/LUTS.

biology that underlies them. Personalization is necessary to use the currently available treatments more wisely as well as to understand the potential of novel therapies to treat subgroups of patients. While we do not yet have the biomarkers to discern personalization, our increased understanding of the genetics, epidemiology, and microenvironmental stress associated with BPH should provide us with valuable tools to begin down this road.

Bibliography

1 Oesterling JE. Benign prostatic hyperplasia: a review of its histogenesis and natural history. *Prostate*. 1996;6:67–73.

2 Graverson PH, Gasser TC, Wasson JH, Hinman F Jr., Bruskewitz RC. Controversies about indications for transurethral resection of the prostate. *J Urol*. 1989;141:475–81.

3 McNeal J. Pathology of benign prostatic hyperplasia. Insight into etiology. *Urol Clin North Am*. 1990; 17(3):477–86.

4 Roehrborn CG, McConnell JD, Saltzman B, Bergner D, Gray T, Narayan P, *et al*. Storage (irritative) and voiding (obstructive) symptoms as predictors of benign prostatic hyperplasia progression and related outcomes. *Eur Urol*. 2002;42:1–6.

5 McVary KT. BPH: Epidemiology and comorbidities. *Am J Manag Care*. 2006;2:S122–8.

6 Taub DA, Wei JT. The economics of benign prostatic hyperplasia and lower urinary tract symptoms in the United States. *Curr Urol Rep*. 2006; 7(4);272–81.

7 Chapple CR. Pharmacological therapy of benign prostatic hyperplasia/lower unirary tract symptoms: an overview for the practising clinician. *BJU Int*. 2004;94:738–44.

8 McConnell JD, Roehrborn CG, Baustista OM, Andriole GL Jr., Dixon CM, Kusek JW, *et al*. The long term effect of doxazosin, finasteride, and combination therapy on the clinical progression of benign prostatic hyperplasia. *N Engl J Med*. 2003; 349:2387–98.

9 Sarma AV, Jacobson DJ, McGree ME, Roberts RO, Lieber M, Jacobsen SJ. A population based study of incidence and treatment of benign prostatic hyperplasia among residents of Olmsted County Minnesota: 1987–1997. *J Urol*. 2003;173:2048–53.

10 Marker PC, Donjacour AA, Dahiya R, Cunha GR. Hormonal, cellular, and molecular control of prostatic development. *Dev Biol*. 2003;253(2):165–74.

11 Lee C. Role of androgen in prostate growth and regression: stromal–epithelial interaction. *Prostate*. 1996;6:52–6.

12 Cunha GR, Fujii H, Neubauer BL, Shannon JM, Sawyer L, Reese BA. Epithelial–mesenchymal interactions in prostatic development. Morphological observations of prostatic induction by urogenital sinus mesenchyme in epithelium of the adult rodent urinary bladder. *J Cell Biol*. 1983;96:1662–70.

13 Cunha GR, Lung B. The importance of stroma in morphogenesis and functional activity of urogenital epithelium. *In Vitro*. 1979;15:50–71.

14 Sar M, Lubahn DB, French FS, Wilson EM. Immuohistochemical localization of the androgen receptor in rat and human tissues. *Endocrinology*. 1990;127:3180–6.

15 Coffey DS. Androgen action and the sex accessory tissues. In: Knobil E, Neill J, *et al*., editors. The physiology of reproduction. New York: Raven Press; 1988. pp. 1081–19.

16 Nicholson TM, Ricke WA. Androgens and estrogens in benign prostatic hyperplasia: past, present and future. *Differentiation*. 2011;82(4–5):184–99.

17 Coffey DS, Walsh PC. Clinical and experimental studies of benign prostatic hyperplasia. *Urol Clin North Am*. 1990;17:461–75.

18 Belanger A, Candas B, Dupont A, Cusan L, Diamond P, Gomez JL, *et al*. Changes in serum concentrations of conjugated and unconjugated steroids in 40- to 80-year old men. *J Clin Endocrinol Metab* 1994;76:1086–90.

19 Lucia MS, Lambert JR. Growth factors in benign prostatic hyperplasia: basic science implications. *Curr Urol Rep.* 2008;9(4):272–8.

20 Alonso-Magdalena P, Brössner C, Reiner A, Cheng G, Sugiyama N, *et al.* A role for epithelial-mesenchymal transition in the etiology of benign prostatic hyperplasia. *Proc Natl Acad Sci USA.* 2009; 106(8):2859–63.

21 Macoska JA. Chemokines and BPH/LUTS. *Differentiation.* 2011;82(4–5):253–60.

22 Wang Z, Olumi AF. Diabetes, growth hormone-insulin-like growth factor pathways and association to benign prostatic hyperplasia. *Differentiation.* 2011;82(4–5):261–71.

23 Vezina CM, Bushman AW. Hedgehog signaling in prostate growth and benign prostate hyperplasia. *Curr Urol Rep.* 2007;8(4):275–80.

24 Sakamoto S, Yokoyama M, Zhang X, Prakash K, Nagao K, Hatanaka T, *et al.* Increased expression of CYR61, an extracellular matrix signaling protein, in human benign prostatic hyperplasia and its regulation by lysophosphatidic acid. *Endocrinology.* 2004; 145(6):2929–40.

25 Chughtai B, Lee R, Te A, Kaplan S. Inflammation and benign prostatic hyperplasia: clinical implications. *Curr Urol Rep.* 2011;12(4):274–7.

26 Robert G, Descazeaud A, Nicolaïew N, Terry S, Sirab N, Vacherot F, *et al.* Inflammation in benign prostatic hyperplasia: a 282 patients' immunohistochemical analysis. *Prostate.* 2009;69(16):1774–80.

27 Willder JM, Walker VC, Halbert GL, Dick CP, Orange C, Qayyum T, *et al.* The prognostic use of inflammation and tissue necrosis in benign prostatic hyperplasia. *Urol Int.* 2013 Jan 10. [Epub ahead of print]

28 Schenk JM, Calip GS, Tangen CM, Goodman P, Parsons JK, Thompson IM, *et al.* Indications for and use of nonsteroidal antiinflammatory drugs and the risk of incident, symptomatic benign prostatic hyperplasia: results from the prostate cancer prevention trial. *Am J Epidemiol.* 2012;176(2): 156–63.

29 Sutcliffe S, Grubb Iii RL, Platz EA, Ragard LR, Riley TL, Kazin SS, *et al.* Non-steroidal antiinflammatory drug use and the risk of benign prostatic hyperplasia-related outcomes and nocturia in the Prostate Lung Colorectal, and Ovarian Cancer Screening Trial. *BJU Int.* 2012;110(7): 1050–9.

30 Lu T, Lin WJ, Izumi K, Wang X, Xu D, Fang LY, *et al.* Targeting androgen receptor to suppress macrophage-induced EMT and benign prostatic hyperplasia (BPH) development. *Mol Endocrinol.* 2012;26(10):1707–15.

31 Fujita K, Ewing CM, Getzenberg RH, Parsons JK, Isaacs WB, Pavlovich CP. Monocyte chemotactic protein-1 (MCP-1/CCL2) is associated with prostatic growth dysregulation and benign prostatic hyperplasia. *Prostate.* 2010;70(5):473–81.

32 Prakash K, Pirozzi G, Elashoff M, Munger W, Waga I, Dhir R, *et al.* Symptomatic and asymptomatic benign prostatic hyperplasia: molecular differentiation by using microarrays. *Proc Natl Acad Sci USA.* 2002;99(11):7598–603.

33 Zeng Y, Gao D, Kim JJ, Shiraishi T, Terada N, Kakehi Y, *et al.* Prostate-associated gene 4 (PAGE4) protects cells against stress by elevating p21 and suppressing reactive oxygen species production. *Am J Clin Exp Urol.* 2013;1(1):39–52.

CHAPTER 2

Lower Urinary Tract Symptoms and Benign Prostatic Hyperplasia: Epidemiology, Correlates, and Risk Factors

Raymond C. Rosen[1] & Benjamin N. Breyer[2]

[1]New England Research Institutes, Watertown, MA, USA
[2]University of California San Francisco, Department of Urology, San Francisco, CA, USA

Key points

- Epidemiologic studies of benign prostatic hyperplasia (BPH)/lower urinary tract symptoms (LUTS) are based primarily on symptom data from recognized scales, such as the American Urological Association Symptom Index (AUA-SI), with scant population data on urodynamic or histologic aspects of BPH.
- Large multinational studies have confirmed the prevalence and age association of LUTS in the general population.
- Numerous studies have suggested a relationship between LUTS and broader health indicators in aging men, including obesity, diabetes, cardiovascular disease, depression, and history of sexually transmitted infection.
- BPH/LUTS and both erectile and ejaculatory dysfunction have been observed and replicated in a growing number of studies. Long-acting phosphodiesterase type 5 (PDE5) inhibitors have been approved to treat both conditions.
- New techniques to expand the scope of the epidemiologic research in BPH/LUTS, such as cluster analysis, hold promise to advance our understanding.

Introduction

BPH is a highly prevalent age-, lifestyle-, and quality-of-life-related condition in aging men. The prevalence of LUTS is expected to grow sharply in the coming decades, as Litman and McKinlay have predicted that 52 million adults will have symptoms by 2025 [1].

The commonly used term "BPH/LUTS" applies to a constellation of physical findings and symptoms in men, and commonly subtyped as obstructive or irritative voiding symptoms [2]. As noted by other reviewers, epidemiologic studies have focused primarily on the symptomatic aspects of the disorder with relatively few population data available on the histology or functional urodynamics of the lower urinary tract. This has not changed significantly in recent years, as most epidemiologic studies reviewed in this chapter have continued to focus predominantly on the symptomatic aspects of the disorder, and the

Male Lower Urinary Tract Symptoms and Benign Prostatic Hyperplasia, First Edition.
Edited by Steven A. Kaplan and Kevin T. McVary.
© 2014 John Wiley & Sons, Ltd. Published 2014 by John Wiley & Sons, Ltd.

relationship of symptoms to other systemic illnesses, risk factors, or correlates of LUTS. Of note, the progression of symptoms and adverse medical outcomes, relative cost in quality of life for affected individuals, and other psychosocial consequences of BPH/LUTS are well substantiated and highly relevant to public health by any measure [3,4]. Medical and surgical complications, including acute urinary retention, are outcomes in most clinical trials [5,6], and the economic cost to society of BPH/LUTS has been estimated to be in the billions of dollars [3,7].

Major advances have been made in recent years in at least three main areas, which are the main focus of this chapter. First is the relationship between LUTS and broader health indicators in aging men, including obesity, diabetes, cardiovascular disease, depression, and history of sexually transmitted infection. Taken together, these findings have led to a more holistic and less organ-centered approach to understanding the signs and symptoms of BPH/LUTS. Second, the specific association of BPH/LUTS with sexual dysfunction in men, including both erectile dysfunction (ED) and ejaculatory dysfunction (EjD), has been observed and replicated in a growing number of studies [8,9]. Moreover, the long-acting PDE5 inhibitor, tadalafil, has been approved as first-line therapy for LUTS, leading to a strong clinical interest in the association between BPH/LUTS and sexual dysfunction in men [10,11]. Third, new measurement methods (e.g. the Visual Prostate Symptom Score) and advanced statistical methods, such as cluster analysis, have been developed and applied. These new measurement approaches challenge existing models and provide opportunities for expanding the scope of epidemiological research on BPH/LUTS in the coming years.

Descriptive epidemiology, risk factors, and correlates

Multiple studies in different population groups provide adequate foundation for our current epidemiologic understanding of BPH/LUTS risk factors and correlates [1,4,12,13]. Of particular importance is the relationship between LUTS and broader health indicators, including obesity, diabetes, cardiovascular disease, depression, and history of sexually transmitted infection.

Metabolic syndrome, obesity, and LUTS

Researchers have postulated the possibility of a link between the metabolic syndrome and BPH/LUTS for nearly 20 years [14]. The Adult Treatment Panel defines the metabolic syndrome to include three or more of the following: central obesity (waist circumference greater than 102 cm), high-density lipoprotein (HDL) less than 40 mg/dl, triglycerides more than 150 mg/dl, blood pressure more than 135/85 mmHg, and fasting plasma glucose more than 110 mg/dl. Hammarsten and Peeker have explored this relationship in depth in a convenience sample of clinic patients who underwent extensive phenotyping. They found increasing plasma insulin level, increased body weight, type 2 diabetes, hypertension, and lower HDL cholesterol to be risk factors for BPH as measured by gland volume [14]. Data from the National Health and Nutrition Examination Survey (NHANES) III demonstrated that any increase in body mass index (BMI) was positively correlated with LUTS [15]. Researchers also examined the placebo arm of the Prostate Cancer Prevention Trial ($n = 5667$) and found that for each 0.05 increase in waist-to-hip ratio, there was an associated 10% increased risk of BPH [16]. However, markedly different results were obtained in an analysis of results from the Olmsted County Study [13], in which:

> There were few significant associations of anthropometric measures with the presence or progression of components of BPH or clinical outcome of BPH, and there were no instances where the point estimates for the BPH components suggested a dose–response effect.

The authors conclude that:

> anthropometric measures are not significantly associated with the presence or progression of BPH as measured by American Urological Association Symptom Index scores, peak urinary flow rate, prostate volume, or acute urinary retention. [13]

On the other hand, a more recent publication from the Olmsted County and Flint Michigan Study [17] reported a significant association between a history of diabetes in both black and white men, and the presence or progression of BPH/LUTS, independent of age and BMI. However, treatment of diabetes in this most recent report from this study was not associated with BPH/LUTS outcomes, thus raising further questions about the nature of the relationship [17].

Additional longitudinal and cross-sectional findings on the association between BPH/LUTS and the metabolic syndrome have been reported in the Boston Area Community Health (BACH) Survey [18–20]. The community-dwelling, population-representative sample included 5503 adults (2301 men, 3202 women; 1767 black, 1877 Hispanic, 1859 white respondents). The BACH Survey is unique among LUTS prevalence studies in the controls provided for effects of gender, race/ethnicity, and socioeconomic status in a random, population-representative sample. The overall prevalence of LUTS (AUA-SI ≥8) in men was 18.7% and increased linearly with age (10.5% for 30–39 years to 25.5% for 70–79 years) but did not differ by gender or race/ethnicity. Metabolic syndrome components (obesity, triglycerides, BP) were correlated with individual symptoms of LUTS and with overall AUA symptom scores in the BACH Survey. Kupelian *et al.* [21] (p. 618) found that a significant increase in the prevalence of metabolic syndrome indicators was noted up to the cutoff point of AUA > 8. With increased severity of LUTS beyond 8, no further increase in metabolic factors was observed, perhaps due to ceiling effects or other unobserved confounders [21].

BPH/LUTS and other health outcomes

Broad health outcomes, including depressed mood and increased inflammatory markers, have been linked in several large studies, including the BACH study, with BPH/LUTS in men. Depressive symptoms and anxiety, in particular, are associated in multiple studies with increased prevalence and odds of LUTS across racial/ethnic groups [22,23]. Storage symptoms (urgency and frequency) appear to have a greater impact on mental health in men than voiding and postmicturition symptoms [24]. Interestingly, the burden of LUTS on mental health rises with the addition of increasing categories of LUTS (storage, voiding, and postmicturition symptoms) [24]. Data from BACH indicate that depressive symptoms have a more robust association with LUTS than any other factor except the AUA-SI quality-of-life item response [23].

Studies that stratified by racial/ethnic group (white/black/Hispanic) found similar risk estimates for the association of mental health and LUTS [22,23]. In the EpiLUTS study, a multinational cross-sectional representative survey, gender, LUTS, and mental health were examined [4,24,25]. Depression and anxiety were assessed using the Hospital Anxiety and Depression Scale; [26] scores of 8 or greater on either subscale were considered indicative of clinically relevant anxiety and/or depression [27]. In men, urinary symptoms predictive of anxiety included nocturia, voiding urgency, incomplete emptying, and bladder pain. Predictors of depressive symptoms in men included urinary frequency and incomplete bladder emptying.

Further evidence for the association of LUTS and depression comes from a large Taiwanese database. Huang and colleagues prospectively examined the relationship between diagnosis of benign prostatic enlargement (BPE) and the 1-year risk of developing a depressive disorder [28]. A total of 16,130 patients diagnosed with BPE and 48,390 matched controls without BPE were followed for 1 year. The risk of developing depressive disorder during this time was 1.87 times higher (adjusted hazard ratio, 95% CI 1.63–2.16) in men receiving a diagnosis of BPE compared with those who did not. This demonstrates a directional relationship with a new onset of depression after preceding BPE. Other investigators have reported single institution convenience samples demonstrating the association of LUTS and depression [29–31].

Systemic factors and inflammation

Markers of inflammation have been associated with BPH/LUTS symptoms in several recent studies. Recent epidemiologic literature supports the hypothesis that inflammation secondary to sexually transmitted infections, for example, plays an important role in LUTS pathogenesis. Sutcliffe and colleagues examined the impact of STIs on LUTS in the large nested Health Professionals Follow-Up Study (HPFS) [32]. The authors found that a history of gonorrhea was associated with any (OR 1.76, CI 1.43–2.15), moderate/severe (OR 1.89, CI 1.51–2.37), and severe (OR 2.69, CI 1.97–3.67) LUTS. History of gonorrhea also correlated to any (OR 1.63, CI 1.14–2.33) and severe

(OR 2.4, CI 1.32–4.38) incident symptoms. Sutcliffe et al. also evaluated the prevalence of viral STIs in male participants of NHANES III [33]. Positive associations were found between serological evidence of several sexually acquired viruses and reporting two or more LUTS symptoms in men age 30–59 years [34]. Of 31,681 men from the HPFS, an ongoing prospective cohort, 16% reported a history of prostatitis or LUTS. History of STI (pathogen not specified) resulted in an 1.8-fold increase in odds of LUTS [34].

Sociodemographic and lifestyle factors

Several studies have addressed LUTS and STI history in African-American men [35,36]. Joseph et al. described a cohort in which over half reported a history of any STI (including gonorrhea, syphilis, genital herpes or genital warts), and this conferred a 1.5-fold increased risk of developing moderate to severe LUTS. Conversely, a population-based sample of African-American men found no significant association between LUTS and history of gonorrhea, syphilis, genital herpes or partner history of cervical cancer [36].

Exercise

Multiple [35,37–39], but not all [40], epidemiologic studies of physical activity and BPH/LUTS have shown a protective association between later-life physical activity and incidence of BPH/LUTS. A meta-analysis reported that compared with the sedentary group, those engaging in light, moderate, or heavy physical activity had up to a 30% reduction in the risk of reported BPH/LUTS [41]. Given the relationship of BPH and metabolic syndrome, individuals with BPH may gain more health benefits from increased activity then men without BPH. The relationship between physical activity and LUTS resolution or symptom reduction in patients who have LUTS is unknown and requires further investigation.

Epidemiologic findings in men who have sex with men

Data from a cross-sectional, Internet-based survey assessed the relationship of LUTS to urinary-tract infection (UTI), prostatitis, and STI prevalence in homosexual men [42]. A relatively young population completed the survey (mean age 39 years). A third of the respondents reported moderate to severe LUTS, and 14.1% reported a history of HIV, 12.6% Chlamydia, and 19% gonorrhea. Multivariate analysis revealed a significant association between positive lifetime history of HIV or gonorrhea and moderate to severe LUTS. Men with HIV were more likely to report moderate to severe LUTS. In an adjusted model, AIDS-defining HIV positive men were 1.79 times more likely to experience moderate to severe LUTS. Gonorrhea was also an independent risk factor for moderate LUTS.

BPH/LUTS and sexual function in men

A large body of epidemiologic data supports the high degree of association and potential causal relationship between BPH/LUTS and sexual dysfunction in men, including both ED and EjD, in addition to decreased frequency of sexual activity and loss of desire in aging men [43,44]. Sexual dysfunction and BPH/LUTS are strongly linked across studies [43,44]. The first large-scale study reporting on an age-independent association between LUTS and male sexual dysfunction was reported by Lukacs *et al.* in 1996 [45]. In this study of 5849 men who participated in a 1-year observational trial with alfuzosin, sexual function was strongly correlated with LUTS incidence and severity. Sexual function status was measured by three questions on sexual desire, quality of erection, and satisfaction with sexual life (sexual score ranging from 0 to 30). The negative effect of LUTS on all three domains was strongly evident. Other studies to show this association are shown in Table 2.1. A comprehensive summary of epidemiologic studies associating LUTS and ED has been reported by Köhler and McVary [44].

Similar findings were reported by Rosen *et al.* in the MSAM-7 study in 2003, in which the relationship between LUTS and key aspects of male sexual function was investigating using validated measures and a large, multinational sample of men [12]. Detailed assessments showed a broader pattern of negative sexual outcomes, including declining

Table 2.1 Relevant epidemiologic studies of the relationship between LUTS and ED [61]

Reference	Country	Patients	Range (years)	ED (%)	LUTS (%)	Risk ratio for ED
Braun et al. [62]	Germany	4,489	30–80	19.2	72.2	2.11
Nicolosi et al. [63]	Brazil, Italy, Japan, Malaysia	2,412	40–70	16.1		2.2–4.9
Rosen et al. [12]	USA and six European countries	12,815	50–80	48.9	30.8	3.7–7.6
Vallancien et al. [64]	Five European countries	1,274	36–92	62	91	1.2–1.9
Boyle et al. [65]	Korea and three European countries	4,800	40–79	21.1		1.1–1.7
Hansen [66]	Denmark	3,700	40–65	28.2	39.1	2.3–3.4
Terai et al. [67]	Japan	2,084	>40	29.9	27.1	1.5

ED, erectile dysfunction; LUTS, lower urinary tract symptoms.
Martinez-Salamanca 2011 [61]. Reproduced with permission of Elsevier.

levels of sexual activity with both age and degree of BPH/LUTS, in addition to a loss of ejaculation and diminished desire, all of which had a linear, dose–effect relationship to LUTS severity. Within each age category, the frequency of ED was strongly related to severity of LUTS with a relative risk increasing from 3.1 (moderate LUTS) to 5.9 (severe LUTS), regardless of the coexistence of comorbid conditions, including diabetes, hypertension, cardiac disease, or hyperlipidemia. Similarly, the association between LUTS and incident ED was examined prospectively in the HPFS. In this study with 3953 incident ED cases among 17,086 men, those with severe LUTS in 1994 or earlier had a statistically significant 40% higher risk of ED subsequently than subjects without LUTS. The risk of ED increased with increasing LUTS severity (P trend <0.0001).

Similar findings were noted in a reanalysis of data from the BACH study [46]. These authors controlled further for effects of comorbidities, race-ethnic and sociodemographic confounder, and other covariates. LUTS, in particular, were associated strongly with sexual function problems in men, such as ED and EjD in several large-scale, community-based studies [8,12,47].

Similar findings were reported in another large observational survey to assess the prevalence LUTS among men and women aged 40 years or older in the USA, the UK, and Sweden [24]. The analysis included 11,834 men with a mean age of 56.1 years, of whom 71% reported being currently sexually active. Twenty-six percent had mild to severe ED, 7% had EjD, and 16% had premature ejaculation. A strong, linearly increasing association was again observed. Almost 30% of men with LUTS reported that their urinary symptoms reduced their enjoyment of sex, and 25% reported that they had decreased

or stopped sexual activity because of their urinary symptoms. Of the 2954 respondents reporting a combination of voiding, storage, and postmicturition symptoms at least sometimes, 28.8% responded that their sexual enjoyment was decreased because of LUTS, and 24.8% reported that they had decreased or stopped sexual activity because of LUTS. By contrast, of the 3326 respondents with no/minimal LUTS, only 1.4% responded that their sexual enjoyment was decreased because of LUTS, and 1.3% reported that they had decreased or stopped sexual activity. Men with multiple LUTS had more severe ED and more frequent EjD and premature ejaculation. In a multivariate analysis, greater age, hypertension, diabetes, depression, urgency with fear of leaking, and leaking during sexual activity were significantly associated with ED. More frequent LUTS were associated with most of the common sexual dysfunctions in men, highlighting again the importance of assessing the sexual health of all men presenting with LUTS.

In summary, the major epidemiologic findings to date include: (1) a consistent dose–response association between the severity of LUTS and prevalence of sexual dysfunction, including both ED and EjD in men, even controlling for all of the known confounders and covariates [43,44,47]. According to these robust findings across studies and considering the magnitude and direction of association observed, a causal, etiological link between LUTS and ED is strongly supported by the available epidemiological data. Moreover, the association between ED and LUTS has biologic plausibility, given the interrelationships of the known pathophysiological mechanisms of these disease states [44,48].

What accounts for this association? Four pathophysiological mechanisms have been proposed to account for the relationship between LUTS and ED [47]. These include the roles of nitric oxide synthase (NOS)/NO, autonomic hyperactivity and the metabolic syndrome, the Rho-kinase activation/endothelin pathway, and pelvic atherosclerosis [47]. These four pathophysiologic processes are not mutually exclusive and may overlap substantially [44].

Measurement and classification of LUTS symptoms in epidemiological research: new concepts and methods

Traditional self-report measures of LUTS, such as the AUA-SI, are lacking in sensitivity and specificity, and have other methodological weaknesses, including lack of applicability to certain populations. Of note, the AUA-SI was developed and validated prior to current concepts for patient-reported outcome (PRO) development. Improved and validated BPH/LUTS directed instruments would be helpful to track voiding symptoms, assess the need for intervention, and compare research results. A sixth-grade reading level is considered necessary to understand the questions asked in the AUA-SI [49], and reduced validity of the AUA-SI compared with actual LUTS is related to lower educational level [50]. To help address the effect of educational level on AUA-SI, visual prostate symptom scores have been developed and validated [51]. The concept of a visual PRO measure is particularly appealing for health-care providers working in areas with low literacy rates and diverse cultures and languages such as inner-city clinics or in underdeveloped countries.

Versions of the visual prostate symptom score (VPSS) include a visual analog scale with pictures of happy to increasingly sad faces for all seven questions in the AUA-SI [52] and a four-question VPSS with pictures demonstrating daytime and night-time urinary frequency and force of urinary stream as well as a visual analog scale to rate quality of life [51]. The four-question version of the VPSS has been validated with regards to both AUA-SI and uroflowmetry measurements.

In addition to new methods for assessing symptoms, innovative and potentially more holistic approaches have also been used for classifying symptoms in epidemiological studies, including the use of cluster analysis [53]. Cluster analysis is a well-defined statistical method for classifying groups of individuals with potentially similar clinical characteristics or properties. The method has been used successfully in other areas of medicine to classify individuals with a broad array of medical and psychiatric disorders into distinct diagnostic and/or etiological clusters [53–56].

Coyne *et al.* conducted a broad symptom cluster analysis of men and women in the European Prospective Investigation into Cancer and Nutrition (EPIC) study, reporting at least one LUTS [57]. Six distinct symptom cluster groups were identified; the largest cluster (56% of men and 57% of women) consisted of respondents reporting minimal symptoms.

Similarly, in an analysis of symptoms in the BACH Survey, five symptom clusters were identified in men that were strongly associated with age, overall health status, major comorbidities, and quality of life in men and women [58–60], supporting the findings of Coyne *et al.* in the EPIC study [57]. Five clusters were identified among symptomatic men. The largest cluster (~50% of symptomatic men) had a low prevalence and frequency of urologic symptoms and a low level of interference with activities of daily living. Men in the second, third, and fourth clusters had mixed patterns of voiding, storage, and postmicturition symptoms with intermediate levels of symptom frequency and prevalence. The remaining cluster included predominantly older men (mean age 58.9 years) with a high prevalence and frequency of urologic symptoms (mean±standard deviation, 9.9 ± 2.1 symptoms) and higher frequency of comorbid conditions (e.g. cardiovascular disease, kidney and bladder infections, prior urologic surgery). Men with more sedentary lifestyles and a larger waist circumference were overrepresented in the more symptomatic clusters. The authors also reported an increased burden of comorbidities (diabetes, obesity, depression, CVD), in the most symptomatic clusters, which was accompanied by a decreased quality of life and greater interference with activities of daily living, as well as increased health-care utilization [58–60].

Summary and conclusion

Epidemiological studies of BPH/LUTS have proliferated in the past 10 years, leading to accumulation of data regarding the prevalence and risk factors for LUTS. There are no population-based studies of histological BPH or urodynamic variables, however, and the current estimates are based on symptoms, usually recorded by means of the AUA symptom index or comparable measures. Despite this limitation, evidence has emerged of the role of BPH/LUTS as a marker or harbinger of men's health, as has been discussed recently in regards to ED. This chapter reviews the growing evidence of association between BPH/LUTS and depression, and between BPH/LUTS and other indicators of systemic illness or inflammation. Further research is needed to elucidate the underlying mechanisms of these associations. A strong link has been established between BPH/LUTS and sexual dysfunction in men, including both EjD and ED in men, in addition to a decrease or discontinuation of sexual activity in older men. Finally, new methods have been developed for investigating symptoms of LUTS and for analyzing epidemiological data on voiding symptoms in men and women. These new methods will add to our understanding of the relationships between voiding symptoms and other health issues in both men and women.

Dos and don'ts

- Epidemiological studies need to be conducted in large, population-representative or randomly selected groups of outpatient participants. Convenience or opportunistic samples have been used in some studies but have potential for misleading generalizations.

- Study measures should be tested and validated prior to use in any epidemiological investigation. Only accepted, validated symptom measures and PROs should be used in large, epidemiological studies.

- The role of confounders and covariates needs to be carefully considered and evaluated. Age is a typical covariate in every epidemiological study of BPH/LUTS. Additionally, body-morphology associations (BMI, waist circumference) should be considered in the analyses, as well as associations with comorbid diseases (e.g. diabetes, depression). Medication effects need to be carefully controlled for.

- Further studies are needed for evaluating the special benefits of new methods and analysis techniques for assessing LUTS impact and severity, and for analyzing effects and consequences of BPH/LUTS in men. Additional studies of LUTS progression and the disease history are also needed. Only one patient registry has been attempted to date, and this was prematurely discontinued.

Bibliography

1 Litman HJ, McKinlay JB. The future magnitude of urological symptoms in the USA: projections using the Boston Area Community Health survey. *BJU Int.* 2007;100(4):820–5.

2 Moul S, McVary KT. Lower urinary tract symptoms, obesity and the metabolic syndrome. *Curr Opin Urol.* 2010;20(1):7–12.

3 DiSantostefano RL, Biddle AK, Lavelle JP. An evaluation of the economic costs and patient-related consequences of treatments for benign prostatic hyperplasia. *BJU Int.* 2006;97(5):1007–16.

4 Coyne KS, Sexton CC, Irwin DE, Kopp ZS, Kelleher CJ, Milsom I. The impact of overactive bladder, incontinence and other lower urinary tract symptoms on quality of life, work productivity, sexuality and emotional well-being in men and women: results from the EPIC study. *BJU Int.* 2008;101(11):1388–95.

5 Milsom I, Kaplan SA, Coyne KS, Sexton CC, Kopp ZS. Effect of bothersome overactive bladder symptoms on health-related quality of life, anxiety, depression, and treatment seeking in the United States: results from EpiLUTS. *Urology.* 2012; 80(1):90–6.

6 Coyne KS, Sexton CC, Thompson CL, Clemens JQ, Chen CI, Bavendam T, *et al.* Impact of overactive bladder on work productivity. *Urology.* 2012;80(1):97–103.

7 Kirby RS, Kirby M, Fitzpatrick JM. Benign prostatic hyperplasia: counting the cost of its management. *BJU Int.* 2010;105(7):901–2.

8 Rosen RC, Giuliano F, Carson CC. Sexual dysfunction and lower urinary tract symptoms (LUTS) associated with benign prostatic hyperplasia (BPH). *Eur Urol.* 2005;47(6):824–37.

9 Rosen RC, Wei JT, Althof SE, Seftel AD, Miner M, Perelman MA, *et al.* Association of sexual dysfunction with lower urinary tract symptoms of BPH and BPH medical therapies: results from the BPH Registry. *Urology.* 2009;73(3):562–6.

10 Porst H, Roehrborn CG, Secrest RJ, Esler A, Viktrup L. Effects of tadalafil on lower urinary tract symptoms secondary to benign prostatic hyperplasia and on erectile dysfunction in sexually active men with both conditions: analyses of pooled data from four randomized, placebo-controlled tadalafil clinical studies. *J Sex Med.* 2013;10(8):2044–52.

11 Porst H, Oelke M, Goldfischer ER, Cox D, Watts S, Dey D, et al. Efficacy and safety of tadalafil 5 mg once daily for lower urinary tract symptoms suggestive of benign prostatic hyperplasia: subgroup analyses of pooled data from 4 multinational, randomized, placebo-controlled clinical studies. *Urology.* 2013 Sep;82(3):667–73.

12 Rosen R, Altwein J, Boyle P, Kirby RS, Lukacs B, Meuleman E, et al. Lower urinary tract symptoms and male sexual dysfunction: the multinational survey of the aging male (MSAM-7). *Eur Urol.* 2003;44(6):637–49.

13 Burke JP, Rhodes T, Jacobson DJ, McGree ME, Roberts RO, Girman CJ, et al. Association of anthropometric measures with the presence and progression of benign prostatic hyperplasia. *Am J Epidemiol.* 2006;164(1):41–6.

14 Hammarsten J, Peeker R. Urological aspects of the metabolic syndrome. *Nature Rev Urol.* 2011 ;8(9):483–94.

15 Rohrmann S, Smit E, Giovannucci E, Platz EA. Associations of obesity with lower urinary tract symptoms and noncancer prostate surgery in the Third National Health and Nutrition Examination Survey. *Am J Epidemiol.* 2004;159(4):390–7.

16 Kristal AR, Arnold KB, Schenk JM, Neuhouser ML, Weiss N, Goodman P, et al. Race/ethnicity, obesity, health related behaviors and the risk of symptomatic benign prostatic hyperplasia: results from the prostate cancer prevention trial. *J Urol.* 2007;177(4):1395–400; quiz 591.

17 Sarma AV, St Sauver JL, Hollingsworth JM, Jacobson DJ, McGree ME, Dunn RL, et al. Diabetes treatment and progression of benign prostatic hyperplasia in community-dwelling black and white men. *Urology.* 2012;79(1):102–8.

18 Kupelian V, McVary KT, Kaplan SA, Hall SA, Link CL, Aiyer LP, et al. Association of lower urinary tract symptoms and the metabolic syndrome: results from the Boston area community health survey. *J Urol.* 2013;189(1 Suppl):S107–14; discussion S15–6.

19 Maserejian NN, Chen S, Chiu GR, Araujo AB, Kupelian V, Hall SA, *et al.* Treatment status and progression or regression of lower urinary tract symptoms among adults in a general population sample. *J Urol.* 2014. doi:10.1016/j.urology.2013.12.016

20 Maserejian NN, Chen S, Chiu GR, Wager CG, Kupelian V, Araujo AB, *et al.* Incidence of lower urinary tract symptoms in a population-based study of men and women. *Urology.* 2013.

21 Kupelian V, McVary KT, Barry MJ, Link CL, Rosen RC, Aiyer LP, et al. Association of C-reactive protein and lower urinary tract symptoms in men and women: results from Boston Area Community Health survey. *Urology*. 2009;73(5):950–7.

22 Laumann EO, Kang JH, Glasser DB, Rosen RC, Carson CC. Lower urinary tract symptoms are associated with depressive symptoms in white, black and Hispanic men in the United States. *J Urol*. 2008;180(1):233–40.

23 Litman HJ, Steers WD, Wei JT, Kupelian V, Link CL, McKinlay JB, et al. Relationship of lifestyle and clinical factors to lower urinary tract symptoms: Results from Boston area community health survey. *Urology*. 2007;70(5):916–21.

24 Coyne KS, Wein AJ, Tubaro A, Sexton CC, Thompson CL, Kopp ZS, et al. The burden of lower urinary tract symptoms: evaluating the effect of LUTS on health-related quality of life, anxiety and depression: EpiLUTS. *BJU Int*. 2009;103 Suppl 3:4–11.

25 Coyne KS, Sexton CC, Thompson C, Kopp ZS, Milsom I, Kaplan SA. The impact of OAB on sexual health in men and women: results from EpiLUTS. *J Sex Med*. 2011;8(6):1603–15.

26 Bjelland I, Dahl AA, Haug TT, Neckelmann D. The validity of the Hospital Anxiety and Depression Scale. An updated literature review. *J Psychosom Res*. 2002;52(2):69–77.

27 Olsson I, Mykletun A, Dahl AA. The Hospital Anxiety and Depression Rating Scale: a cross-sectional study of psychometrics and case finding abilities in general practice. *BMC Psychiatry*. 2005;5:46.

28 Huang CY, Chiu KM, Chung SD, Keller JJ, Huang CC, Lin HC. Increased risk of depressive disorder following the diagnosis of benign prostatic enlargement: one-year follow-up study. *J Affect Disord*. 2011;135(1–3):395–9.

29 Wong SY, Woo J, Leung JC, Leung PC. Depressive symptoms and lifestyle factors as risk factors of lower urinary tract symptoms in Southern Chinese men: a prospective study. *Aging Male*. 2010; 13(2):113–9.

30 Wong SY, Woo J, Hong A, Leung JC, Kwok T, Leung PC. Risk factors for lower urinary tract symptoms in southern Chinese men. *Urology*. 2006;68(5):1009–14.

31 Johnson TV, Abbasi A, Ehrlich SS, Kleris RS, Chirumamilla SL, Schoenberg ED, et al. Major depression drives severity of American Urological Association Symptom Index. *Urology*. 2010;76(6): 1317–20.

32 Sutcliffe S, Giovannucci E, De Marzo AM, Willett WC, Platz EA. Sexually transmitted infections, prostatitis, ejaculation frequency, and the odds of lower urinary tract symptoms. *Am J Epidemiol*. 2005;162(9):898–906.

33 Sutcliffe S, Rohrmann S, Giovannucci E, Nelson KE, De Marzo AM, Isaacs WB, et al. Viral infections and lower urinary tract symptoms in the third national health and nutrition examination survey. *J Urol*. 2007;178(5):2181–5.

34 Collins MM, Meigs JB, Barry MJ, Walker Corkery E, Giovannucci E, Kawachi I. Prevalence and correlates of prostatitis in the health professionals follow-up study cohort. *J Urol*. 2002;167(3): 1363–6.

35 Joseph MA, Harlow SD, Wei JT, Sarma AV, Dunn RL, Taylor JM, et al. Risk factors for lower urinary tract symptoms in a population-based sample of African-American men. *Am J Epidemiol*. 2003; 157(10):906–14.

36 Wallner LP, Clemens JQ, Sarma AV. Prevalence of and risk factors for prostatitis in African American men: the Flint Men's Health Study. *The Prostate*. 2009;69(1):24–32.

37 Platz EA, Kawachi I, Rimm EB, Colditz GA, Stampfer MJ, Willett WC, et al. Physical activity and benign prostatic hyperplasia. *Arch Intern Med*. 1998;158(21):2349–56.

38 Dal Maso L, Zucchetto A, Tavani A, Montella M, Ramazzotti V, Polesel J, et al. Lifetime occupational and recreational physical activity and risk of benign prostatic hyperplasia. *Int J Cancer*. 2006;118(10):2632–5.

39 Prezioso D, Catuogno C, Galassi P, D'Andrea G, Castello G, Pirritano D. Life-style in patients with LUTS suggestive of BPH. *Eur Urol*. 2001;40 Suppl 1:9–12.

40 Lacey JV, Jr., Deng J, Dosemeci M, Gao YT, Mostofi FK, Sesterhenn IA, et al. Prostate cancer, benign prostatic hyperplasia and physical activity in Shanghai, China. *Int J Epidemiol*. 2001;30(2):341–9.

41 Parsons JK, Kashefi C. Physical activity, benign prostatic hyperplasia, and lower urinary tract symptoms. *Eur Urol*. 2008;53(6):1228–35.

42 Breyer BN, Vittinghoff E, Van Den Eeden SK, Erickson BA, Shindel AW. Effect of sexually transmitted infections, lifetime sexual partner count, and recreational drug use on lower urinary tract

symptoms in men who have sex with men. *Urology*. 2012;79(1):188–93.

43 Gacci M, Eardley I, Giuliano F, Hatzichristou D, Kaplan SA, Maggi M, et al. Critical analysis of the relationship between sexual dysfunctions and lower urinary tract symptoms due to benign prostatic hyperplasia. *Eur Urol*. 2011;60(4):809–25.

44 Köhler TS, McVary KT. The relationship between erectile dysfunction and lower urinary tract symptoms and the role of phosphodiesterase type 5 inhibitors. *Eur Urol*. 2009;55(1):38–48.

45 Lukacs B, Leplege A, Thibault P, Jardin A. Prospective study of men with clinical benign prostatic hyperplasia treated with alfuzosin by general practitioners: 1-year results. *Urology*. 1996;48(5): 731–40.

46 Travison TG, Hall SA, Fisher WA, Araujo AB, Rosen RC, McKinlay JB, et al. Correlates of PDE5i use among subjects with erectile dysfunction in two population-based surveys. *J Sex Med*. 2011;8(11):3051–7.

47 McVary K. Lower urinary tract symptoms and sexual dysfunction: epidemiology and pathophysiology. *BJU Int*. 2006;97 Suppl 2:23–8; discussion 44–5.

48 Sarma AV, Wei JT. Clinical practice. *Benign prostatic hyperplasia and lower urinary tract symptoms. The N Engl J Med*. 2012;367(3):248–57.

49 MacDiarmid SA, Goodson TC, Holmes TM, Martin PR, Doyle RB. An assessment of the comprehension of the American Urological Association Symptom Index. *J Urol*. 1998;159(3):873–4.

50 Johnson TV, Abbasi A, Ehrlich SS, Kleris RS, Schoenberg ED, Owen-Smith A, et al. Patient misunderstanding of the individual questions of the American Urological Association symptom score. *J Urol*. 2008;179(6):2291–4; discussion 4–5.

51 van der Walt CL, Heyns CF, Groeneveld AE, Edlin RS, van Vuuren SP. Prospective comparison of a new visual prostate symptom score versus the international prostate symptom score in men with lower urinary tract symptoms. *Urology*. 2011;78(1): 17–20.

52 Ushijima S, Ukimura O, Okihara K, Mizutani Y, Kawauchi A, Miki T. Visual analog scale questionnaire to assess quality of life specific to each symptom of the International Prostate Symptom Score. *J Urol*. 2006;176(2):665–71.

53 Clatworthy J, Buick D, Hankins M, Weinman J, Horne R. The use and reporting of cluster analysis in health psychology: a review. *Br J Health Psychol*. 2005;10(Pt 3):329–58.

54 Barsevick AM, Whitmer K, Nail LM, Beck SL, Dudley WN. Symptom cluster research: conceptual, design, measurement, and analysis issues. *J Pain Symptom Manage*. 2006;31(1):85–95.

55 Everitt B. Cluster analysis is a generic term for a wide range of numerical methods for examining data. *Stat Meth Med Res*. 2004;13(5):343–5.

56 Tolan PH, Henry D. Patterns of psychopathology among urban poor children: comorbidity and aggression effects. *J Consult Clin Psychol*. 1996; 64(5):1094–9.

57 Coyne KS, Matza LS, Kopp ZS, Thompson C, Henry D, Irwin DE, et al. Examining lower urinary tract symptom constellations using cluster analysis. *BJU Int*. 2008;101(10):1267–73.

58 Hall SA, Cinar A, Link CL, Kopp ZS, Roehrborn CG, Kaplan SA, et al. Do urological symptoms cluster among women? Results from the Boston Area Community Health Survey. *BJU Int*. 2008;101(10):1257–66.

59 Cinar A, Hall SA, Link CL, Kaplan SA, Kopp ZS, Roehrborn CG, et al. Cluster analysis and lower urinary tract symptoms in men: findings from the Boston Area Community Health Survey. *BJU Int*. 2008;101(10):1247–56.

60 Rosen RC, Coyne KS, Henry D, Link CL, Cinar A, Aiyer LP, et al. Beyond the cluster: methodological and clinical implications in the Boston Area Community Health survey and EPIC studies. *BJU Int*. 2008;101(10):1274–8.

61 Martinez-Salamanca JI, Carballido J, Eardley I, Giuliano F, Gratzke C, Rosen R, et al. Phosphodiesterase type 5 inhibitors in the management of non-neurogenic male lower urinary tract symptoms: critical analysis of current evidence. *Eur Urol*. 2011;60(3):527–35.

62 Braun M, Wassmer G, Klotz T, Reifenrath B, Mathers M, Engelmann U. Epidemiology of erectile dysfunction: results of the "Cologne Male Survey." *Int J Impot Res*. 2000;12(6):305–11.

63 Nicolosi A, Moreira ED, Jr., Shirai M, Bin Mohd Tambi MI, Glasser DB. Epidemiology of erectile dysfunction in four countries: cross-national study of the prevalence and correlates of erectile dysfunction. *Urology*. 2003;61(1):201–6.

64 Vallancien G, Emberton M, Harving N, van Moorselaar RJ, Alf-One Study G. Sexual dysfunction in 1,274 European men suffering from lower urinary tract symptoms. *J Urol*. 2003;169(6): 2257–61.

65 Boyle P, Robertson C, Mazzetta C, Keech M, Hobbs R, Fourcade R, et al. The association between lower urinary tract symptoms and erectile dysfunction in four centres: the UrEpik study. *BJU Int.* 2003;92(7):719–25.

66 Hansen BL. Lower urinary tract symptoms (LUTS) and sexual function in both sexes. *Eur Urol.* 2004;46(2):229–34.

67 Terai A, Ichioka K, Matsui Y, Yoshimura K. Association of lower urinary tract symptoms with erectile dysfunction in Japanese men. *Urology.* 2004;64(1):132–6.

CHAPTER 3

Clinical Assessment and Diagnosis of Lower Urinary Tract Dysfunction: United States

Christopher P. Filson & John T. Wei

University of Michigan, Department of Urology, Division of Health Services Research, Ann Arbor, MI, USA

Key points

- Men who present with lower urinary tract symptoms (LUTS) should undergo a thorough medical history to characterize symptoms and rule out other nonprostate-related etiologies for their symptoms, such as urinary tract infection (UTI).
- All men with lower urinary tract dysfunction (LUTD) that may be related to benign prostatic hyperplasia (BPH) and/or benign prostatic enlargement (BPE) should have baseline symptoms characterized with a validated instrument and an assessment of urinary bother, such as the American Urological Association (AUA) Symptom Score or International Prostate Symptom Score.
- Physical examination, including digital rectal examination (DRE), is critical to rule out diagnoses that require additional testing or treatment.
- Frequency–volume charts are recommended to rule out polyuria as a cause of LUTS.
- Uroflowmetry and assessments of postvoid residual urine volume are optional for patients with severe LUTS or persistently bothersome LUTS after basic treatment.
- Pressure–flow urodynamic studies should be reserved for select patients who are being considered for surgical management of their BPH/BPE or those with other conditions requiring complex care.

Introduction

LUTD due to BPH/BPE is manifested clinically in a variety of ways. Classically, men with BPH/BPE exhibit LUTS, including urinary frequency and hesitancy. As BPH/BPE and bladder outlet obstruction (BOO) become more severe, patients can develop bladder dysfunction characterized by either detrusor overactivity or urinary retention. Advanced cases of BPH/BPE can cause recurrent UTI, gross hematuria, or renal insufficiency secondary to urinary obstruction. Quality of life is adversely affected with progression of disease and with more severe LUTS [1]. Patients who are older, with progressive symptoms, and with moderate or severe symptoms are significantly more likely to seek care [2]. Though the majority of patients with LUTS receive initial care from a primary care physician, it is

Male Lower Urinary Tract Symptoms and Benign Prostatic Hyperplasia, First Edition.
Edited by Steven A. Kaplan and Kevin T. McVary.
© 2014 John Wiley & Sons, Ltd. Published 2014 by John Wiley & Sons, Ltd.

recommended that more complex cases be referred to a urologist [3,4].

As a background, it is important to review the comprehensive history of guideline-driven management of men with LUTS. In the United States, initial guidelines were formulated by the Agency for Health Care Policy and Research (AHCPR) in 1994 [5]. Before the dissemination of these guidelines, a group of researchers in the 1980s sought to establish a critical evaluation of LUTD and BPH/BPE management for men and standardize treatment recommendations [6]. Work accomplished by this group, with collaboration with the AUA, eventually led to the establishment of treatment guidelines for the management of men with LUTD and BPH/BPE by AHCPR in 1994 [5,7].

Subsequently, the turn of the century brought a series of guidelines around the world. The European Association of Urology (EAU) established their initial guidelines in 2001, with frequent updates since then [8,9]. The AUA generated their initial guidelines in 2003, which drew heavily upon the initial AHCPR guidelines and incorporated additional clinical trial data [10]. Soon after, the International Consultation on Urologic Diseases (ICUD) formulated and published their own set of guidelines in 2006 [11]. More recently, the AUA updated their guidelines with a more detailed algorithm that specifies basic and complex management of patients with LUTD, paralleling the algorithms found in the ICUD guidelines (Figure 3.1) [12].

Initial evaluation of men presenting with LUTS

The first goal of the evaluation of men complaining of LUTS is to classify symptoms in one of four categories: LUTS with minimal bother, polyuria, bothersome LUTS, or complicated LUTS. LUTS with minimal bother does not merit a significant workup and often can be managed expectantly. On the other hand, patients with complicated LUTS [e.g., associated with hematuria or an abnormal prostate-specific antigen (PSA)] require a more detailed workup, which will be discussed below. Finally, patients with bothersome LUTS then need to be evaluated to determine whether polyuria (vs BOO) can account for their symptoms.

Medical history

All current guidelines recommend that an in-depth medical history be obtained from the male patient with LUTS [5,10,12]. The primary focus of this evaluation is to confirm the presence of symptoms secondary to BPH/BPE and to rule out other nonprostatic causes of voiding dysfunction. The secondary focus of the medical history is to evaluate for conditions that may make medical or surgical interventions less optimal (e.g. medical comorbidity or poor functional status).

Characterization of LUTS and quality of life

Men with BPH/BPE can exhibit a wide spectrum of LUTS at the initial presentation. These include storage symptoms (e.g. urinary frequency, urgency), voiding symptoms (e.g. slow stream, intermittency, hesitancy), and/or postmicturition symptoms (e.g. incomplete emptying) [13]. An objective, validated assessment of a patient's symptom profile is a crucial step in the clinical assessment of men with LUTD.

International Prostate Symptom Score

Current guidelines recommend using the International Prostate Symptom Score (IPSS) to characterize baseline LUTS for a patient

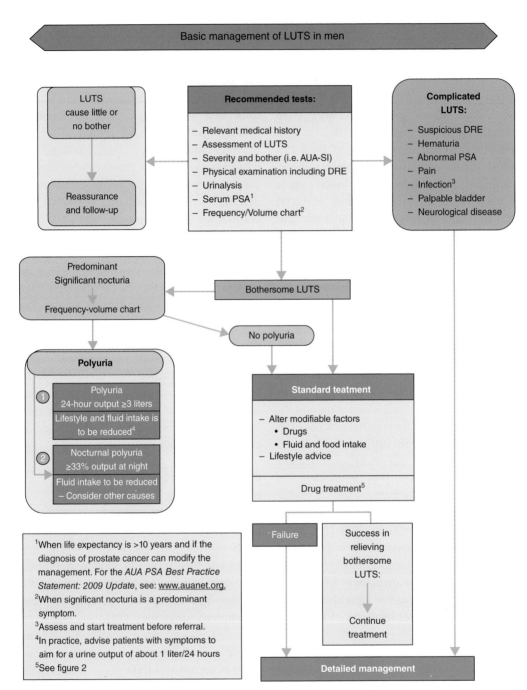

Figure 3.1 Algorithms for diagnosis and management of lower urinary tract dysfunction (LUTD). AUA-SI, American Urological Association-Symptom Index; DRE, digital rectal examination; LUTS, lower urinary tract symptoms. Professor Paul Abrams International Consultation on Urological Diseases (ICUD). Reproduced with permission of Paul Abrams.

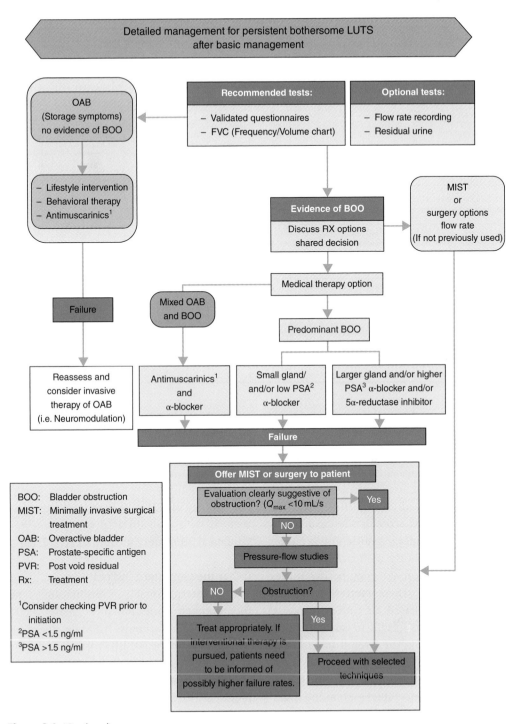

Figure 3.1 (*Continued*).

Patient name: _____ DOB: _____ ID: _____ Date of assessment: _____

Initial assessment ( ) Monitor during: _____ Therapy ( ) after: _____ Therapy/surgery ( ) _____

AUA BPH symptom score

	Not at all	Less than 1 time in 5	Less than half the time	About half the time	More than half the time	Almost always	
1. Over the past month, how often have you had a sensation of not emptying your bladder completely after you finished urinating?	0	1	2	3	4	5	
2. Over the past month, how often have you had to urinate again less than two hours after you finished urinating?	0	1	2	3	4	5	
3. Over the past month, how often have you found you stopped and started again several times when you urinated?	0	1	2	3	4	5	
4. Over the past month, how often have you found it difficult to postpone urination?	0	1	2	3	4	5	
5. Over the past month, how often have you had a weak urinary stream?	0	1	2	3	4	5	
6. Over the past month, how often have you had to push or strain to begin urination?	0	1	2	3	4	5	
	None	1 time	2 times	3 times	4 times	5 or more times	
7. Over the past month, how many times did you most typically get up to urinate from the time you went to bed at night until the time you got up in the morning?	0	1	2	3	4	5	
						Total symptom score	

Figure 3.2 American Urological Association (AUA) Symptom Index [15]. This is the breakdown of the AUA Symptom Index. The index comprises seven questions that address voiding symptoms, storage symptoms, and nocturia. Patients are classified as having mild (0–7), moderate (8–16), or severe (17–35) urinary-tract symptoms. The International Prostate Symptom Score also includes a question assessing the degree of bother related to urinary symptoms. BPH, benign prostatic hyperplasia. (Permission granted by Elsevier Publishing).

with LUTD related to BPE/BPH [5,10,12] (Figure 3.2). This score is identical to the American Urological Association-Symptom Index (AUA-SI; shown in Figure 3.2) with an additional question assessing bother related to LUTS [14,15]. These metrics generate a composite score based on patient responses to seven questions specific to various urinary symptoms [14,15]. The overall score can be divided between irritative (i.e. frequency, urgency, and nocturia questions) and obstructive (i.e. incomplete emptying, intermittency, weak stream, and straining questions) domains [16]. By itself, the IPSS cannot rule in the diagnosis of BPH/BPE as the etiology of LUTD, as high IPSS scores are seen in men with urethral obstruction and women with urinary incontinence [17,18].

Other measurement indices

The International Consultation on Incontinence Questionnaire Male LUTS (ICIQ-MLUTS, formerly ICSMale questionnaire) [19] and the Danish Prostatic Symptom Score [20] are both validated tools that AUA guidelines describe as options for measurement of LUTS. In addition, the Benign Prostatic Hyperplasia Impact Index (BPH-II) assesses health-related quality of life (HRQoL) in men with LUTS that may be related to BPH/BPE [21]. It consists of four questions directed at specific health domains (i.e. physical discomfort, worry, bother, and interference with daily activities). Higher scores on the BPH-II reflect a greater impact on QoL [21]. For patients who have storage complaints suggestive of an overactive bladder (OAB), other instruments exist that have been validated among men with symptoms consistent with OAB. These include the Kings' Health Questionnaire [22], OAB Questionnaire (OAB-q) [23], and Patient Perception of Bladder Condition index [24].

Although the IPSS is the most commonly used standard among validated instruments for measuring LUTS in men, there is a continued effort to fine-tune measurements among individual subgroups (e.g. those with OAB). The recent Meeting on Measurement of Urinary Symptoms held by the National Institute of Diabetes and Digestive and Kidney Diseases was focused on this effort [25]. The report from this meeting highlights the limitations of existing metrics, including a lack of specificity for BOO, suboptimal retest reliability, overemphasis of voiding symptoms, poor correlation between reported nocturia and actual voiding patterns, among others [25].

Physical examination

The original AHCPR guidelines also recommended a "physical examination, including DRE and focused neurologic examination" for the initial evaluation of men with LUTS. This recommendation is echoed by the most recent AUA guidelines [3,10].

The most important portion of the physical examination for a patient with LUTS is the focused genitourinary exam. Palpation of the lower abdomen can elicit evidence of a distended bladder and raise concern for urinary retention. Furthermore, examination of the foreskin (if present) and urethral meatus can reveal signs of phimosis or meatal stenosis, respectively. The DRE is also a crucial component of the physical examination, in that it can help rule out prostate cancer and help guide therapy. The DRE is 53% sensitive and 85% specific for identifying underlying prostate cancer when abnormalities (i.e. induration or nodule) are present [26]. Furthermore, abnormal rectal tone can raise suspicion of an occult neurologic disorder that may be contributing to a patient's symptoms.

Although the DRE can also provide a rough estimate of the size of the prostate, these measurements are unreliable. Specifically, DREs performed by urologists tend to underestimate the size of the prostate gland, particularly for patients with larger prostates [27,28]. Nevertheless, the size of the prostate is important to acknowledge during the workup of the BPH patient for multiple reasons. Although data are mixed [29], prostate size is correlated (albeit weakly) with severity of LUTS [30]. Patients with larger prostates are at higher risk of experiencing acute urinary retention and progression of symptoms [15,31]. Finally, men with larger prostate glands can respond better to certain medication regimens. For instance, the Medical Therapy of Prostatic Symptoms trial demonstrated that men with prostates larger than 25 g had a treatment response and decreased progression when treated with a combination of doxazosin and finasteride, compared with doxazosin alone [32].

Initial diagnostic tests
Urinalysis

All patients undergoing an evaluation for LUTS due to BPH should have a urinalysis performed to evaluate for UTIs or other uropathology. The most significant findings would include evidence of pyuria, bacteriuria, and/or hematuria. Leukocyte esterase on a dipstick urinalysis

Table 3.1 Example of frequency/volume chart and voiding diary

Date	Time (AM/PM)	Voided urine volume (mL or ounces)	Catheterized urine volume (mL or ounces)	Amount leaked (1 = drops/damp; 2 = wet-soaked; 3 = emptied)	Pad change? (Yes/no)	Activity during leak	Urgency (1 = mild; 2 = moderate; 3 = severe)	Sensation and/or pain (1 = mild; 2 = moderate; 3 = severe)	Fluid intake and type
1/1/2006	7.00 AM	250 mL							
1/1/2006	7.30 AM			2	Yes	Running	2	1	
1/1/2006	8.00 AM								8 oz tea, 4 oz OJ

This is an example of the voiding diary utilized at the University of Michigan Department of Urology. The diary is kept over 3 days and characterizes fluid intake, urine volume, urinary frequency, the nature and volume of urinary incontinence, and urinary urgency.

is up to 98% sensitive and 96% specific for a UTI [33]. Furthermore, the presence of nitrites is up to 45% sensitive and 98% specific for a UTI [33]. Any single episode of microscopic hematuria (i.e. 3–5 red blood cells per high-power field) mandates an in-depth workup for other sources of hematuria besides BPH (including genitourinary malignancy) [34].

PSA testing

According to AUA guidelines, not all men who undergo an evaluation for BPH-related LUTS require additional PSA testing. PSA testing, in general, should be reserved for patients with a life expectancy of over 10 years, and withheld for patients over the age of 75 [35]. However, the test should be considered if the diagnosis of prostate cancer would alter management [10]. Importantly, a single PSA test is only 72% sensitive and 93% specific for the presence of prostate cancer, based on a meta-analysis of published data [26]. Prostatic trauma (e.g. biopsy), urinary retention, and infection can all spuriously elevate PSA values, and PSA testing should be repeated 6–8 weeks after any of these events [36]. PSA values correlate directly with prostate size, with patients with larger prostates typically having abnormally elevated PSA values [37].

Voiding diaries

The most recent guidelines recommend that patients who complain of nocturia undergo an evaluation with a frequency/volume diary (Table 3.1; as opposed to questionnaires, which are subject to recall bias) [38]. Voiding diaries can differentiate men experiencing polyuria from those with LUTD due to BPH/BPE, which is an integral part of the diagnostic algorithm in the most recent guidelines [10]. Of note, 3-day voiding diaries are as accurate as 7-day diaries and likely more convenient for patients [39].

Differential diagnosis after the initial evaluation
Carcinoma of the bladder

The classic clinical presentation of patients with carcinoma *in situ* (CIS) of the bladder includes hematuria (gross or microscopic) associated with urinary frequency and/or urgency. Nearly half of patients with bladder CIS present with irritative voiding symptoms [40]. These urinary symptoms are more prevalent (and more severe) with multifocal and diffuse CIS [41]. Importantly, up to 15% of patients with CIS do not have hematuria. It is crucial to evaluate for history of tobacco exposure (both past and current) and other risk factors for malignancies of the bladder during the workup of a man with irritative LUTS.

UTI

UTIs in men that can mimic LUTD due to BPE/BPH include urethritis, cystitis, and prostatitis. Other symptoms typically associated with UTIs include fever, malodorous urine, urethral discharge, and flank pain. It is important to assess the patient's sexual history and any prior history of UTIs, in addition to checking results of the urinalysis and urine culture.

Bladder calculi

Patients with bladder calculi can exhibit LUTS similar to those with LUTD due to BPH/BPE, including urinary retention, hematuria, and dysuria [42]. Nearly 90% of bladder calculi are related to BOO [43].

Urethral stricture disease

Over half of patients who have anterior urethral strictures present with the primary complaint of LUTS, particularly a weak stream and incomplete emptying [44,45]. Risk factors for urethral strictures include trauma (particularly straddle injuries), gonococcal urethritis, balanitis xerotica obliterans, and prior urethral/prostatic surgery [46].

Neurologic disorders

Patients with underlying neurologic disorders can present initially with LUTS. These disorders include Parkinson's disease, multiple system atrophy, and multiple sclerosis, among others [47]. Diabetic uropathy can also present commonly with nocturia and urinary frequency [48]. Signs and symptoms of end-stage disease (e.g. diabetic neuropathy, renal dysfunction, diabetic retinopathy) can increase suspicion of detrusor hypoactivity due to diabetes.

Nocturia, polyuria, and nocturnal polyuria

Nocturia occurs when a patient awakens multiple times to void in the midst of sleeping at night [13]. A number of factors contribute to nocturia, including reduced bladder capacity, detrusor overactivity, and increased urine production (i.e. nocturnal polyuria) [11]. Importantly, frequent awakenings from a condition such as sleep apnea can also mimic nocturia, and should be ruled out [49]. Polyuria is the production of ≥40 mL/kg of urine volume over 24 h (approximately 2.8 L for a 70 kg individual) [13]. Nocturnal polyuria is the production of a majority of the urine volume (>33%) at night [13]. A number of conditions can cause polyuria, including polydipsia, congestive heart failure, and diabetes insipidus, among others [50]. Patients complaining of nocturia are recommended to complete frequency–volume charts, and try fluid restriction if diagnosed with polyuria (nocturnal or otherwise) [12].

Evaluation of the persistent or complicated LUTS in the male patient with LUTD

A more involved evaluation of men with LUTD is indicated for a number of reasons. First, men who exhibit signs of non-BPH-related disease processes (e.g. malignancy) require additional evaluation. Second, men may fail initial medical management of bothersome LUTS. Finally, patients may not have subjective complaints or bother but present with other evidence of clinically significant BOO due to BPH (e.g. renal insufficiency, bladder calculi). In all of these cases, further investigation is directed towards evaluating a patient's candidacy for surgical intervention.

Diagnostic tests for patients with complicated LUTD
Uroflowmetry

The most recent AUA guidelines list uroflowmetry as an option in the evaluation of men with persistently bothersome LUTS that does not respond to initial management [12]. Uroflowmetry measures the volume of urine flow over time, usually in milliliters per second. Pertinent measures from uroflowmetry include maximal urinary flow (Q_{max}), average urinary flow (Q_{ave}), and the volume voided [51]. In order to be reliable, the voided volume needs to exceed at least 150 mL [5]. Theoretical examples of uroflowmetry results are shown in Figure 3.3. The average Q_{max} for men decreases with age [52,53]. Although a Q_{max} of <10 mL/s can suggest BOO due to BPH, uroflowmetry cannot distinguish between BPH or detrusor inactivity as a basis for decreased urinary flow [11,54]. Furthermore, due to the variability between individual measurements, it is recommended that more than one test be performed [55]. Current AUA guidelines for performance of urodynamics state that uroflowmetry "may be used" as a diagnostic tool for the workup of men with urinary symptoms consistent with voiding dysfunction [56].

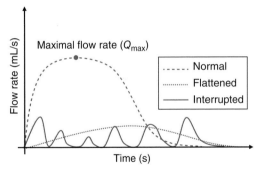

Figure 3.3 Examples of uroflowmetry curves. This schematic shows three theoretical examples of uroflowmetry curves. The *y*-axis represents flow rate (in milliliters per second), and the *x*-axis is time (in seconds). The area under the curve represents the volume voided. A "normal" uroflow curve tends to resemble a "loaf of bread" with a rapid rise in flow rate, followed by constant flow for a time period, until a rapid drop-off in flow at the completion of the void. Patients with obstruction or detrusor underactivity tend to exhibit flattened or interrupted uroflow curves with prolonged voiding times.

Postvoid residual urine volume

Measurement of postvoid residual urine volume (PVR) can provide an insight into the patient's capability of emptying the bladder to completion and help rule out the presence of chronic urinary retention. The sensitivity and specificity of a PVR over 50 mL for diagnosing BOO are 72% and 42%, respectively [57]. Measurement of PVR can be done either by ultrasonography or with urethral catheterization. The advantage of ultrasonography is its noninvasive nature, but it is subject to operator error and inaccuracy in certain clinical scenarios (i.e. ascites or morbid obesity). However, modern bladder scanners are more accurate and comparable with urethral catheterization [58,59]. Urethral catheterization also increases the risk of urethral trauma and UTI. Furthermore, a number of factors can contribute to a variation in PVR readings, including the time of day [60]. There can be significant variation between repeated measurements for individual patients [60].

In addition, PVR is not a predictive measure for response to treatment (particularly surgery) and cannot differentiate between outlet obstruction and detrusor underactivity [61].

Despite its marginally predictive nature for response to treatment, measurement of PVR can help rule out chronic urinary retention. "Urinary retention" encompasses a diverse group of clinical scenarios varying in presentation and time course. Acute urinary retention (AUR) is the sudden onset of an inability to empty the bladder adequately. This is characterized by symptoms (e.g. pelvic pain and urgency) and often requires catheterization for treatment. Chronic urinary retention is characterized by a longer time course (i.e. months to years) and a variable presentation, ranging from a lack of symptoms (i.e. occult or silent retention) to bothersome obstructive LUTS (e.g. hesitancy, weak stream, subjectively incomplete emptying). Although the cutoff volume to define chronic urinary retention is generally accepted to be 300 mL, varying definitions exist [13,62]. Risk factors for urinary retention include increasing age [63,64], prior episodes of urinary retention [65], and a prior diagnosis of BPE/BPH [63]. Interestingly, elevated PVR is not a predictor of subsequent AUR [66]. Chronic urinary retention requires further investigation with pressure–flow studies to rule out detrusor underactivity. There are currently insufficient data to recommend routine measurement of PVR in the workup of a male patient presenting with LUTS.

Pressure–flow studies

Pressure–flow studies can assess and confirm adequate bladder function in the setting of obstructive urinary symptoms (i.e. confirming BOO). Thus, these studies are reserved for patients being considered for surgical management of the bladder outlet with other conditions (e.g. neurologic disease or diabetes) that can mimic BOO [9,12]. The ICUD for LUTD recommends pressure–flow studies for all patients being considered for surgery who have maximal urine flow on uroflowmetry greater than 10 mL/s [11].

Additional selected diagnostic tests for complex BPH patients

Flexible cystoscopy

Cystoscopy is reserved for select patients and should not be standard in any BPH evaluation. Cystoscopy can also be considered in patients who are to undergo definitive surgery to map out the appearance of the prostate and to determine if a median lobe is present [10,12]. Patients who demonstrate either microscopic or gross hematuria require cystoscopic evaluation of their bladder to rule out the presence of bladder cancer [34]. Patients who have risk factors for urethral stricture disease are also candidates for cystoscopy.

Transrectal ultrasound of the prostate

Similar to cystoscopy, a transrectal ultrasound of the prostate is only indicated to assist with operative planning for patients who have failed medical therapy. Although the PSA level (if checked) correlates well with prostate size and response to certain medical therapies (i.e.

finasteride), knowing a more accurate size may be crucial in deciding between different surgical modalities (e.g. transurethral resection of the prostate versus open prostatectomy; laser ablation vs laser enucleation). There is no role for transrectal ultrasound in the assessment of a basic BPH patient [5,10,12].

Imaging

Routine imaging of the upper tracts is currently not recommended during a basic evaluation of a patient with BPH, unless there is an indication of UTI, renal dysfunction, or a prior history of nephrolithiasis [5,10,12].

Serum creatinine

Though the AHCPR and the initial AUA guidelines initially described serum creatinine as a recommended test during the basic evaluation of patients with suspected BPH [5, 10], the most recent guidelines do not recommend serum creatinine as a part of the standard workup for a patient being evaluated for BPH [12]. This is in contrast to the current EAU guidelines, which recommend checking serum creatinine for all men undergoing an evaluation for LUTD [9].

Dos and don'ts

- Practitioners should rely on clinical guidelines to assist with assessment and diagnosis of men with LUTS due to BPH.
- All patients should undergo a thorough medical history, physical examination (including DRE), and assessment of baseline symptoms with a validated measurement tool for LUTS (i.e. AUA-SI).
- PSA testing should be restricted to those with a life expectancy over 10 years or where a diagnosis of prostate cancer would influence management.
- Serum creatinine is no longer a recommended test for all patients being assessed for a diagnosis of BPH.
- Frequency–volume charts should be administered to patients complaining primarily of nocturia or patients with persistent LUTS after basic treatment.
- Uroflowmetry and PVR do not have to be checked on all patients with LUTS, but are an option for patients with complicated LUTS or persistently bothersome LUTS after basic management.

Bibliography

1 Welch G, Weinger K, Barry MJ. Quality-of-life impact of lower urinary tract symptom severity: results from the Health Professionals Follow-up Study. *Urology*. 2002;59:245–50.

2 Jacobsen SJ, Girman CJ, Guess HA, Rhodes T, Oesterling JE, Lieber MM. Natural history of prostatism: longitudinal changes in voiding symptoms in community dwelling men. *J Urol*. 1996; 155:595–600.

3 Hollingsworth JM, Hollenbeck BK, Daignault S, Kim SP, Wei JT. Differences in initial benign prostatic hyperplasia management between primary care physicians and urologists. *J Urol*. 2009; 182:2410–14.

4 Wei JT, Sarma AV. Benign prostatic hyperplasia and lower urinary tract symptoms. *N Eng J Med*. 2012;367:248–57.

5 McConnell JD, Barry MJ, Bruskewitz RC, *et al*. Clinical Practice Guideline: Number 8. Benign prostatic hyperplasia: diagnosis and treatment. Rockville, MD: United States Department of Health and Human Services, 1994.

6 Wennberg JE. On the status of the Prostate Disease Assessment Team. *Health Serv Res*. 1990; 25:709–16.

7 Wennberg JE. AHCPR and the strategy for health care reform. *Health Aff*. 1992;11:67–71.

8 De la Rosette, JJ, Alivizatos G, Madersbacher S, Perachino M, Thomas D, Desgrandchamps F, *et al*. EAU guidelines on benign prostatic hyperplasia (BPH). *Eur Urol*. 2001;40:256–63.

9 Madersbacher S, Alivizatos G, Nordling J, Sanz CR, Emberton M, de la Rosette JJ. EAU 2004 guidelines on assessment, therapy and follow-up of men with lower urinary tract symptoms suggestive of benign prostatic obstruction (BPH Guidelines). *J Urol*. 2004;46:547–54.

10 AUA Practice Guidelines Committee. AUA guideline on management of benign prostatic hyperplasia [2003]. Chapter 1: Diagnosis and treatment recommendations. *J Urol* 2003; 170:530–47.

11 Mcconnell JD, Abrams P, Denis L, Khoury S, Roehrborn CG, editors. International Consultation on Urological Diseases. Male lower urinary tract dysfunction: evaluation and management. 2006 ed. Paris: Health Publications; 2006.

12 McVary KT, Roehrborn CG, Avins AL, Barry MJ, Bruskewitz RC, Donnell RF, *et al*. Update on AUA guideline on the management of benign prostatic hyperplasia. *J Urol*. 2011; 185:1793–803.

13 Abrams P, Cardozo L, Fall M, Griffiths D, Rosier P, Ulmsten U, *et al*. The standardisation of terminology of lower urinary tract function: report from the Standardisation Subcommittee of the International Continence Society. *Neurourol Urodyn*. 2002; 21:167–78.

14 Cockett ATK, Khoury S, Aso Y, Chatelain C, Denis L, Griffiths K, *et al*., editors. Recommendations of the International Consensus Committee concerning: International Prostate Symptom Score (I-PSS) and quality of life assessment. The 2nd International Consultation on Benign Prostatic Hyperplasia (BPH). Scientific Communication International; 1994.

15 Barry MJ, Fowler FJ Jr, O'Leary MP, Bruskewitz RC, Holtgrewe HL, Mebust WK, *et al*. The American Urological Association symptom index for benign prostatic hyperplasia. *J Urol*. 1992; 148:1549–57.

16 Barry MJ, Williford WO, Fowler FJ, Jones KM, Lepor H. Filling and voiding symptoms in the American Urological Association Symptom Index: the value of their distinction in a Veterans Affairs randomized trial of medical therapy in men with a clinical diagnosis of benign prostatic hyperplasia. *J Urol*. 2000;164[5]: 1559–64.

17 Roberts RO, Jacobsen SJ, Jacobson DJ, Reilly WT, Talley NJ, Lieber MM. Natural history of prostatism: high American Urological Association Symptom scores among community-dwelling men and women with urinary incontinence. *Urology*. 1998;51:213–9.

18 Chancellor MB, Rivas DA, Keeley FX, Lotfi MA, Gomella LG. Similarity of the American Urological Association Symptom Index among men with benign prostate hyperplasia (BPH), urethral obstruction not due to BPH and detrusor hyperreflexia without outlet obstruction. *Br J Urol*. 1994;74:200–3.

19 Donovan JL, Abrams P, Peters TJ, Kay HE, Reynard J, Chapple C, *et al*. The ICS-"BPH" Study: the psychometric validity and reliability of the ICSmale questionnaire. *Br J Urol*. 1996;77: 554–62.

20 Hansen BJ, Flyger H, Brasso K, Schou J, Nordling J, Thorup Andersen J, *et al.* Validation of the self-administered Danish Prostatic Symptom Score (DAN-PSS-1) system for use in benign prostatic hyperplasia. *Br J Urol.* 1995;76: 451–8.

21 Barry MJ, Williford WO, Chang Y, Machi M, Jones KM, Walker-Corkery E, *et al.* Benign prostatic hyperplasia specific health status measures in clinical research: how much change in the American Urological Association Symptom Index and the Benign Prostatic Hyperplasia Impact Index is perceptible to patients? *J Urol.* 1995;154: 1770–4.

22 Okamura K, Nojiri Y, Osuga Y. Reliability and validity of the King's Health Questionnaire for lower urinary tract symptoms in both genders. *BJU Int.* 2009;103:1673–8.

23 Coyne KS, Revicki D, Hunt T, Corey R, Stewart W, Bentkover J, *et al.* Psychometric validation of an overactive bladder symptom and health-related quality of life questionnaire: The OAB-q. *Qual Life Res.* 2002;11:563–74.

24 Coyne KS, Matza LS, Kopp Z, Abrams P. The validation of the Patient Perception of Bladder Condition (PPBC): a single-item global measure for patients with overactive bladder. *Eur Urol.* 2006;49:1079–86.

25 National Institute of Diabetes and Digestive and Kidney Diseases (NIDDK) Meeting on Measurement of Urinary Symptoms (MOMUS) Summary Report [Internet]. National Institutes of Diabetes and Kidney Diseases: Bethesda, MD. [updated November 11, 2011; cited February 1, 2013]. Available from: http://www3.niddk.nih.gov/fund/other/MOMUS.pdf

26 Mistry K, Cable G. Meta-analysis of prostate-specific antigen and digital rectal examination as screening tests for prostate carcinoma. *J Am Board Fam Med.* 2003;16:95–101.

27 Roehrborn CG, GIrman CJ, Rhodes T, Hanson KA, Collins GN, Sech SM, *et al.* Correlation between prostate size estimated by digital rectal examination and measured by transrectal ultrasound. *Urology.* 1997;49:548–57.

28 Roehrborn CG, Sech S, Montoya J, Rhodes T, Girman CJ. Interexaminer reliability and validity of a three-dimensional model to assess prostate volume by digital rectal examination. *Urology.* 2001;57:1087–92.

29 Eckhardt MD, van Venrooij GEPM, Boon TA. Symptoms and quality of life versus age, prostate volume, and urodynamic parameters in 565 strictly selected men with lower urinary tract symptoms suggestive of benign prostatic hyperplasia. *Urology.* 2001;57:695–700.

30 Girman CJ, Jacobsen SJ, Guess HA, Oesterling JE, Chute CG, Panser LA, *et al.* Natural history of prostatism: relationship among symptoms, prostate volume and peak urinary flow rate. *J Urol.* 1995;153:1510–5.

31 Roehrborn CG, McConnell JD, Lieber M, Kaplan S, Geller J, Malek GH, *et al.* Serum prostate-specific antigen concentration is a powerful predictor of acute urinary retention and need for surgery in men with clinical benign prostatic hyperplasia. *Urology.* 1999;53:473–80.

32 Kaplan SA, McConnell JD, Roehrborn CG, Meehan AG, Lee MW, Noble WR, *et al.* Combination therapy With doxazosin and finasteride for benign prostatic hyperplasia in patients with lower urinary tract symptoms and a baseline total prostate volume of 25 mL or greater. *J Urol.* 2006;175:217–20.

33 Wilson ML, Gaido L. Laboratory diagnosis of urinary tract infections in adult patients. *Clin Infect Dis.* 2004;38:1150–8.

34 Davis R, Jones JS, Barocas DA, Castle EP, Lang EK, Leveillee RJ, *et al.* Diagnosis, evaluation and follow-up of asymptomatic microhematuria (AMH) in adults: AUA guideline. *J Urol.* 2012;188: 2473–81.

35 Greene KL, Albertsen PC, Babaian RJ, Carter HB, Gann PH, Han M, *et al.* Prostate specific antigen Best Practice Statement: 2009 update. *J Urol.* 2009;182:2232–41.

36 Tchetgen MN, Oesterling JE. The effect of prostatitis, urinary retention, ejaculation, and ambulation on the serum prostate specific antigen concentration. *Urol Clin N Am.* 1997;24: 283–91.

37 Collins GN, Lee RJ, McKelvie GB, Rogers AC, Hehir M. Relationship between prostate specific antigen, prostate volume and age in the benign prostate. *Br J Urol.* 1993;71:445–50.

38 Ku JH, Hong SK, Kim HH, Paick JS, Lee SE, Oh SJ. Is questionnaire enough to assess number of nocturic episodes? Prospective comparative study between data from questionnaire and frequency–volume charts. *Urology.* 2004;64:966–9.

39 Dmochowski RR, Sanders SW, Appell RA, et al. Bladder-health diaries: an assessment of 3-day vs 7-day entries. *BJU Int.* 2005;96: 1049–54.

40 Cheng L, Cheville JC, Neumann RM, Nitti VW, Davila GW. Survival of patients with carcinoma in situ of the urinary bladder. *Cancer.* 1999;85: 2469–74.

41 Hudson MA, Herr HW. Carcinoma in situ of the bladder. *J Urol.* 1995;153:564–72.

42 Hammad FT, Kaya M, Kazim E. Bladder calculi: Did the clinical picture change? *Urology.* 2006; 67:1154–8.

43 Douenias R, Rich M, Badlani G, Mazor D, Smith A. Predisposing factors in bladder calculi: review of 100 cases. *Urology.* 1991;37: 240–3.

44 Rourke K, Hickle J. The clinical spectrum of the presenting signs and symptoms of anterior urethral stricture: detailed analysis of a single institutional cohort. *Urology.* 2012;79:1163–7.

45 Nuss GR, Granieri MA, Zhao LC, Thum DJ, Gonzalez CM. Presenting symptoms of anterior urethral stricture disease: a disease specific, patient reported questionnaire to measure outcomes. *J Urol.* 2012;187:559–62.

46 Fenton AS, Morey AF, Aviles R, Garcia CR. Anterior urethral strictures: etiology and characteristics. *Urology.* 2005;65:1055–8.

47 Magari T, Fukabori Y, Ogura H, Suzuki K. Lower urinary tract symptoms of neurological origin in urological practice. *Clin Auton Res.* 2012;1: 1–6.

48 Kaplan SA, Te AE, Blaivas JG. Urodynamic findings in patients with diabetic cystopathy. *J Urol.* 1995;153:342–4.

49 Pressman MR, Figueroa WG, Kendrick-Mohamed J, Greenspon LW, Peterson DD. Nocturia—a rarely recognized symptom of sleep apnea and other occult sleep disorders. *Arch Int Med* 1996; 156:545–50.

50 Van Kerrebroeck P, Weiss J. Standardization and terminology of nocturia. *BJU Int.* 1999;84: 1–4.

51 Siroky MB, Olsson CA, Krane RJ. The flow rate nomogram: I. Development. *J Urol.* 1979;122: 665–8.

52 Jorgensen JB, Jensen KME, Bille-Brahe NE, Mogensen P. Uroflowmetry in asymptomatic elderly males. *Br J Urol.* 1986;58:390–5.

53 Jensen KME. Uroflowmetry in elderly men. *World J Urol.* 1995;13:21–3.

54 Chancellor MB, Blaivas JG, Kaplan SA, Axelrod S. Bladder outlet obstruction versus impaired detrusor contractility: the role of outflow. *J Urol.* 1991;145:810–2.

55 Feneley MR, Dunsmuir WD, Pearce J, Kirby RS. Reproducibility of uroflow measurement: experience during a double-blind, placebo-controlled study of doxazosin in benign prostatic hyperplasia. *Urology.* 1996;47:658–63.

56 Winters JC, Dmochowski RR, Goldman HB, Herndon CD, Kobashi KC, Kraus SR, et al. Urodynamic studies in adults: AUA/SUFU Guideline. *J Urol.* 2012;188:2464–72.

57 Oelke M, Höfner K, Jonas U, de la Rosette JJ, Ubbink DT, Wijkstra H. Diagnostic accuracy of noninvasive tests to evaluate bladder outlet obstruction in men: detrusor wall thickness, uroflowmetry, postvoid residual urine, and prostate volume. *Eur Urol.* 2007;52:827–35.

58 Kelly CE. Evaluation of voiding dysfunction and measurement of bladder volume. *Rev Urol.* 2004;6:S32.

59 Byun S-S, Kim HH, Lee E, Paick JS, Kamg W, Oh SJ. Accuracy of bladder volume determinations by ultrasonography: are they accurate over entire bladder volume range? *Urology.* 2003;62: 656–60.

60 Griffiths DJ, Harrison G, Moore K, McCracken P. Variability of post-void residual urine volume in the elderly. *Urol Res.* 1996;24:23–6.

61 Bruskewitz RC, Reda DJ, Wasson JH, et al. Testing to predict outcome after transurethral resection of the prostate. *J Urol.* 1997;157: 1304–8.

62 Kaplan SA, Wein AJ, Staskin DR, Roehrborn CG, Steers WD. Urinary retention and post-void residual urine in men: separating truth from tradition. *J Urol.* 2008;180:47–54.

63 Verhamme KMC, Dieleman JP, van Wijk MAM, Bosch JL, Stricker BH, Sturkenboom MC. Low incidence of acute urinary retention in the general male population: The Triumph project. *J Urol.* 2005;47:494–8.

64 Meigs JB, Barry MJ, Giovannucci E, Rimm EB, Stampfer MJ, Kawachi I. Incidence rates and risk factors for acute urinary retention: the health professionals followup study. *J Urol.* 1999;162: 376–82.

65 Klarskov P, Andersen JT, Asmussen CF, Brenøe J, Jensen SK, Jensen IL, *et al*. Symptoms and signs predictive of the voiding pattern after acute urinary retention in men. *Scand J Urol Nephrol.* 1987;21:23–8.

66 Roehrborn CG, Kaplan SA, Lee MW, *et al*. Baseline post void residual urine volume as a predictor of urinary outcomes in men with BPH in the MTOPS study. *J Urol.* 2005;173(Suppl):443.

CHAPTER 4

Clinical Assessment and Diagnosis of Lower Urinary Tract Symptoms/Benign Prostatic Hyperplasia: Europe

Stavros Gravas[1] & Jean J. M. C. H. de la Rosette[2]

[1]Department of Urology, University of Thessalia, Larissa, Greece
[2]Department of Urology, Academic Medical Center, University of Amsterdam, Amsterdam, The Netherlands

Key points

- Lower urinary tract symptoms (LUTS) may have a multifactorial etiology, and so European Guidelines focus on male LUTS and not only on benign prostatic hyperplasia (BPH).
- In order to diagnose BPH, a systematic diagnostic work-up should exclude other diseases or conditions also associated with LUTS.
- All men with LUTS should be formally assessed prior to starting any form of treatment in order to define the clinical profile of patient and select the appropriate management.
- The level of evidence for the investigational test used in the assessment of male LUTS is low and based on expert opinion, so the strength of those recommendations is weak.
- Diagnostic investigations (recommended or under conditions) of patients with LUTS include medical history, symptom score questionnaires, physical examination, digital rectal examination, frequency–volume charts, bladder diaries, urinalysis, serum creatinine, prostate-specific antigen (PSA), postvoid residual urine, imaging of urinary tract, endoscopy, uroflowmetry, and pressure–flow studies.
- There is a significant disparity in clinical assessment and diagnosis of BPH among European countries that seem to be based upon personal experience and choice rather than evidence-based management of LUTS.

Although, it is well known that LUTS can result from several pathophysiologic conditions, LUTS in men were traditionally attributed to the prostate gland, and terms such as BPH, benign prostatic enlargement (BPE), benign prostatic obstruction (BPO), and bladder outlet obstruction (BOO) have been used to describe the underlying etiology. However, it is only in recent years that urologists have begun to acknowledge that factors other than the enlarged prostate are of equal importance for the development of LUTS in a proportion of men over 40 years of age.

This multifactorial view of the etiology of LUTS has led most experts to regard the whole urinary tract as a single functional unit [1]. In our daily practice, patients seek professional help for LUTS, and not for an underlying attribute of the prostate. This fact led the European Association of Urology

Male Lower Urinary Tract Symptoms and Benign Prostatic Hyperplasia, First Edition.
Edited by Steven A. Kaplan and Kevin T. McVary.
© 2014 John Wiley & Sons, Ltd. Published 2014 by John Wiley & Sons, Ltd.

(EAU) to develop the "EAU Guidelines on Non-Neurogenic Male LUTS, including BPO" that reflect the European perspective in the management of male LUTS. These European Guidelines aim to provide a more realistic and practical approach to the management of men who complain about a variety of bladder storage, voiding, and/or postmicturition symptoms [2]. Interestingly, the American Urological Association Guidelines on BPH use the Index Patient [3]. The Index Patient is a male aged 45 or older who is consulting a qualified health-care provider for his LUTS and does not have a history suggesting non-BPH causes of LUTS, and his LUTS may or may not be associated with an enlarged prostate gland, BOO, or histological BPH. Therefore, the EAU and AUA Guidelines use a different approach and underline the lack of a global assessment of male LUTS.

Aim of the assessment

Investigational tests are useful for diagnosis, monitoring of the condition, prognosis of disease progression, treatment planning, and prediction of treatment outcome. The clinical assessment of patients with LUTS has two main objectives.

The first objective is to exclude other conditions that cause LUTS and diagnose BPH. Causes of male LUTS include BPO, bladder stones, detrusor overactivity – overactive bladder, detrusor underactivity, distal ureteral stones, foreign bodies, neurological diseases, nocturnal polyuria, prostatitis, urinary incontinence, urethral strictures, urinary tract infections, and others. The assessment may be interrupted or stopped when pathologies other than BPH have been identified. In this case, the guidelines on the management of specific conditions should be followed [2].

The second objective is to define the clinical profile of patient with LUTS due to BPH in order to provide the best care. The assessment should be able to allocate patients for watchful waiting, medical or surgical treatment [based on severity of symptoms and degree of bother and the presence of recurrent or refractory urinary retention, overflow incontinence, recurrent urinary tract infections, bladder stones or diverticula, treatment-resistant macroscopic hematuria due to BPH/BPE, or dilatation of the upper urinary tract due to BPO, with or without renal insufficiency, and insufficient relief of LUTS or postvoid residual urine volume (PVR) after conservative or medical treatment] and to discriminate men at risk of progression (older men with larger prostates, higher serum PSA concentrations, larger PVR and low Q_{max}) [2,4].

Specifically, for BPH, it should be emphasized that there are no strong data to support (or not) the use of some of those investigational tests. It is very difficult to perform randomized studies to evaluate the use of investigational tests; therefore, evidence comes from large observational studies or as indirect (secondary) conclusions from randomized studies with different primary objectives. As a result, most of the recommendations on LUTS/BPH tests are of a low level of evidence and based on expert opinion, and consequently the strength of those recommendations is weak.

Investigational tests

The diagnostic investigations of patients with LUTS are detailed below.

Medical history
Medical history is an inevitable part of clinical assessment with the aim to (1) identify the

nature of patient's LUTS, and their duration, progression, severity and bother; (2) identify other conditions responsible for LUTS; (3) assess the lifestyle, including alcohol consumption, fluid-intake habits, smoking, and exercise; (4) evaluate the sexual-function status; (5) review previous surgical interventions (especially those affecting genitourinary tract and pelvic floor) and current medication (drugs that may contribute to LUTS); and (6) evaluate the patient's fitness for possible surgical procedures and identify comorbidities that may affect treatment choice.

Symptom score

Existing guidelines on male LUTS and/or BPH recommend the use of a validated symptom score questionnaire as a routine part of the assessment [2,3].

The International Prostate Symptom Score (IPSS) with the quality-of-life question is an eight-item (seven symptom questions plus the quality-of-life question), self-administered questionnaire validated in several languages [5]. It is considered the international standard and represents a very useful tool to assess and quantify LUTS. The IPSS can be used to assess the storage symptoms (frequency, urgency, nocturia, or questions 2, 4, and 7) and voiding symptoms (feeling of incomplete emptying, intermittency, weak stream, straining, or questions 1, 3, 5, and 6). It is sensitive to post-treatment changes with a high volume of data to be available, since almost all the studies use IPSS. However, IPSS is not disease or condition specific and is poorly correlated with peak urinary flow, postvoid residual urine, prostate volume, and BOO [6,7]. Another limitation is that IPSS does not evaluate urgency incontinence, postmicturition symptoms, and sexual function.

Other questionnaires that can be used include the Danish Prostatic Symptom Score, the International Consultation on Incontinence Questionnaire for Male LUTS, and the BPH Impact Index [8,9].

Physical examination and digital rectal examination

A physical examination should be performed, focusing on the suprapubic area to rule out bladder distention, and on external genitalia to identify conditions that may contribute to LUTS (e.g. urethral discharge). A focused neurological examination is also recommended.

A digital rectal examination (DRE) is a subjective test and can be used to (1) exclude the presence of prostate cancer (PCa), (2) evaluate the anal sphincter tone, and (3) estimate the prostate volume. However, DRE has a low sensitivity and specificity for PCa detection. A suspect DRE alone leads to PCa diagnosis in about 18% of patients, irrespective of PSA level [10]. A suspect DRE has a positive predictive value (PPV) of 5–30% for a PSA level of ≤4 ng/mL [11], and as high as 50% for a PSA level of ≥3.0 ng/mL [12]. DRE is the simplest way to assess the prostate volume, but correct estimation of the prostatic volume by DRE has been questioned. Data from four studies comparing estimations of prostate volume by DRE were compared with those determined by transrectal ultrasound (TRUS) and showed that underestimation of DRE increased with increasing TRUS volume, particularly if the volume was greater than 30 mL [13]. In a community-based study, it was found that DRE overestimates the volume in smaller prostates and underestimates the volume in larger prostates [14]. It was concluded that DRE is good in distinguishing between prostate volumes greater or smaller than 50 mL [14].

Frequency–volume charts and bladder diaries

Frequency–volume charts (FVC) record the volume and time of each void and are simple for the patient to complete. A bladder diary captures additional information such as fluid intake or symptom scores [15]. These can provide useful and objective clinical information and identify patients with polyuria, nocturnal polyuria, or excessive fluid intake. There is a close correlation between LUTS, as assessed by symptom scores, and data generated by voiding charts, such as frequency and nocturia. There remains a lack of consensus about how long a diary should be kept, but FVCs of 3–7 days' duration are a reliable tool for the objective measurement of mean voided volume, daytime and night-time frequency, and incontinence-episode frequency [16]. FVC is recommended in the assessment of nocturia and storage LUTS.

Urinalysis (dipstick)

Dipstick urinalysis can be used to identify conditions that may cause LUTS (e.g. urinary-tract infections, bladder carcinoma, diabetes mellitus, etc.), based on abnormal findings (e.g. hematuria, proteinuria, pyuria, glucosuria, ketonuria, positive nitrite test). Despite its low specificity, urinalysis is recommended for the initial evaluation of patients presenting with LUTS.

Serum creatinine

No clinical or economic studies were identified regarding the impact of measuring renal function on patient outcomes in men with LUTS versus not measuring serum creatinine. In addition, in the Medical Therapy of Prostatic Symptoms study, less than 1% of men with LUTS presented with renal insufficiency due to BPH [4]. Creatinine measurement in initial assessment of patients with LUTS is recommended when renal impairment is suspected based on history or presence of hydronephrosis, and when considering surgical treatment. In other situations, creatinine measurement is optional.

PSA

The chance of having prostate cancer is strongly related to the serum PSA. However, the benefits and risks of using serum PSA as a marker for PCa should be discussed with the patient with LUTS. Several reports have also demonstrated the reliability of PSA as a proxy for prostate volume. An analysis of placebo-controlled multicenter BPH trials and a safety study (4627 patients) showed that PSA had good predictive value for assessing prostate volume, with areas under the curve ranging from 0.76 to 0.78 for various prostate volume cutoff points [17]. PSA level seems to be a highly significant predictor of clinical progression [18] and a strong predictor of the risk of acute urinary retention and the need for BPH-related surgery in men with LUTS [19,20]. PSA has also been significantly associated with BOO [21,22].

Postvoid residual urine

Measurement of postvoid residual urine (PVR) is a simple, inexpensive, and non-invasive method. It is not necessarily associated with obstruction, since high PVR volumes can be a consequence of both obstruction and poor detrusor function. High baseline PVR has been associated with an increased risk of symptom deterioration [19,20]. Monitoring of PVR over time could predict the occurrence of acute urinary retention (AUR), since patients with a steady increase in PVR subsequently develop AUR [20]. This is important for the treatment of patients using anticholinergic medication and is recommended by the EAU Guidelines. A large PVR may predict a poor response to treatment and especially to watchful waiting.

Imaging of urinary tract

In daily practice, imaging of the prostate is currently performed by TRUS, or by trans-abdominal ultrasound. Reasons for such investigation in patients with LUTS include primarily the determination of prostatic size and shape (presence of middle protruding lobe). Assessment of prostate size is important for the diagnosis of BPE and selection of the appropriate interventional treatment (open prostatectomy vs transurethral resection vs transurethral incision of the prostate vs minimally invasive therapies) or prior to treatment with a 5a-reductase inhibitor [2]. The size of the prostate gland may also predict which patients with LUTS are at risk for progression of symptoms, AUR, and need for BPH-related surgery. The presence of a middle protruding lobe may guide the choice of therapy in patients scheduled for a minimally invasive treatment. A large body of evidence has documented the accuracy of TRUS over transabdominal ultrasound in calculating the volume of the prostate [23,24]. However, transabdominal ultrasound can measure PVR at the same time.

Routine imaging of the upper urinary tract in men with LUTS is not recommended at the initial evaluation of those patients. Renal ultrasound is indicated in patients with an elevated serum creatinine level and/or increased PVR [25]. Imaging of the upper urinary tract should also be performed when kidney pathology is suspected.

Endoscopy

Urethrocystoscopy is not recommended as a routine test in the initial evaluation of patients with LUTS. Urethrocystoscopy is indicated prior to minimal invasive/surgical therapies if findings (e.g middle lobe) may change the respective treatment modality and as part of the assessment to exclude any bladder pathology.

Uroflowmetry

Uroflowmetry is the most commonly performed urodynamic test, due to its non-invasive nature. Uroflowmetry is unable to distinguish between BOO and detrusor underactivity, but the sensitivity and specificity of uroflowmetry for diagnosis of BOO are greater if the maximum flow rate is less than 10 mL/s [26,27]. It can be used to predict the progression of the disease and monitor changes during a follow-up after treatment.

Pressure–flow studies

Pressure–flow studies can help to diagnose BOO and detrusor overactivity accurately. According to the EAU Guidelines, filling cystometry and pressure–flow measurement are optional tests usually indicated before surgical treatment in men who: cannot void ≥150 mL, have a maximum flow rate ≥10 mL/s, are <50 or >80 years of age, can void but have a PVR of >300 mL, suspect having a neurogenic bladder dysfunction, had radical pelvic surgery, or had previous unsuccessful (invasive) treatment [2]. Figure 4.1 shows an algorithm that was developed based on the above recommendations.

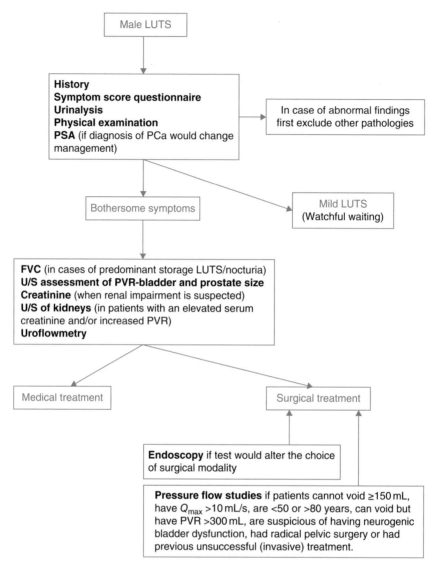

Figure 4.1 Algorithm of male lower urinary tract symptoms (LUTS) assessment. FVC, frequency–volume charts; PCa, prostate cancer; PVR, postvoid residual urine volume; PSA, prostate-specific antigen.

What happens in real life in Europe?

Several surveys have attempted to investigate if health-care professionals comply with the recommendations of evidence-based guidelines regarding the diagnostic evaluation of patients with LUTS. Despite the fact that these surveys were conducted in different periods of time and not in all European countries, they can display useful information about the trends in clinical assessment and diagnosis of BPH in Europe. It should be underlined that a patient may first consult with either his general practitioner (GP) or an office-based urologist depending on the national health system of each country reflecting the disparity in clinical assessment of LUTS in Europe.

A French survey (published in 2004) focusing on the modalities of prescription of subsequent examinations in BPO demonstrated an important inconsistency between clinical guidelines (both French and European) and routine attitudes in clinical practice [28]. It was found that the initial management of LUTS due to BPH in France was nationally similar among urologists regardless of their age or type of practice. Clinical interview and DRE were performed by all urologists, but IPSS was used by 23.3% of the participants. Detailed results are presented in Table 4.1. The TransEuropean Research Into the Use of Management Policies for LUTS Suggestive of BPH in Primary Health Care Project was an observational study intended to provide comparative information on the management of LUTS/BPH in real-life practice in six European countries. Primary care provision differed among countries. Patients in France, Italy, and the UK initially consult GPs, those in Poland and Spain initially consult office-based urologists, and those in Germany may consult either. Data from 4979 patients demonstrated that the initial assessment varied significantly between countries [29]. Overall, the most common test was DRE (85% of cases), although 37% of Italian patients did not receive a DRE. On the other hand, transrectal ultrasound of prostate was the less frequently performed examination (overall 12.3%), ranging from 0.2% in the UK to 21.6% in Germany (Table 4.1). On average, urologists carried out twice as many tests as

Table 4.1 Investigational tests used in the clinical assessment of lower urinary tract symptoms in Europe (mean values and range) based on surveys

Investigational test	France Uro (%)	Triumph Uro or GPs (%)	BPH usage Uro or GPs (%)	Five EU countries GPs (%)
History	100	NA	NA	66.2[a] (7.8–85.1)
Digital rectal examination	100	84.90 (62.5–97.9)	74.40 (52–96.9)	63.80 (20–91.6)
International Prostate Symptom Score	23.30	Obligatory per protocol	45 (6–77.2)	15.40 (3.2–82.1)
Urinalysis	72.70	NA	73.30 (50–100)	60.80 (2.2–81.9)
Serum creatinine	44.70	49.30 (32.8–57)	NA	43.20 (34.1–63.1)
Prostate-specific antigen	98	67.80 (48.6–83.4)	83.80 (81.3–90)	87.90 (45.3–94.7)
Postvoid residual urine	89.90	44.00 (9.9–77.4)	NA	NA
Imaging of prostate			63.8 (36.8–92)	
Transrectal US	54.2	12.3 (0.2–21.6)	NA	27.9 (2.3–51.1)
Abdominal US	61.8	42.3 (1.1–75.9)	NA	29.8 (12.2–36.3)
Imaging of upper tract	80.8	NA	NA	NA
Endoscopy	4.7	NA	NA	NA
Uroflowmetry	65	19.5 (0.4–35.9)	23.8 (6.4–51)	16.8 (15.1–55.9)
Pressure–flow studies	NA	NA	NA	9.5 (6.3–13.4)

Countries participating in the studies: benign prostatic hyperplasia (BPH) usage: France, Germany, Portugal, and Spain; five EU countries: France, Germany, Italy, Spain, and UK; Triumph: France, Germany, Italy, Poland, Spain, and UK.

GP, general practitioner; NA, not available; US, ultrasound.

[a]Description of symptoms.

GPs. Another observational study recorded the management of LUTS/BPH patients by primary care physicians in four European countries (GPs in France, Spain, and Portugal, and office-based urologists in Germany) [30]. In line with previous surveys, adherence to the Guidelines was low, and examinations were carried out disparately depending on the country (Table 4.1). Recently, a selected cohort of 455 GPs in Europe were asked to report information on BPH patients with LUTS [31]. Large differences in BPH diagnostic work-up across the five European countries were reported (Table 4.1). In addition, this survey on LUTS in primary care in Europe has shown that there was a varying degree of application of clinical guidelines in daily practice; for example, the EAU-recommended IPSS questionnaire was used by a minority of GPs (from 3.2% to 14.5%) except in Spain (57.1%) [31].

Reasons for the observed discrepancy between evidence-based guidelines and clinical practice in Europe include the lack of a high level of evidence for the investigational tests, the existence of numerous clinical guidelines (both national and international) on LUTS/BPH that may confuse urologists or GPs, differences in primary care provision, beliefs, costs, availability, and reimbursement policy, practice of defensive medicine, and uncertainty about how to proceed with specific patients [32]. Compliance of clinicians with evidence-based recommendations should overcome negative perceptions on clinical guidelines. Strategies to inform and educate both urologists and GPs in their respective countries should be carried out and should focus mainly on training of residents. There are fewer barriers to the adoption of guidelines by residentsl these are related to knowledge and are not related to changes in existing routines and habits, and to fears for declining autonomy in making decisions.

The development of algorithms may make evidence-based medicine easily accessible and comprehensible. The Diagnosis IMprovement in PrimAry Care Trial (D-IMPACT) study was a prospective, multicenter epidemiological study in three European countries (France, Italy, and Spain) to evaluate the accuracy of simple tests used to diagnose symptomatic BPH in a primary care setting when compared with gold-standard diagnosis by a urologist. In a logistic regression model including age, IPSS, PSA and probability of BPH (based on physical examination and symptoms), PPV was 77.1%. Exclusion of BPH probability resulted in a PPV of 75.7%. The D-IMPACT study has shown that an algorithm based on models using simple tests, which are recommended in European guidelines, had an acceptable diagnostic accuracy for BPH in men spontaneously presenting with LUTS and could be implemented in a standard practice for the initial evaluation [33].

In conclusion, clinical assessment of patients with LUTS includes a number of potential diagnostic investigations. The initial evaluation comprises specific recommended tests, and interpretation of test results together with the evaluation of a patient's need will help to gauge the necessity for additional tests. The diagnosis of BPH as the cause of male LUTS is mainly made by exclusion of all other non-neurogenic benign forms of LUTS. The current diagnostic process seems to be based upon personal experience and choice rather than evidence-based management of LUTS. This underlines the need for the development of training and for the diffusion of guidelines in order to establish optimal management for patients with LUTS.

Dos and don'ts

- Take a structured medical history, ask patients to complete an IPSS, do a physical examination and DRE, and offer a dipstick urinalysis as part of the initial evaluation of all patients with LUTS.

- Measurement of PVR and prostate size, and performance of uroflowmetry are useful in the initial assessment of male bothersome LUTS, especially when treatment is being planned. These can be used to identify patients at risk of progression and to monitor patients during treatment.

- Frequency–volume charts and bladder diaries are recommended in the assessment of nocturia and storage LUTS.

- Imaging of the upper urinary tract, endoscopy, and pressure–flow studies are not recommended as routine tests in the initial evaluation of male LUTS

Bibliography

1 Chapple CR, Wein AJ, Abrams P, Dmochowski RR, Giuliano F, Kaplan SA, et al. Lower urinary tract symptoms revisited: a broader clinical perspective. Eur Urol. 2008;54:563–9.

2 Oelke M, Bachmann A, Descazeaud A, Emberton M, Gravas S, Michel MC, et al. EAU guidelines on the treatment and follow-up of non-neurogenic male lower urinary tract symptoms including benign prostatic obstruction. Eur Urol. 2013;64:118–40.

3 McVary KT, Roehrborn CG, Avins AL, Barry MJ, Bruskewitz RC, Donnell RF, et al. Update on AUA guideline on the management of benign prostatic hyperplasia. J Urol. 2011;185:1793–803.

4 McConnell JD, Roehrborn CG, Bautista OM, Andriole GL Jr, Dixon CM, Kusek JW, et al. The long-term effect of doxazosin, finasteride, and combination therapy on the clinical progression of benign prostatic hyperplasia. N Engl J Med. 2003; 349:2387–98.

5 Barry MJ, Fowler FJ, Jr., O'Leary MP, Bruskewitz RC, Holtgrewe HL, Mebust WK, et al. The American Urological Association symptom index for benign prostatic hyperplasia. The Measurement Committee of the American Urological Association. J Urol. 1992;148:1549–57; discussion 1564.

6 Nitti VW, Kim Y, Combs AJ. Correlation of the AUA symptom index with urodynamics in patients with suspected benign prostatic hyperplasia. Neurourol Urodyn. 1994;13:521–7.

7 Barry MJ, Cockett AT, Holtgrewe HL, McConnell JD, Sihelnik SA, Winfield HN. Relationship of symptoms of prostatism to commonly used physiological and anatomical measures of the severity of benign prostatic hyperplasia. J Urol. 1993;150:351–8.

8 Schou J, Poulsen AL, Nordling J. The value of a new symptom score (DAN-PSS) in diagnosing uro-dynamic infravesical obstruction in BPH. Scand J Urol Nephrol. 1993;27:489–92.

9 Donovan JL, Peters TJ, Abrams P, Brookes ST, de la Rosette JJ, Schafer W. Scoring the short form ICSmaleSF questionnaire. International Continence Society. J Urol. 2000;164:1948–55.

10 Richie JP, Catalona WJ, Ahmann FR, Hudson MA, Scardino PT, Flanigan RC, et al. Effect of patient age on early detection of prostate cancer with serum prostate-specific antigen and digital rectal examination. Urology. 1993;42:365–74.

11 Carvalhal GF, Smith DS, Mager DE, Ramos C, Catalona WJ. Digital rectal examination for detecting prostate cancer at prostate specific antigen levels of 4ng/ml or less. J Urol. 1999;161:835–9.

12 Gosselaar C, Kranse R, Roobol MJ, Roemeling S, Schroder FH. The interobserver variability of digital rectal examination in a large randomized trial for the screening of prostate cancer. Prostate. 2008;68:985–93.

13 Roehrborn CG. Accurate determination of prostate size via digital rectal examination and transrectal ultrasound. Urology. 2001;51:19–22.

14 Bosch JL, Bohnen AM, Groeneveld FP. Validity of digital rectal examination and serum prostate specific antigen in the estimation of prostate volume in community-based men aged 50 to 78 years: the Krimpen Study. Eur Urol. 2004;46:753–9.

15 Abrams P, Cardozo L, Fall M, Griffiths D, Rosier P, Ulmsten U, et al. The standardisation of terminology of lower urinary tract function: report from the Standardisation Sub-committee of the International Continence Society. Neurourol Urodyn. 2002;21:167–78.

16 Lucas MG, Bedretdinova D, Bosch JLHR, Burkhard F, Cruz F, Nambiar AK, *et al.* EAU guidelines on urinary incontinence; Uroweb 2013 [cited May 1, 2013]. Available from: http://www.uroweb.org/guidelines/online-guidelines/

17 Roehrborn CG, Boyle P, Gould AL, Waldstreicher J. Serum prostate specific antigen as a predictor of prostate volume in men with benign prostatic hyperplasia. *Urology.* 1999;53:581–9.

18 Djavan B, Fong YK, Harik M, Milani S, Reissigl A, Chaudry A, *et al.* Longitudinal study of men with mild symptoms of bladder outlet obstruction treated with watchful waiting for four years. *Urology.* 2004;64:1144–8.

19 McConnell JD, Roehrborn CG, Bautista OM, Andriole GL Jr, Dixon CM, Kusek JW, *et al.* The long-term effect of doxazosin, finasteride, and combination therapy on the clinical progression of benign prostatic hyperplasia. *N Engl J Med.* 2003;349:2387–98.

20 Roehrborn CG. Alfuzosin 10 mg once daily prevents overall clinical progression of benign prostatic hyperplasia but not acute urinary retention: results of a 2-year placebo-controlled study. *BJU Int.* 2006;97:734–41.

21 Laniado ME, Ockrim JL, Marronaro A, Tubaro A, Carter SS. Serum prostate-specific antigen to predict the presence of bladder outlet obstruction in men with urinary symptoms. *BJU Int.* 2004;94:1283–6.

22 Kang MY, Ku JH, Oh SJ. Non-invasive parameters predicting bladder outlet obstruction in Korean men with lower urinary tract symptoms. *J Korean Med Sci.* 2010;25:272–5.

23 Loch AC, Bannowsky A, Baeurle L, Grabski B, König B, Flier G, *et al.* Technical and anatomical essentials for transrectal ultrasound of the prostate. *World J Urol.* 2007;25:361–6.

24 Stravodimos KG, Petrolekas A, Kapetanakis T, Vourekas S, Koritsiadis G, Adamakis I, *et al.* TRUS versus transabdominal ultrasound as a predictor of enucleated adenoma weight in patients with BPH: a tool for standard preoperative work-up? *Int Urol Nephrol.* 2009;41:767–71.

25 Koch WF, Ezz el Din K, de Wildt MJ, Debruyne FM, de la Rosette JJ. The outcome of renal ultrasound in the assessment of 556 consecutive patients with benign prostatic hyperplasia. *J Urol.* 1996;155:186–9.

26 Siroky MB, Olsson CA, Krane RJ. The flow rate nomogram: I. Development. *J Urol.* 1979;122:665–8.

27 Siroky MB, Olsson CA, Krane RJ. The flow rate nomogram: II. Clinical correlation. *J Urol.* 1980;123:208–10.

28 De la Taille A, Desgrandchamps F, Saussine C, Lukacs B, Haillot O. Do urologists apply benign prostatic hyperplasia clinical practice guidelines? Survey on the complementary investigation request modalities in France. *Prog Urol.* 2004;14:320–5.

29 Hutchison A, Farmer R, Chapple C, Berges R, Pientka L, Teillac P, *et al.* Characteristics of patients presenting with LUTS/BPH in six European countries. *Eur Urol.* 2006;50:555–61.

30 Fourcade RO, Theret N, Taieb C, BPH USAGE Study Group. Profile and management of patients treated for the first time for lower urinary tract symptoms/benign prostatic hyperplasia in four European countries. *BJU Int.* 2008;101:1111–8.

31 Montorsi F, Mercadante D. Diagnosis of BPH and treatment of LUTS among GPs: a European survey. *Int J Clin Pract.* 2013;67: 114–19.

32 Gravas S, Tzortzis V, Melekos MD. Translation of benign prostatic hyperplasia guidelines into clinical practice. *Curr Opin Urol.* 2008;18:56–60.

33 Carballido J, Fourcade R, Pagliarulo A, Brenes F, Boye A, Sessa A, *et al.* Can benign prostatic hyperplasia be identified in the primary care setting using only simple tests? Results of the Diagnosis IMprovement in PrimAry Care Trial. *Int J Clin Pract.* 2011;65:989–96.

CHAPTER 5

Clinical Assessment and Diagnosis of Lower Urinary Tract Symptoms/Benign Prostatic Hyperplasia: Primary Care

Matt T. Rosenberg[1], John B. Riley[1] & Marty M. Miner[2]
[1] Mid Michigan Health Centers, Jackson, MI, USA
[2] Warren Alpert School of Medicine, Brown University, Providence, RI, USA

Key points

- The primary care provider (PCP) is the first point of contact for the patient with prostate-related lower urinary tract symptoms (LUTS) .
- The diagnosis of prostate-related LUTS can be made in the office of the PCP without specialized equipment.
- Abnormalities of the prostate are generally seen as flow disturbances.
- Bladder dysfunction is generally seen as the inability to hold adequate volumes.
- LUTS can be caused or worsened by medical conditions, medications, surgeries, or physical abnormalities.
- The bladder diary can be very useful in identifying behaviors or habits affecting LUTS.
- The physical examination of the patient with LUTS must include an adequate assessment of the genitals and prostate.
- Prostate-specific antigen (PSA) is a surrogate marker for prostate size, and a level of 1.5 ng/mL equates to a minimum prostate size of 30 g.

As the first line of defense in healthcare, the PCP is generally the first to encounter a patient with symptoms consistent with a problematic prostate. However, identification of the symptoms, the origin, or validation of the bother may elude both of them. One can speculate on the reasons for this, but there are two realities that support this occurrence. First, the training for the PCP in urologic issues is minimal at best. During residency, there may be some limited exposure during rotations, but after residency, continuing education opportunities are few. This has the potential result of the evaluation of prostate problems or LUTS being limited and highly variable. A 2013 European study verified that this inconsistent urological education of the providers resulted in assessments lacking uniformity [1]. Second, the patient may simply relegate the symptoms to the idea that things do not work as well as he ages, so he does not inform the provider of them. Many patients believe that certain medical ailments are their destiny, as they witnessed their

Male Lower Urinary Tract Symptoms and Benign Prostatic Hyperplasia, First Edition.
Edited by Steven A. Kaplan and Kevin T. McVary.
© 2014 John Wiley & Sons, Ltd. Published 2014 by John Wiley & Sons, Ltd.

parents suffer from them as they aged. Unfortunately, they do not understand what to expect from their body, and no one has ever explained to them what is normal as they age. An additional hurdle is that many of the same symptoms that are consistent with benign prostatic hyperplasia (BPH) can be found with other problems. In fact, LUTS may be a result not only of problems with the prostate or the bladder, but also of medical conditions, surgeries, or medications [2]. Since the PCP generally has the global view of the patient, they are in the optimal position to tease away the comorbid conditions in order to discover the true etiology of the symptoms.

As we begin the evaluation of the patient with symptomatic BPH, there are a few crucial ideas to keep in mind:

1 The PCP is the first contact for the symptomatic patient.

2 It is not a normal part of aging to suffer from urinary difficulties.

3 The evaluation and diagnosis of BPH can be efficiently and safely done in the office of the PCP.

Why should primary care be concerned?

Prevalence and impact are discussed in other chapters, so the importance of evaluation of prostate-related LUTS by the PCP need not be debated here. However, it would be prudent to mention that the complications of prostate-related LUTS, although infrequent, may include acute urinary retention (AUR), impaired bladder emptying, the need for corrective surgery, recurrent urinary tract infections (UTIs), renal failure, stones, or gross hematuria [3]. For years, the prostate had been the domain of the urologist, and

surgical reduction was the primary mode of treatment. With effective medications now available for the treatment of prostate-related LUTS, the PCP should be able to offer satisfactory treatment to the majority of patients, and surgical intervention is then left for the refractory patients or those with disease progression. Part of the disconnect is that there is a significant difference between how the PCP and the urologist view the disease. In a study in 2009, Miner noted this discrepancy and speculated that this was due to the fact that PCPs view LUTS predominantly as a quality-of-life issue, without considering that it could progress [4]. The goal for the PCP is then to be able to identify the correct patient with symptom distress or who is asymptomatic but at risk for progression. In addition, they must recognize the need for referral when appropriate. The urological community has done an extraordinary job in developing an understanding of the prostate, the symptoms of its dysfunction, and the progression potential of these, which in turn makes it more reasonable for the PCP to be the gatekeeper. The needs of the PCP in regard to prostate care can be summed up in three words: "simple," "effective," and "safe." A "simple" way to evaluate the at-risk patient, "effective" treatment options that can be prescribed within the primary care setting, and, most importantly, a "safe" approach to patient management that minimizes the chance of a poor outcome for the patient.

Definitions

There are many terms and abbreviations that are used to describe the prostate, and unfortunately, this word soup can make it confusing for the provider. That being said, some clarification here would be useful. BPH is the benign proliferation of the prostatic stroma and epithelium. Over the years, it has become synonymous with the "troublesome prostate"; however, it is only when it affects urinary flow that it is in fact pathologic. This pathologic condition is known as benign prostatic obstruction. Another term commonly seen is benign prostatic enlargement (BPE). This is when the prostate growth is diagnosed by clinical or ultrasound examination. A final term that has been used in the literature is enlarged prostate (EP), which refers to symptomatic BPE. Though differences in terminology are important when reviewing the literature, they are largely irrelevant in clinical practice. For the sake of clarity, throughout this chapter, we will use the term "BPH" in dealing with the complex of symptoms experienced by the affected patient as a result of his prostate.

What are LUTS?

The International Continence Society classifies LUTS into voiding, storage, and postmicturition symptoms [5]. Voiding symptoms may be experienced as a result of a blocked outlet (prostate or urethra) or an underactive detrusor, whereas storage symptoms are generally related to the bladder alone. Postmicturition symptoms are experienced right after voiding. In order to understand the pathology associated with these symptoms, it is useful to review the function of the main elements: the prostate and the bladder.

Normal function of the prostate

The prostate itself is a gland that produces fluid for seminal emission. In the unaffected male, the urethra is wide open through the prostate, thereby allowing a free flow of urine and a good urinary stream. Experts have defined this good flow as a smooth arc-shaped curve with high amplitude and without interruption [6]. As the male ages, there is proliferation and expansion of cells within the gland. This normal occurrence makes BPH the most common benign neoplasm among American men [7].

Abnormal function of the prostate

When the growth is outside of the prostatic urethra, it generally causes minimal issues, unless the prostate becomes so massive that it puts pressure on the bladder. The problems generally seen with prostatic growth happen via two possible routes. The first is direct bladder outlet obstruction (BOO), which is considered the "static" component. The second is due to increased smooth muscle tone and resistance within the prostatic urethra, which is called the "dynamic component." Either of these possible mechanisms would cause a blockage of urine and, subsequently, a poor urinary flow. Symptoms are variable but include a slow or intermittent stream, hesitancy, straining, or a terminal dribble [3]. Quite frequently, the patient and the provider associate nocturia with obstruction caused by the prostate, but that is not necessarily correct. Nocturia is the complaint that the individual has to wake at night one or more times to void. When nocturia occurs with a normal urinary stream, obstruction is less likely a causative factor. It is when nocturia is associated with a poor stream that we think about the prostate.

Normal function of the bladder

The bladder is a storage and emptying vehicle. The properly functioning bladder holds about 300–500 mL and empties the same amount. Filling should be gradual and comfortable, and emptying should follow a gentle urge or awareness to void, giving the patient adequate time to prepare for voluntary micturition [8].

Abnormal function of the bladder

Holding less than the normal capacity of 300 mL indicates compromised function of the bladder. This premature signaling to empty the bladder is generally consistent with an overactive bladder (OAB). OAB is a syndrome in which the patient experiences urinary urgency with or without frequency, nocturia, and incontinence [5]. It is important to emphasize that these symptoms are abnormal when they occur before the bladder is full. Experiencing these symptoms when bladder capacity is reached is normal. Voiding frequently of normal amounts means the bladder is functioning normally but too much fluid is being filtered. Feeling the need to hurry and empty (urgency) when the bladder is full is expected. Getting up at night to void (nocturia) is also expected when the bladder has reached capacity. Voiding large amounts at night could be a sign of nocturnal polyuria and should be evaluated.

History, physical, and laboratory evaluation

The initial challenge for the provider is to identify LUTS. The patient presenting with LUTS associated with the prostate does not come with the diagnosis in hand. Since he may not freely offer pertinent information, the identification can be quite difficult for the provider. The reality is that the symptoms are, more often than not, nonspecific and could originate from many sources. Though screening tools exist, they may not always be practical in the office of the busy PCP. In one study, it was shown that two thirds of PCPs were aware of the American Urological Association (AUA) symptom score, but only a third used it [9]. Another screening tool, the International Prostate Symptom Score (IPSS) sheet, is valuable in that it is universal and has been validated [10] (Table 5.1). The difference between the AUA score and the IPSS is that the latter added a quality-of-life question (question 8); the other seven questions are the same. Both tools are helpful in obtaining a thorough history, but they are not diagnostic, as other conditions can produce similar symptoms [11].

Although practice constraints may result in only a few providers using the questionnaires, all providers should be familiar with them. In many cases, a few simple questions can provide helpful direction. No questionnaire can absolutely establish a definitive diagnosis, but a thoughtful history will provide a guide for evaluation and eventual treatment [5]. Table 5.2 shows the symptoms consistent with LUTS as it is associated with BPH or OAB [8,12,13]. Questions directed at these symptoms will assist in clarifying the diagnosis.

Once the LUTS are identified, the provider should focus on other causative factors. These include certain behaviors, medical problems, medications, or physical abnormalities. The next step is to proceed with a focused history and physical, as well as a few laboratory tests. The goal is to identify other factors that may cause or contribute to BPH symptoms, including reversible issues or comorbidities that may complicate treatment. Table 5.3 lists the possible causes of LUTS [8,14,15]. The PCP often has a distinct advantage in having prior knowledge of the patient, thereby making this information readily available.

It is useful at this junction to keep in mind the temporal relationship of the symptoms the patient is describing to any change in his life or daily habits. As with many other

Table 5.1 International Prostate Symptom Score Questionnaire

	Not at all	Less than 1 time in 5	Less than half the time	About half the time	More than half the time	Almost always	Your score
1. Incomplete emptying: Over the past month, how often have you had a sensation of not emptying your bladder completely after you finished urinating?	0	1	2	3	4	5	
2. Frequency: Over the past month, how often have you had to urinate again less than two hours after you finished urinating?	0	1	2	3	4	5	
3. Intermittency: Over the past month, how often have you found you stopped and started again several times when you urinated?	0	1	2	3	4	5	
4. Urgency: Over the past month, how often have you found it difficult to postpone urination?	0	1	2	3	4	5	
5. Weak Stream: Over the past month, how often have you had a weak urinary stream?	0	1	2	3	4	5	
6. Straining: Over the past month, how often have you had to push or strain to begin urination?	0	1	2	3	4	5	

	None	1 time	2 times	3 times	4 times	5 times or more	
7. Nocturia: Over the past month, how many times did you most typically get up to urinate from the time you went to bed at night until the time you got up in the morning?	0	1	2	3	4	5	
Total International Prostate Symptom Score			_____mild BPH (1–7), moderate BPH (8–19), or severe BPH (20–35).				

	Delighted	Pleased	Mostly satisfied	Mixed	Mostly dissatisfied	Unhappy	Terrible
1. Quality of Life Due to Urinary Symptoms: If you were to spend the rest of your life with your urinary condition just the way it is now, how would you feel about that?	0	1	2	3	4	5	6

BPH, benign prostatic hyperplasia.
Barry 1992 [10]. Reproduced with permission of Elsevier.

diseases, certain behaviors can be a major cause of the bothersome symptoms of BPH. Urinary hygiene is a term that has been used to describe voiding habits [16]. Good habits include relaxing the pelvic musculature and taking the time to void to completion. For some males, this may involve taking a little extra time to void or sitting on the toilet as opposed to standing. An example of poor urinary hygiene may be found in the work place when a patient is given limited time at the toilet and is not able to void to completion [16]. Limiting the time per episode for the patient may decrease the volume he

is able to void, resulting in more frequent trips to the toilet.

Awareness of the patient's medical and surgical history is essential to the provider seeking to identify a cause of the LUTS or an associated temporal relationship. A few examples are in order here for further clarification.

A poor stream that is infrequent may not, in fact, be of much concern for the patient. However, the polyuria of the poorly controlled diabetic may increase the voiding frequency enough that the symptoms become markedly more bothersome. The patient with congestive heart failure may find that night-time output is increased as a result of elevating his legs. This may worsen as his disease worsens, resulting in more frequent trips to the bathroom.

There are several medications that can affect urinary function (Table 5.3). Polyuria associated with a diuretic could increase output. The alpha antagonism of an average cold medication may tighten the prostatic urethra enough to obstruct flow. The clue that the medication is exacerbating or causing the condition may be the temporal relationship between when the medication regimen was started and when the symptoms began.

Table 5.2 Male lower urinary tract symptoms

Benign prostatic hyperplasia (obstructive)	Overactive bladder (irritative)
Hesitancy	Urgency
Poor flow/weak stream	Frequency
Intermittency	Nocturia
Straining to void	Urge incontinence
Terminal dribble	Stress incontinence
Prolonged urination	Mixed incontinence
Urinary retention	Overflow incontinence

Table 5.3 Lower urinary tract symptoms: differential diagnosis and other causes

Differential diagnosis	Medications	Other risk factors
Consider: • prostate cancer • prostatitis • bladder stones • interstitial cystitis • radiation cystitis • urinary tract infection • diabetes mellitus • Parkinson's disease • primary bladder neck hypertrophy • congestive heart failure • lumbosacral disc disease • multiple sclerosis	May cause or exacerbate lower urinary tract symptoms: • tricyclic antidepressants • anticholinergic agents • diuretics • narcotics • 1st generation antihistamines • decongestants	Consider: • obesity • cigarette smoking • regular alcohol consumption • elevated blood pressure

Recent genitourinary surgery may cause LUTS for obvious reasons, but the effects from other surgeries may not be so apparent. For instance, recent orthopedic surgery may cause mobility constraints that result in the patient delaying voiding until the last minute. The patient may also have difficulty maneuvering, thereby hindering the ability to relax the pelvic musculature enough to void completely. Opioids given in the postoperative period may cause constipation and subsequent voiding difficulty. Regardless of the cause, identifying the temporal relationship of the voiding issue with the prior surgery can provide essential information.

The physical examination should be focused. The abdominal examination is necessary to check for masses or an enlarged bladder. A brief neurological examination is needed to evaluate a patient's mental and ambulatory status as well as neuromuscular function. The provider should conduct a thorough examination of the genitalia, including the meatus and the foreskin. Meatal stenosis or a phimotic foreskin can mimic the EP by impeding flow. A digital rectal examination (DRE) can provide information about the anal sphincter tone as well as prostate size, shape, and consistency [11]. BPH usually results in a smooth EP that is not tender to palpation [17]. The gland may have a rubbery consistency, similar to the thenar eminence of the hand, and has often lost the median furrow [18]. In contrast, a nodular prostate raises the suspicion of carcinoma, and a tender, possibly indurated, gland may indicate infection (prostatitis) [18,19]. It is useful to keep in mind what information the DRE actually provides. It does offer a basic idea about the size, shape, and consistency of the gland, but it is only an estimate. The DRE can lead the provider to underestimate prostate size, as the digital exam cannot assess the full length or anterior portion of the gland [20].

Furthermore, size alone does not correlate with symptom severity because obstruction is dependent on growth into the prostatic urethra [21].

The physical examination, as just reviewed, describes what should be included in the basic evaluation of LUTS in the male. However, much of this may have been done at prior visits with the PCP, so that reexamination (i.e. prostate exam) may not be necessary if it is up to date.

The necessary laboratory tests are minimal, and most have probably been done during the routine or yearly examination of the patient. A urinalysis performed by dipstick or microscopic examination is strongly recommended to check for blood, protein, glucose, or any signs of infection. This may prompt treatment or referral [22]. Although hematuria or pyuria is not always found in conditions such as bladder cancer, stones, or infection, a normal urinalysis makes these diagnoses less likely [22]. It is not adequate to use the urinalysis to rule out the possibility of diabetes as the serum blood sugar must be over 180 mg/dl before glucose is spilled into the urine [8]. Consequently, a dipstick urinalysis may fail to pick up on intermittently high sugars or mild diabetics. Therefore, although this is not part of the AUA guidelines, there is a good argument for testing blood sugar, either random or fasting [22].

Assessment of renal function by measurement of electrolytes, blood urea nitrogen (BUN), and creatinine is useful in screening for chronic renal insufficiency in patients with a high postvoid residual (PVR) bladder volume [23]. However, they are not universally recommended in the initial evaluation of LUTS [22,24–26].

There is significant controversy surrounding the benefits of checking the PSA [27]. Recent studies have mixed results about its ability to assist in decreasing morbidity or mortality where prostate cancer is involved [28,29]. As a result of these studies and other supportive information, in 2012 the United States Preventative Task Force (USPTF) recommended against widespread use of the PSA for prostate cancer screening. This has led to a very vibrant discussion among healthcare providers and patients. Regardless of the provider's view on this lab value, it must be remembered that the PSA is prostate specific and not cancer specific. When used appropriately, it can assist the provider and the patient in making an educated decision about care.

Studies have found that PSA, along with IPSS score and age, are factors that show a statistically significant correlation to diagnosis of BPH [30]. In 1999, Roehrborn demonstrated how the PSA correlates to the size or volume of the prostate and, in fact, is a more accurate predictor of the volume of the gland than DRE [31]. It was shown in the Roehrborn paper that a PSA value of 1.5 ng/mL, in a male of any age, correlates to a minimal volume of 30 mL. A review of the placebo arm of MTOPS (Medical Therapy of Prostatic Symptoms) revealed that an increase in size of the prostate is directly related to increased risk of progression or worsening of LUTS caused by the prostate [32]. The prostate volume that put the patient at this risk was 31 mL. Understanding this well-researched fact allows the conscientious provider to utilize the PSA to assist in the evaluation of BPH and the development of treatment options for prostate-related LUTS. It is not the purpose of this chapter to debate the merits or concerns surrounding the PSA as a cancer-screening tool, but the controversy itself makes it vital to discuss with the patient the reasons and implications of checking the PSA. In any case, the PSA remains a useful prostate volume proxy.

Knowing this information can be a critical factor in deciding which medical therapy to pursue.

Other modalities in assessment

A bladder or voiding diary is an irreplaceable tool in the evaluation of LUTS. On the surface, it simply documents the frequency and timing of voids, the volume of intake, and the volume of output. Its key benefit, however, may be that of revealing the voiding habits that the patient has developed. For example, some patients may have symptoms that occur only during a certain time of the day, or week for that matter. It may be related to a time that they drink copious amounts of fluid or are unable to readily access a toilet. Thus, the diary may offer a clue to behaviors that can be altered to minimize symptoms. Certainly, there may be an issue with compliance in obtaining this information, but the PCP is in an optimal position to encourage the patient to follow through with this. Furthermore, most patients are likely relieved to find out that certain simple behavioral changes can help decrease their symptoms, as they may be reluctant to take medications or have surgery.

The PVR is the volume of urine remaining in the bladder after a normal voiding effort. While there is no across-the-board consensus on a safe PVR, for the PCP it is generally considered that a value of less than 50 mL represents reasonable voiding and over 200 mL is consistent with inadequate emptying [3]. In regard to the patient with BPH, a large residual urine volume is consistent with a significant risk of disease progression. This volume can be checked via direct catheterization or ultrasound scanning, neither of which is likely available in the office of the

PCP. However, checking the PVR is not necessary in the initial evaluation, but rather it should be considered when the patient is refractory to therapy, and the provider is trying to check for retention as a result of obstruction. An increased PVR may not be a problem unless it leads to UTIs or causes a significant decrease in functional bladder capacity. A UTI may not be eradicated in the presence of a residual that remains infected, and decreased capacity may lead to symptoms of urgency, frequency, or nocturia [33].

In the initial evaluation of the prostate, ultrasonography (abdominal, renal, transrectal) and intravenous urography are generally not indicated. If needed, they could be useful in helping determine the size of the prostate or bladder and the degree of hydronephrosis (if suspected) in patients with urinary retention or signs of renal impairment.

Reasons for referral

The role of the PCP in the evaluation noted in this chapter is not only to treat the prostate, if appropriate, but also to identify other possible causes of the LUTS. Behavioral modifications, medication alterations, and medical treatment are all within the realm of the PCP. Those diagnoses that cannot be addressed by the clinician should be referred. Indications for referral include the following [3,34]:
- history of recurrent UTIs or other infection;
- microscopic or gross hematuria;
- prior genitourinary surgery;
- elevated PSA;
- abnormal prostate exam (nodules);
- suspicion of neurologic cause of symptoms;
- findings or suspicion of urinary retention;
- meatal stenosis;
- history of genitourinary trauma;
- uncertain diagnosis;
- desire to see a specialist.

Assessing bother

If the evaluation reveals the prostate as a likely cause of the LUTS, the next step is to assess bother. As mentioned earlier, there are tools to assist in assessment of symptoms and bother, and it is acknowledged that the validated scores (IPSS or AUA Symptom Index) are superior to an unstructured interview [22]. Nevertheless, as mentioned earlier, the practicality of these tools in the primary care office can be debated [3]. In practice, patients often feel that taking medications and risk of surgery are of greater concern than symptoms of LUTS or even some of the associated quality-of-life issues [35]. One simple question at this point may be enough: "Are your symptoms bad enough that it would justify taking a medication each day or having a surgical procedure?" In the clinical opinion of the authors, most patients will answer honestly and appreciate being part of the process. This should be asked in such a way that the patient is aware that he can come back at any time if, and when, he is ready for intervention.

If assessment reveals minimal bother, then informed surveillance might be appropriate. Informed surveillance refers to the idea that the patient is knowledgeable about the symptoms or the complications that may occur. We prefer this term because it denotes a shared responsibility between the provider and the patient. Although treatment will be discussed in other chapters, it is useful to mention this concept briefly, as it may be commonly discussed in the office of the PCP during the evaluation. Informed surveillance is recommended if symptoms are not bothersome to the patient, and he has not developed complications of BPH, such as BOO, hydroureter, hematuria, hydronephrosis, AUR, UTIs, bladder hypertrophy, or others [36]. It is critical for the PCP to explain that BPH is a progressive disease and emphasize that the patient should speak to the provider if the symptoms worsen. In his MTOPS evaluation, Crawford identified five factors that put the patient at risk of progression. These include total prostate volume ≥31 mL, PSA ≥1.6 ng/mL, Q_{max} (flow rate) < 10.6 mL/s, PVR ≥39 mL, or age ≥62 [32]. It is understood that not all of these values may be attained in the office of the PCP; however, the patient should be made aware of what risk factors have been identified in his evaluation.

The reasons why some patients choose treatment, whereas others do not, is certainly an interesting issue about which one can speculate. Patients will often acknowledge their symptoms and seek to verify that a fatal disease is not the cause (e.g. prostate cancer). It is interesting to note that many men are reluctant to bring up LUTS due to fear that these symptoms represent a serious or life-threatening problem. An education from his PCP regarding the cause of his symptoms can be enlightening and relieving for the patient. The downside of waiting is that some patients' symptoms will progress. In a longitudinal study, Djaven *et al.* found that over a 4-year time span, 87% of men with mild symptoms went on to experience worsening symptoms, while 13% of men with mild symptoms experienced stability or improvement of their symptoms [37]. Informed surveillance may only delay treatment and not prevent it. Understanding the risk factors, as mentioned earlier, puts the patient and the provider in good position to anticipate future issues.

Those patients who opt for informed surveillance may benefit from lifestyle changes. Limitations of fluids, bladder training focused on timed and complete voiding, and treatment of constipation may help the patient regulate urinary symptoms. Similarly, a review of the patient's medication list will help identify opportunities to modify (i.e. change the timing of diuretics) or avoid (i.e. decongestants) medications that may impact symptoms of BPH [16].

Summary

The evaluation of LUTS can be done without a tremendous time investment or need for equipment outside of what is available in the typical PCP office. Knowing that, the fact that so many men suffer in silence is more likely a result of the lack of identification and awareness by both the patient and the provider. Empowering the patient means that he must understand normal function so that he can identify the problem and bring it to the attention of the provider. Empowering the PCP means this process needs to be streamlined. Understanding that the education may not be uniform reveals that an opportunity to teach exists. It is not simply a matter of telling the provider to "do this" or to "do that"; it is a matter of teaching the provider why to do certain things. It is for this reason that we outlined why this information is necessary and how it should be interpreted. If the pathology and the evaluation behind prostate-related LUTS are understood, the process becomes simple, effective, and safe. Most importantly, the patient does not suffer needlessly and in silence [1].

Dos and don'ts

- Patients may believe that worsening urinary function is to be expected as they age. Take the time to explain normal function of the bladder and prostate.

- There can be many causes of LUTS that are not associated with the bladder or prostate. A careful history and medication review may help reveal the cause.

- Frequently, the patient may unknowingly develop poor bladder (or urinating habits). Behavioral changes may alleviate some of the bothersome symptoms associated with LUTS.

- Regardless of one's view of the PSA in screening for cancer, the PSA is a surrogate marker for prostate size and should be used in the evaluation of prostate-related LUTS.

- Many patients may wish to postpone intervention and take a "wait and see" approach to their LUTS. Educating the individual on the risks of progression is essential.

Bibliography

1 Montorsi F, Mercadante D. Diagnosis of BPH and treatment of LUTS among GPs: a European survey. *Int J Clin Pract.* 2013;67(2):114–9.

2 Hyman M, Groutz A, Blaivas J. Detrusor instability in men: correlation of lower urinary tract symptoms with urodynamic findings. *J Urol.* 2001;166:550–3.

3 Rosenberg MT, Miner MM, Riley PA, Staskin DR. STEP: Simplified Treatment of the Enlarged Prostate. *Int J Clin Pract.* 2010;64(4):488–96.

4 Miner M. Primary care physician versus urologist: how does their medical management of LUTS associated with BPH differ? *Curr Urol Rep.* 2009;10:254–60.

5 Abrams P, Cardozo L, Fall M, Griffiths D, Rosier P, Ulmsten U, *et al.* The standardisation of terminology of lower urinary tract function: report from the Standardisation Sub-committee of the International Continence Society. *Neurourol Urodyn.* 2002; 187:167–78.

6 Abrams P. Urodynamics. 3rd edn. London: Springer; 2005.

7 Wei JT, Calhoun E, Jacobsen SJ. Urologic diseases in America project: benign prostatic hyperplasia. *J Urol.* 2005;173:1256–61.

8 Rosenberg MT, Staskin DR, Kaplan SA, MacDiarmid SA, Newman DK, Ohl DA. A practical guide to the evaluation and treatment of male lower urinary tract symptoms in the primary care setting. *Int J Clin Pract.* 2007;61:1535–46.

9 Fawzy A, Fontenot C, Guthrie R, Baudier MM. Practice patterns among primary care physicians in benign prostatic hyperplasia and prostate cancer. *Fam Med* 1997;29:321–5.

10 Barry M, Fowler FJ, O'Leary M, Bruskewitz RC, Holtgrewe HL, Mebust WK, *et al.* Association at MCotAU. The American Urological Association symptom index for benign prostatic hyperplasia. *J Urol.* 1992;148:1549–57.

11 Speakman M, Kirby R, Joyce A, Abrams P, Pocock R. Guideline for the primary care management of male lower urinary tract symptoms. *BJU Int.* 2004;93:985–90.

12 Lukacz ES, Sampselle C, Gray M, Macdiarmid S, Rosenberg M, Ellsworth P, *et al.* A healthy bladder: a consensus statement. *Int J Clin Pract.* 2011;65(10): 1026–36.

13 Wein AJ. Pathophysiology and categorization of voiding dysfunction. In: Wein, AJ, Kavoussi LR, Novick AC, *et al.* editors. Campbell's urology. 9th ed. Philadelphia: WB Saunders Elsevier; 2007. pp. 1973–85.

14 Haidinger G, Temml C, Schatzl G, Brössner C, Roehlich M, Schmidbauer CP, *et al.* Risk factors for lower urinary tract symptoms in elderly men. For the Prostate Study Group of the Austrian Society of Urology. *Eur Urol.* 2000;37:413–20.

15 Gades N, Jacobson D, Girman C, Roberts RO, Lieber MM, Jacobsen SJ, *et al.* Prevalence of conditions potentially associated with lower urinary tract symptoms in men. *BJU Int.* 2005;95:549–53.

16 Burgio KL, Newman DK, Rosenberg MT, Sampselle C. Impact of behavior and lifestyle on bladder health. *Int J Clin Pract.* 2013;67(6):495–504.

17 Stoller ML, Carroll PR. Urology. In: Tierney LM Jr, McPhee SJ, Papadakis MA, editors. Current medical diagnosis and treatment. 43rd ed. New York: Lange Medical Books/McGraw Hill; 2004. pp. 899–940.

18 Beers MH, Berkow R, editors. Benign prostatic hyperplasia. In: The Merck manual. 17th ed. Whitehouse Stastion, NJ: Merck Research Laboratories; 1999. pp. 1829–31.

19 Scher HI. Hyperplastic and malignant diseases of the prostate. In: Braunwald E, Fauci AS, Kasper DL, et al., editors. Harrison's principles of internal medicine. 15th ed. New York: McGraw-Hill; 2001. pp. 608–16.

20 Roehrborn CG, Girman CJ, Rhodes T, Hanson KA, Collins GN, Sech SM, et al. Correlation between prostate size estimated by digital rectal examination and measured by transrectal ultrasound. Urology. 1997;49:548–57.

21 Narayan P: Diagnosis and evaluation. In: Narayan P, editor. Benign prostatic hyperplasia. Gainesville, FL: Churchill Livingstone; 2000. pp. 80–7.

22 AUA Practice Guidelines Committee. AUA Guideline on Management of Benign Prostatic Hyperplasia. Chapter 1: Diagnosis and treatment recommendations. J Urol. 2003;170:530–47.

23 McVary KT, Roehrborn CG, Avins AL, Barry MJ, Bruskewitz RC, Donnell RF, et al. Update on AUA guideline on the management of benign prostatic hyperplasia. J Urol. 2011;185(5):1793–803.

24 de la Rosette J, Alivizatos G, Madersbacher S, Perachino M, Thomas D, Desgrandchamps F, et al. Guidelines on benign prostatic hyperplasia. Arnhem, The Netherlands: European Association of Urology, 2008.

25 Kaplan SA. Editorial comment on: effect of discontinuation of 5alpha-reductase inhibitors on prostate volume and symptoms in men with BPH: a prospective study. Urology. 2009;73:2417.

26 Madersbacher S, Alivizatos G, Nordling J, Sanz CR, Emberton M, de la Rosette JJ. EAU 2004 guidelines on assessment, therapy and follow-up of men with lower urinary tract symptoms suggestive of benign prostatic obstruction (BPH guidelines). Eur Urol. 2004;46:547–54.

27 Rehsia S, Shayegan B. PSA implications and medical management of prostate cancer for the primary care physician. Can J Urol. 2012;19 Suppl 1:28–35.

28 Andriole GL, Crawford D, Grubb RL, Buys SS, Chia D, Church TR, et al. Mortality results from a randomized prostate-cancer screening trial. N Engl J Med. 2009;360(13):1310–9.

29 Eckersberger E, Finkelstein J, Sadri H, Margreiter M, Taneja SS, Lepor H, et al. Screening for prostate cancer: a review of the ERSPC and PLCO trials. Rev Urol. 2009;11(3):127–33.

30 Carballido J, Fourcade R, Pagliarulo A, Brenes F, Boye A, Sessa A, et al. Can benign prostatic hyperplasia be identified in the primary care setting using only simple tests? Results of the Diagnosis IMprovement in PrimAry Care Trial. Int J Clin Pract. 2011;65(9):989–96.

31 Tanguay S, Awde M, Brock G, Casey R, Kozak J, Lee J, et al. Diagnosis and management of benign prostatic hyperplasia in primary care. Can Urol Assoc J. 2009;3:S92–100.

32 Crawford ED, Wilson SS, McConnell JD, Slawin KM, Lieber MC, Smith JA, et al. Baseline factors as predictors of clinical progression of benign prostatic hyperplasia in men treated with placebo. Urology. 2006;175:1422–7.

33 Kaplan SA, Wein AJ, Staskin DR, Roehrborn CG, Steers WD. Urinary retention and post-void residual urine in men: separating truth from tradition. J Urol. 2008;180(1):47–54.

34 Kapoor A. Benign prostatic hyperplasia (BPH) management in the primary care setting. Can J Urol. 2012;19 Suppl 1:10–7.

35 Emberton M, Cornel EB, Bassi PF, Fourcade RO, Gómez JM, Castro R. Benign prostatic hyperplasia as a progressive disease: a guide to the risk factors and options for medical management. Int J Clin Pract. 2008;62(7):1076–86.

36 Levy A, Samraj GP. Benign prostatic hyperplasia: when to "watch and wait," when and how to treat. Cleve Clin J Med. 2007;74:S15–20.

37 Djavan B, Fong YK, Harik M, Milani S, Reissigl A, Chaudry A, et al. Longitudinal study of men with mild symptoms of bladder outlet obstruction treated with watchful waiting for four years. Urology. 2004;64(6):1144–8.

CHAPTER 6

Watchful Waiting

Reginald Bruskewitz

University of Wisconsin, Madison, WI, USA

Key points
- Development of urinary retention develops in around 1–3% of men on watchful waiting. The risk is higher for men with large prostates.
- Benign prostatic hyperplasia (BPH) progresses to bladder or renal dysfunction in a small but clinically significant percentage of men on watchful waiting.
- Bother from urinary symptoms is the primary determinant in selecting watchful waiting over treatment.
- Spontaneous urinary retention has a greater probability of recurring than precipitated retention.

Introduction

To provide the best advice to patients electing watchful waiting, an understanding of the natural history or progression is necessary. While projections on likelihood of a given scenario playing out for the individual patient are imprecise, general estimates are helpful. The mode of presentation has considerable bearing on the chance of BPH progression (Table 6.1). Some modes of presentation are upfront indicators for a recommendation to intervene and not watch. And some outcomes may be merely inconvenient, while others can be severe or even life threatening. Therefore, individualization for watchful waiting based on patient preferences and risk is appropriate.

Our understanding of what may lie ahead for the patient is found in community-based longitudinal evaluations of community-dwelling men not presenting for care or evaluation, patients followed by single institutions in a clinical setting over longer periods of time, and the placebo arms of larger drug studies of BPH. These different data sources might lead to different conclusions regarding probability of watchful waiting outcomes. A patient attending a clinic may have a greater chance of BPH progression than a man living in the community and not seeking medical attention, and the double-blinded drug trials may measure the placebo effect, not pure watching, with the patient's knowledge that he may be on a drug.

Main sources of information on BPH natural history

- community-dwelling older men;
- clinic patients;
- placebo arms of BPH drug trials.

Male Lower Urinary Tract Symptoms and Benign Prostatic Hyperplasia, First Edition.
Edited by Steven A. Kaplan and Kevin T. McVary.
© 2014 John Wiley & Sons, Ltd. Published 2014 by John Wiley & Sons, Ltd.

Table 6.1 Various modes of presentation and possible outcomes reflecting benign prostatic hyperplasia progression

Presentation	Clinical outcome
Bother from benign prostatic hyperplasia	Increased bother from benign prostatic hyperplasia
Lower urinary tract symptoms	Decision to treat: drug or procedure
Residual urine	Acute urinary retention
Urine flow rate	Increased lower urinary tract symptoms
Prostate size	Renal disease
Elevated prostate-specific antigen	Increased residual urine
Retention	Bladder dysfunction
Urinary tract infection	Urinary tract infection
Renal disease	Prostatic bleeding
Bladder dysfunction	
Prostatic bleeding	
Obstruction (urodynamic)	

Note that some entities appear as presentation and outcome. The more severe the presentation, the greater the risk of benign prostatic hyperplasia progression.

Symptom progression

BPH-related urinary tract symptoms, now generally referred to as lower urinary tract symptoms (LUTS), are often measured by symptoms scores such as the American Urological Association Symptom Index (AUA-SI) and the International Prostate Symptom Score (IPSS). These have been widely used to quantify symptoms in published studies. While these symptom scores have been validated to correspond well with symptoms emanating from BPH, symptoms often attributed to prostate cases may in fact not be prostate related. One example is nocturia, which is generally defined as getting up with the need to void on more than one occasion per night. Excessive night-time urine production from large bedtime fluid intake, congestive heart failure, medications, and other causes may account for nocturia, and treating nocturia as prostate induced may not result in an improvement or may miss an important alternate diagnosis. For both surgical and medical treatment, nocturia tends to be the most refractory to improvement.

The Olmsted County, Minnesota evaluation of the natural history in community-dwelling men looked at longitudinal changes in voiding symptoms men aged 40–79. The study revealed a slow, mild, and steady increase on average in the AUA symptom index of 0.18 point per year [1]. The worsening of symptoms was more marked in older men, men with larger prostates, and those presenting with a reduced urine flow rate.

The issue of symptom progression was addressed in a study of 500 men at five clinics in the United States who were candidates for transurethral prostatectomy and followed initially nonoperatively over 4 years [2].

As shown in Table 6.2, for patients presenting with moderate symptoms and followed for 4 years, 13% then had mild symptoms after 4 years, 46% continued with moderate symptoms, 17% had severe symptoms, and 24% had undergone surgical intervention.

Table 6.2 Watchful waiting outcomes at 4 years

Presenting with moderate symptoms – outcome
4 years later

Mild	Moderate	Severe	Surgery
13%	46%	17%	24%

Presenting with severe symptoms – outcome
4 years later

Mild	Moderate	Severe	Surgery
2%	21%	38%	29%

For those initially presenting with severe symptoms, after 4 years 2% had mild symptoms and 21% moderate, 38% continued with severe symptoms, and 29% had surgery to deal with BPH. This illustrates that patient symptom level is subject to change. More often, the symptoms increase, and bother may increase to the point of electing intervention, but some patients spontaneously improve.

Acute urinary retention

The sudden inability to urinate is painful, feared by patients, and a sign of progression indicating a need to change the course of management. Unlike some signs of BPH progression such as worsening symptoms or bother, retention requires prompt action and an immediate review of the watchful waiting treatment plan. In the literature, the exact magnitude of the problem is often blurred. Some articles confuse an elevated postvoid residual of urine in a patient able to void with complete retention.

Retention can be brought on by precipitating factors such as hospitalization with bed rest, alcohol consumption, nonurologic surgery with anesthesia, and decongestant medication. Anticholinergic and antihistamine meds are often mentioned, but these are likely less often implicated than decongestants, and prostatic infarct is cited as a cause of retention in some reports, but the evidence for this is mixed.

Present-day estimates of the annual rate of urinary retention with untreated BPH are related to symptom severity and on average range from 0.5 to 2.5% per year. The risk is cumulative and increases with advancing age. The cumulative risk for a man in his fifties with more than mild symptoms, if he lives to be 80, is 20%. For a man in his seventies, the risk is 30% [3]. In a substantial minority of men, urinary retention is the initial BPH-related development, and around 40% of retention episodes are precipitated by medical or medication events.

The urodynamic impact of acute urinary retention was evaluated in 78 patients who underwent transurethral resection of the prostate (TURP) because of LUTS or acute retention [4]. Thirty-two percent of these patients presented with acute retention. While TURP led to a sustained and clinically relevant improvement in pressure–flow parameters in both groups, those with acute retention had a comparable symptom result, but an impaired urodynamic outcome with less recovery of detrusor function. Al-Hayek *et al.* studied 196 patients for a minimum of 10 years with baseline and follow-up pressure–flow studies and found no statistical difference in bladder contractility in patients treated by TURP compared with those untreated [5]. For this group of patients, relieving obstruction did not improve bladder contractility.

The rate of retention over time varies by study. In the Physicians Health Study, a study of 15,851 men, a subset of 6100 men self-reported urinary retention, and 4.5 episodes of retention per 1000 patient years were recorded [6].

In the Physicians Health Study, increasing age, greater baseline symptom score severity, and a prior diagnosis of BPH made retention more likely. In an older study, the Veterans Affairs (VA) Cooperative study of watchful waiting versus surgery, retention occurred at a rate of 9.6/1000 patient years in the watchful waiting group [7]. In this VA study of over 500 men lasting 3.5–5.5 years, around a third of men in the watchful waiting group crossed over to TURP, so this cross-over reduced the chance these men would have retention, and yet the rate was twice that of the Health Professionals Study.

At the other extreme for the average retention rate for a study is the Proscar Long-Term Efficacy and Safety Study. In the placebo arm of this study, the retention rate was 18/1000 patient years [8], and men with greater symptoms, larger prostates, and lower baseline flow rates were above the average rate of retention. In the Olmsted County Study of community-dwelling men, the retention rate was 6.8/1000 patient years [9].

The Olmsted County Study examined factors that increased the chance for retention. In addition to the increasing effect of age above age 60, lower baseline flow rates, worse symptoms, and larger prostates each independently increased the chance of acute retention by factors of 3 to 4. When multiple adverse factors are considered together, such as older, worse symptoms, larger prostate, and lower flow, the risk might increase by as much as 15 times. A large prostate seems to be the greatest of these risk factors, other than age.

After sorting through the various studies, a fair general conclusion is that a man who has signs and symptoms suggesting BPH as the cause has an annual rate of retention of about 1–2%. The circumstances during which the retention occurs will help in advising the patient on

Table 6.3 Acute urinary risk factors

Increased retention risk	Sign or symptom
Age	Over 60 years; more marked over 70 years
Uroflow	Less than 12 mL/s
Prostate size	Greater than 30 mL
Worse symptoms	Symptom score: moderate or severe
Prostate-specific antigen	Greater than 3

what to do if retention does develop. Should the patient continue watching once the retention episode has been dealt with or should he seek intervention beyond the initial retention management? If a patient develops spontaneous retention without any discernible cause, he is much more likely to have recurring episodes of retention than if the retention was precipitated by such factors as medication, illness, or unrelated surgery [10].

The factors that increase the risk of retention are moderate and severe symptoms, larger prostate, and older age (Table 6.3). However, in the BPH age group, a younger male with milder symptoms and a smaller prostate still runs a risk of retention, albeit a substantially lower risk.

Prostate size and growth

In that prostate size and growth over time play a significant role in the outcome of watchful waiting, just what is the growth rate? The consideration of prostate size for a patient considering his options is important because an estimate of size is an easy bit of information to obtain, particularly when considering prostate-specific antigen (PSA) as a surrogate for size measurement.

Prostate size has traditionally been measured by a digital rectal exam. This is inaccurate

Table 6.4 Prostate measurement options

Test	Accuracy	Cost	Other issue
Digital exam	Poor	Lowest	
Transrectal ultrasound	High	Moderate	
Prostate-specific antigen	High	Low	
MRI	High	High	
CT	High	High	Radiation exposure

compared with more objective options. Other measures such as an MRI or CT can be used and are accurate, but are cost prohibitive for routine use (Table 6.4). The Olmsted County Study tracked prostate size over 4 years and recorded an annual growth rate of 1.9% [11]. A subset of the full group of community-dwelling men had their prostates measured by transrectal ultrasound. A look at the placebo arm of a finasteride drug study documented an average size increase of 14% over 4 years [8]. Again, transrectal ultrasound measurements were used in this finasteride versus placebo study to serially measure the prostate size and growth. In addition, in this finasteride study, PSA was a powerful predictor of BPH progression [12].

For the patient initially presenting for consideration of watchful waiting for BPH, the baseline PSA predicts future prostatic growth [13]. The Medical Treatment of Prostate Symptoms (MTOPS) confirmed that prostate volume, measured by transrectal ultrasound scan (TRUS), and PSA were predictors of both future prostate growth and the eventual need for prostate surgery or the development of acute urinary retention [14,15]. Simply put, the larger the prostate, as determined by either transrectal ultrasound or PSA, the faster the prostate grows; and the larger the prostate, the greater the risk of BPH progression.

While the overall retention and surgery risk was 14% over 4 years, the risk increased from 9% to 22% as the baseline prostate size increased, as measured by TRUS. The risk of this progression increased 8–20% when stratified by increasing PSA. PSA correlated to ultrasound determined prostate size and was a predictor of acute urinary retention and the need for BPH surgery. Also, there was a linear increase in retention risk for both spontaneous and precipitated retention.

Bladder function changes in men over time

Thomas *et al.* observed the natural history of lower urinary tract dysfunction in older men over a period of 10 or more years [16]. Bladder outlet obstruction and detrusor dysfunction progress with age. Maximum urine flow declines with age from prostatic enlargement or declining detrusor function. Urodynamics changes include a reduction in detrusor contractility and increased detrusor overactivity. The overall failed watchful-waiting rate in this conservatively managed group was 17.1%, with an acute urinary retention (AUR) rate of 4.12% over the mean 14-year follow-up. Patients with untreated bladder outlet obstruction (BOO) do not significantly deteriorate urodynamically in the long-term.

These findings serve to justify a conservative approach to men with LUTS associated with BOO. Styles *et al.* investigated 41 English men with chronic urinary retention secondary to BOO [17]. The authors compared convention cystometry with long-term cystometry bladder monitoring and found that detrusor instability was found in 51% during conventional and 88% during long-term monitoring. Unstable detrusor contractions on long-term observation were associated with upper tract dilation and impairment of glomerular filtration. De Nunzio evaluated 101 obstructed men with BPH initially and after a mean of 2 years [18].

In a watchful-waiting subgroup, detrusor overactivity was present in 45% at baseline and 55% at follow-up. For medical therapy with alpha blockers, it was 35% and 30%, reductase inhibitor 62.5% before and after 2 years, TURP 68% at baseline, and 31% detrusor overactivity after surgery. Only surgery significantly reduced detrusor overactivity.

One hundred and sixty one men with LUTS were evaluated for BOO, detrusor instability, and reduced bladder compliance [19]. Bladder dysfunction was correlated with abnormalities in blood urea nitrogen (BUN) or serum creatinine. Outlet obstruction with or without detrusor instability did not appear to be risk factors for elevated BUN or creatinine, but when decreased bladder compliance was associated with outlet obstruction and instability, the risk of elevated BUN or creatinine was substantially increased.

The issue of whether delaying treatment while continuing watchful waiting was addressed in several studies. In the VA Cooperative Study on Transurethral Resection of the Prostate versus watchful waiting, men who were initially randomized to watch, and then elected to cross over to TURP, had a less favorable improvement in symptom score and bother from urinary issues than those who underwent immediate TURP [20,21]. The finding of an elevated baseline postvoid residual urine was associated with a poorer outcome following surgery. This suggests that bladder deterioration with watching played a role. In a drug-versus-placebo study, there were findings similar to the VA surgery study. Men who were initially randomized to placebo in a dutasteride versus placebo study did not report any appreciable improvement in symptoms compared with those who started dutasteride immediately [22]. The 2-year delay until crossover likely played a role. In this study, there are no data conveyed to suggest that the bladder was the reason.

Renal disease and benign prostatic hyperplasia

A population-based report by Rule *et al.* on 2115 men in Olmstead County Minnesota found that end-stage renal disease (ESRD) is associated with diminished peak urinary flow, moderate to severe LUTS, and chronic urinary retention. A significant cross-sectional relationship between BOO and chronic kidney disease was found in community-dwelling men [23].

Rule *et al.* also explored the association of renal disease and BPH, and found publications citing chronic larger volume urinary retention, detrusor instability, and decreased bladder compliance to be associated with chronic renal failure. Episodic retention and secondary hypertension may be factors as well [24]. A clinic referral-based population in Korea was evaluated for an association of BPH and chronic kidney disease [25]. In 2741 consecutive clinic visits, chronic kidney disease was associated with reduced maximum urinary flow, hypertension, and diabetes, but not PSA level, prostate volume, postvoid residual volume, or symptom score.

Associations in common between chronic kidney disease and benign prostatic hyperplasia

Might BPH alter renal function through mechanisms other than obstruction and bladder dysfunction leading to renal dysfunction? Common conditions might increase the risk for both renal disease and BPH, or prostate-related abnormalities might lead to renal dysfunction independent of obstruction and bladder dysfunction. Associations do not necessarily imply causation. However, in other systems, common conditions may cause disease in another system. For example, low-grade systemic inflammation is associated with vascular and cardiac disease [26]. There is considerable overlap in conditions associated with BPH and renal disease, but a listing provides conditions for consideration of other prostatic mechanisms that might cause renal disease. Diabetes, hypertension, central adiposity, the metabolic syndrome, and dyslipidemia are associated with renal disease [27]. BPH is associated with diabetes, central adiposity, inflammation, and the metabolic syndrome.

Inflammation

Prostatic inflammation has been associated with BPH progression and pathogenesis. Mishra *et al.* evaluated 374 men and found that 70% with urinary retention versus 45% of men with LUTS had chronic prostatic inflammation [28]. St Sauver *et al.* studied men in Olmstead County, Minnesota and found that physician-diagnosed prostatitis was associated with a 2.4-fold increase of a later diagnosis of prostatism, enlarged prostate, or BPH and increased the odds of undergoing BPH treatment [29]. AUR was increased in those with a prostatitis diagnosis but not to a significant level.

Diabetes

Another evaluation of 170 diabetic men in Olmstead County found that nocturia and irritative urinary symptoms, but not prostate volume, PSA, or peak urinary flow rate, were associated with diabetes [30]. The authors speculate that diabetes may be less associated with prostatic growth and more associated with lower urinary tract dysfunction. (The lower tract dysfunction could contribute to renal disease.)

Hypertension

Michel *et al.* evaluated 9857 men diagnosed with and seeking treatment for BPH, looking for associations with blood pressure, maximum urinary flow rate, and IPSS. An association of LUTS, but not urinary flow, and hypertension was identified [31]. In evaluating 1019 men with BPH in the Massachusetts male Aging Study, heart disease increased, and cigarette smoking and high levels of physical activity decreased the risk of BPH [32]. In addition, waist–hip ratio, diastolic blood pressure, diabetes, hypertension, and serum androgens or estrogens did not individually predict BPH.

Metabolic syndrome

The metabolic syndrome is associated with cardiovascular disease, sexual dysfunction, and diabetes. Lee *et al.* studied 409 men and found that waist circumference was positively associated with prostate volume, PSA, and IPSS [33]. They confirmed that a greater waist circumference was associated with hypertension, coronary artery disease, type 2 diabetes, and erectile and ejaculatory dysfunction. In a case–control study in India of 85 men with a diagnosis of BPH compared with 115 men without BPH, an association of increased waist-to-hip circumference and elevated triglyceride and decreased high-density lipoprotein was found in the BPH group [34].

Autonomic nervous system

McVary *et al.* studied 38 men from the 3047 men enrolled in the MTOPS study with autonomic nervous system studies including measurements of heart rate, blood pressure, circulatory response to a tilt table, and plasma and urinary catecholamines [35]. These measurements were compared with AUA SI, BPH Impact Index, prostate size, and maximum urinary flow. They found an association of AUA SI, BPH Impact Index, and change in systolic and diastolic blood pressure after tilt-table testing.

Monitoring renal function in men with benign prostatic hyperplasia

The 2010 BPH AUA Guidelines state: "baseline renal insufficiency appears to be no more common in men with BPH than in men of the same age group in the general population" [36]. Accordingly, the current AUA Guidelines do not recommend routine measurement of serum creatinine in the initial evaluation of men with LUTS secondary to BPH. This conclusion, drawn by the AUA Guidelines panel, was largely gleaned from observations on impairment of renal function in the placebo arms of large randomized BPH drug trials. In these trials, patients were selected by relatively stringent inclusion and exclusion criteria. Roberts *et al.* compared the placebo arm of the MTOPS trial with community-dwelling men [37]. They concluded: "Compared to community-dwelling men, men in the placebo arm of clinical trials of BPH treatments had a substantially lower risk of BPH-related outcomes." The use of clinical trials to describe the natural history of BPH should be done with caution. Literature on BPH and renal disease suggests that BOO plus bladder dysfunction such as the development of urinary retention, reduced bladder capacity or compliance, and bladder instability are key elements in increased risk of renal dysfunction.

End-stage renal disease

More than 485,000 Americans are being treated for kidney failure, also called ESRD (Table 6.5). Of these, more than 341,000 are dialysis patients, and more than 140,000 have a functioning kidney transplant. Over the last 5 years, the number of new patients with ESRD has averaged more than 90,000 annually. The current annual cost of treating ESRD in the US is approximately $23 billion. In 2005, 85,790 patients died as a result of ESRD.

Table 6.5 End-stage renal disease in the US

	Number	Percent
Sex		
Males	270,524	55.8
Females	214,466	44.2
Age		
Below 19 years	7362	1.5
20–44 years	95,208	19.6
45–64 years	211,985	43.7
65–74 years	94,353	19.5
75 years or more	76,171	15.7
Disorders		
Diabetes	179,157	36.9
High blood pressure	117,438	24.2
Glomerulonephritis	78,345	16.2
Cystic kidney	22,458	4.6
Other urologic	13,581	2.8
Other/unknown causes	86,905	17.9

Source: National Kidney Foundation, March 2008, US Renal Data System Annual Data Report for 2005.

> **Dos and don'ts**
>
> - Monitor renal function for men with increased risk of renal deterioration.
> - Assess prostate size (PSA is more accurate than a digital rectal examination) to help stratify risk for BPH progression.
> - Consider measurement of postvoid residual, especially in men with marked frequency, nocturia, or insensible urine loss.
> - Don't fail to watch men electing to wait with periodic in-office follow-up.

Approximately 11% of US adults have ESRD, as documented in the National Health and Nutrition Examination Survey III [38]. A report from England compared the prevalence of renal impairment in 382 consecutive patients undergoing prostatectomy in 1985 compared with 191 patients undergoing herniorrhapy or cholecystectomy [39]. The prostatectomy patients had a rate of renal impairment of 7.7% compared with 3.7% in the controls.

Conclusion

Most men are well served by an initial strategy of watchful waiting. For most, BPH progression is gradual and not associated with long-term harmful outcomes. For a minority, negative systemic health outcomes may result. Although BPH progression can be predicted with some degree of certainty, men with pre-existing comorbid conditions may actually be the subgroup that is at greatest risk of harm from BPH.

Bibliography

1 Jacobsen SL, Girman CJ, Guess HA, Rhodes T, Oesterling JE, Lieber MM. Natural history of prostatism: longitudinal changes in voiding symptoms in community dwelling men. *J Urol.* 1996;155:595.

2 Barry MJ, Fowler FJ, Bin L, Pitts JC 3rd, Harris CJ, Mulley AG Jr. The natural history of patients with benign prostatic hyperplasia as diagnosed by North American urologists. *J Urol.* 1997;157:10–5.

3 Roehrborn CG. The epidemiology of acute urinary retention in benign prostatic hyperplasia. *Rev Urol.* 2001;3:187–92.

4 Wagenlehner FM, Bescherer K, Wagenlehner C, Zellner M, Weidner W, Naber KG. Urodynamic impact of acute urinary retention in patients with benign prostatic hyperplasia: a 2-year follow-up after transurethral resection of the prostate. *Urol Int.* 2011;86:73.

5 Al-Hayek S, Thomas A, Abrams P. Natural history of detrusor contractility-minimum ten-year urodynamic follow-up in men with bladder outlet obstruction. *Scand J Urol Nephrol.* Suppl 2004; 21:101.

6 Meigs JB, Barry MJ, Giovannucci E, Rimm EB, Stampfer MJ, Kawachi I. Incidence rates and risk factors for acute urinary retention: the Health Professionals Followup Study. *J Urol.* 1999;162: 376–82.

7 Wasson JH, Reda DJ, Bruskewitz RC, Elinson J, Keller AM, Henderson WG. A comparison of transurethral surgery with watchful waiting for moderate symptoms of benign prostatic hyperplasia. The Veterans Affairs Cooperative Study Group on Transurethral Resection of the Prostate. *N Engl J Med.* 1995;332:75–9.

8 McConnell JD, Bruskewitz R, Walsh P, Andriole G, Lieber M, Holtgrewe HL, *et al.* The effect of finasteride on the risk of acute urinary retention and the need for surgical treatment among men with benign prostatic hyperplasia. Finasteride Long-Term Efficacy and Safety Study Group. *N Engl J Med.* 1998;338:557–63.

9 Jacobsen SJ, Jacobsen DJ, Girman CJ, Roberts RO, Rhodes T, Guess HA, *et al.* Natural history of prostatism: risk factors for acute urinary retention. *J Urol.* 1997;158:481–7.

10 Roehrborn CG, Bruskewitz R, Nickel GC, Glickman S, Cox II C, Anderson R, *et al.* Urinary retention in patients with BPH treated with finasteride or placebo over 4 years. Characterization of patients and ultimate outcome. The PLESS Study group. *Eur Urol.* 2000;37:528–36.

11 Rhodes T, Girman CJ, Jacobsen DJ, Roberts RO, Lieber MM, Jacobsen SJ. Longitudinal prostate volume in a community- based sample: 7 year followup in the Olmsted County Study of urinary symptoms and health status among men. *J Urol.* 2000;163(Suppl 4):249 (Abstract 1105).

12 Roehrborn CG, McConnell JD, Lieber M, Kaplan S, Geller J, Malek GH, et al. Serum prostate-specific antigen is a powerful predictor of acute urinary retention and the need for surgery in men with benign prostatic hyperplasia. *Urology.* 1999;53:473–80.

13 Roehrborn CG, McConnell JD, Bonilla J, Rosenblatt S, Hudson PB, Malek GH, et al. Serum prostate specific antigen is a strong predictor of future prostate growth in men with benign prostatic hyperplasia: Proscar Long-Term Efficacy and Safety study. *J Urol.* 2000;163:13–20.

14 Roehrborn CG, McConnell JD, Jacobs S, Slawin K, Kreder K, Foley J, et al. Baseline prostate volume and serum PSA predict rate of prostate growth: analysis of the MTOPS data. *J Urol.* 2003(Suppl 4):364 (Abstract 1361).

15 McConnell JD, Roehrborn CG, Slawin KM, Lieber MM, Smith JA, Kaplan SA, et al. Baseline measures predict the risk of benign prostatic hyperplasia clinical progression in placebo-treated patients. *J Urol.* 2003;169(Suppl 4):332 (Abstract 1287).

16 Thomas AW, Cannon A, Bartlett E, Ellis-Jones J, Abrams P. The natural history of lower urinary tract dysfunction in men: minimum 10-year urodynamic followup of untreated bladder outlet obstruction. *BJU Int.* 2005;96:1301.

17 Styles RA, Neal DE, Griffiths CJ, Ramsden PD. Long-term monitoring of bladder pressure in chronic retention of urine; the relationship between detrusor activity and upper tract dilation. *J Urol.* 1988;140:330.

18 De Nunzio C, Franco G, Rocchegiani A, Iori F, Leonardo C, Laurenti C. The evolution of detrusor activity after watchful waiting, medical therapy and surgery in patients with bladder outlet obstruction. *J Urol.* 2003;169:535.

19 Comiter CV, Sullivan MP, Schacterie RS, Cohen LH, Valla SV. Urodynamic risk factors for renal dysfunction in men with obstructive and non obstructive voiding dysfunction. *J Urol.* 1997;158:181.

20 Flanigan RC, Reda DJ, Wasson, JH, Anderson RJ, Abdellatif M, Bruskewitz RC. 5-year outcome of surgical resection and watchful waiting for men with moderately symptomatic benign prostatic hyperplasia: a Department of Veterans Affairs cooperative study. *J Urol.* 1998;160(1):12–6.

21 Wasson JH Reda DJ, Bruskewitz RC, Elinson J, Keller AM, Henderson WG. A comparison of transurethral surgery with watchful waiting for moderate symptoms of benign prostatic hyperplasia. The Veterans Affairs Cooperative Study Group on Transurethral Resection of the Prostate. *N Engl J Med.* 1995;332(2):75–9.

22 Roehrborn CG, Lukkarinen O, Mark S, Siami P, Ramsdell J, Zinner N. Long-term of sustained improvement in symptoms of benign prostatic hyperplasia with the dual 5 alpha reductase inhibitor dutasteride: results of 4-year studies. *BJU Int.* 2005;96:572–7.

23 Rule AD, Jacobsen DJ, Roberts RO, Girman CJ, McGree ME, Lieber MM, et al. The association between benign prostatic hyperplasia and chronic kidney disease. *Kidney Int.* 2005;67:2376.

24 Rule Ad, Lieber MM, Jacobsen SJ. Is benign prostatic hyperplasia risk factor for chronic renal failure? *J Urol.* 2001;173:691.

25 Hong SK, Lee ST, Jeong SJ, Byun SS, Hong YK, Park DS, et al. Chronic kidney disease among men with lower urinary tract symptoms due to benign prostatic hyperplasia. *BJU Int.* 2012;105:1424.

26 Buckley DI, Fu R, Freeman M, Rogers K, Helfand M. C-reactive protein as a risk factor for coronary heart disease: a systematic review and meta-analysis for the U.S. Preventive Services Task Force. *Ann Inter Med.* 2009;151(7):483.

27 National Kidney Foundation. Clinical practice Guidelines for chronic kidney disease: evaluation, classification, and stratification. Kidney Disease Outcome Quality Initiative. *Am J Kidney Dis.* 2002;39:S1–46.

28 Mishra VC, Allen DJ, Nicolaou C, Sharif H, Hudd C, Karim OM, et al. Does prostatic inflammation have a role in the pathogenesis and progression in benign prostatic hyperplasia? *BJU Int.* 2007;100:327.

29 St Sauver JL, Jacobsen SJ, McGree ME, Girman CJ, Lieber MM, Jacobsen SJ. Longitudinal association between prostatitis and development of benign prostatic hyperplasia. *Urology.* 2008;71:475.

30 Sarma AV, Burke JP Jacobsen SJ, McGree ME, St Sauver J, Girman CJ, *et al.* Associations between diabetes and clinical markers of benign prostatic hyperplasia among community dwelling Black and White men. *Diabetes Care.* 2008;31:476.

31 Michel MC, Heeman U, Schumacher H, Mehlburger L, Goepel M. Association of hypertension with symptoms of benign prostatic hyperplasia. *J Urol.* 2004;172:1390.

32 Meigs JB, Mohr B, Barry MJ, Collins MM, McKinlay JB. Risk factors for clinical benign prostatic hyperplasia in a community-based population of healthy aging men. *J Clin Epidemiol.* 2001;54:939.

33 Lee RK, Chung D, Chughtai B, Te AE, Kaplan SA. Central obesity as measured by waist circumference is predictive of severity of lower urinary tract symptoms. *BJU Int.* 2012;110(4):540–5.

34 Tewari R, Prabhat P, Natu SM, Dalela D, Goel A, Goel MM, et al. Association of benign prostatic hyperplasia (BPH) with the metabolic syndrome (MS) and its components—"a growing dilemma." *J Men's Health* 2011;8:66.

35 McVary KT, Rademaker A, Lloyd GL, Gann P. Autonomic nervous system overactivity in men with lower urinary tract symptoms secondary to benign prostatic hyperplasia. *J Urol.* 2005; 174:1327.

36 McVary KT, Roehrborn CG, Alvins AL, Barry MJ, Bruskewitz RC, Donnell RF, et al. Update on AUA guidelines on the management of benign prostatic hyperplasia. *J Urol.* 2011;185:1793.

37 Roberts RO, Lieber MM, Jacobsen DJ, Girman CJ, Jacobsen SJ. Limitations of using outcomes in the placebo arm of a clinical trial of benign prostatic hyperplasia to quantify those in the community. *Mayo Clin Proc.* 2005;80:759.

38 Coresh J, Astor BC, Greene T, Levey AS. Prevalence of chronic kidney disease and decreased renal function in the adult US population: third National Health and Nutrition Examination Survey. *Am J Kidney Dis.* 2003;41:1.

39 Hill AM, Philpott N, Kay LDS, Smith JC, Fellows GJ, Sacks SH. Prevalence and outcome of renal impairment at prostatectomy. *Br J Urol.* 1993;71:464.

α-Adrenergic Antagonists for Lower Urinary Symptoms Secondary to Benign Prostatic Hyperplasia

Nathaly François, Raunak D. Patel & Kevin T. McVary

Division of Urology, Southern Illinois University School of Medicine, Springfield, IL, USA

Key points

- Symptomatic benign prostatic hyperplasia (BPH) is primarily due to prostate enlargement, and secondarily due to the increase in prostate smooth muscle tone mediated by the α-adrenergic system.
- Selective α-blockers are safe, effective treatment options for symptomatic BPH.
- Nonselective α-blockers are not recommended for treatment of BPH/lower urinary tract symptoms.
- The most common side effects of the α-blockers include dizziness and hypotension, which occur less frequently with the more α_1-selective blockers such as tamsulosin and silodosin.
- Sexual side effects are also noted with α-blockers, notably ejaculatory dysfunction, which occurs more frequently with the more α_1-selective blockers tamsulosin and silodosin.
- Combination therapy with α-blockers and 5α-reductase inhibitors is effective for treatment of BPH/lower urinary tract symptoms (LUTS) and recommended in patients with an enlarged prostate gland (i.e. >35 mL).

Introduction

BPH, a prostate stromal proliferative process, is a familiar problem among aging men, often giving rise to bothersome LUTS. These symptoms can be classified as obstructive/voiding symptoms including urinary hesitancy, a weak urinary stream, incomplete bladder emptying, and straining; or irritative/storage symptoms including nocturia, urinary frequency, and urinary urgency [1].

Symptomatic BPH results from the obstruction attributed largely to a static or anatomical component of prostate growth related to the physiologic enlargement of the prostate gland with age, and is secondarily due to a dynamic or functional component related to the increase in smooth muscle tone in the prostate stroma and capsule, and the bladder neck, mediated by the autonomic nervous system. Although there is a wide variability in prostate growth among individuals, one study did identify a steady increase in prostate volume among randomly selected community men of about 1.6% per year [2]. In another study, the prostate gland was found to increase steadily in volume with a percent change from baseline of 12.5–16.6% for men

Male Lower Urinary Tract Symptoms and Benign Prostatic Hyperplasia, First Edition.
Edited by Steven A. Kaplan and Kevin T. McVary.
© 2014 John Wiley & Sons, Ltd. Published 2014 by John Wiley & Sons, Ltd.

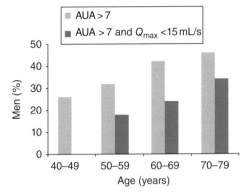

Q_{max} = Peak urinary flow rate.

Figure 7.1 Prevalence of moderate-to-severe lower urinary tract symptoms and lower urinary tract symptoms with a Q_{max} of <15 mL/s, by age. AUA, American Urological Association. Fawzy A, Pool JL. Benign Prostatic Hypertrophy and the Role of Alpha-Adrenergic Blockade. MEDSCAPE 2002. Reproduced with permission of Ahmed Fawzy, MD.

aged 50–59 years to those aged 70–79 years [3]. Also, about 50% of the male population aged 51–60 years is found to develop symptomatic BPH [4]. Moreover, nearly 50% of men 70 years or older have an American Urological Association Symptom Index/International Prostate Symptom Score (AUA-SI/IPSS) score suggestive of moderate-to-severe LUTS (≥8), and the possibility of a peak urinary flow rate indicative of obstruction (<15 mL/s) increases significantly in men 50 years or older (Figure 7.1) [5].

While about 53% of total urethral pressure is due to static pressure from the enlarged prostate with resulting bothersome LUTS from BPH, up to 40% of this pressure is related to α-adrenergic tone [6]. Prostatic smooth muscle cells contract under the influence of adrenergic sympathetic nerves, and subsequently constrict the urethra with resulting impairment in urine flow. Our focus is on the effect of the adrenergic sympathetic system, as α-antagonists have been developed to target this system with success-

ful medical management of LUTS/BPH given their effect to relax the prostate smooth muscle tone, possibly also to mitigate central nervous system (CNS) effects, with an increase in urinary flow and improvement in LUTS in patients with symptomatic BPH [7].

The prostate gland contains high levels of α_1- and α_2-adrenergic receptors (AR) [6,8–10]. However, the stromal elements of the prostate are predominantly associated with α_1-ARs, with the greatest influence on prostatic and urethral tone. Therefore, α_1-AR blockade would be expected to relax prostatic smooth muscle, relieve bladder outlet obstruction (BOO), and improve uroflow, as it has indeed been demonstrated to do.

Of note, the α_{1D}-subtype of ARs is primarily located in the bladder body and dome. Stimulation of these receptors may result in detrusor instability. Blockade of these receptors has been shown in animal models to reduce irritative LUTS [11].

Multiple α-AR antagonists have been developed for treatment of patients with bothersome LUTS. When symptomatic, BPH can have a profound impact on a patient's quality of life. For example, nocturia is known to be associated with higher rates of depression [12] and work absenteeism [13], decreased self-rated physical and mental health [14], as well as increased rates of accidental falls in the very old [15]. Community-based investigations of the natural history of BPH, and symptomatic LUTS due to BPH, indicate that if left untreated, the disease progresses over time with variable frequency. In a large, 5-year prospective investigation, men with moderate LUTS due to BPH who underwent watchful waiting were found to have worse outcomes than those who received treatment [i.e. via transurethral resection of the prostate (TURP)], with significantly higher incidences observed for acute urinary retention (AUR), for an elevated postvoid residual (PVR) urine volume, and for development of severe LUTS [16].

α-Adrenergic receptors in the prostate

α_1-Receptor subtypes, the α_{1A}, α_{1B}, and α_{1D}, are each present in the prostate (Figure 7.2), but among these the prostate smooth muscle cells predominantly express α_{1A}-receptors, which are more specifically concentrated in the urinary bladder neck, capsule of the prostate, fibromuscular stroma of the prostate, and the urethra [17]. Stimulation of these adrenoreceptors, therefore, results in an increased resistance to urine flow. Furthermore, afferent α_1-receptor stimulation in the spinal cord contributes to an increased frequency of the reflex to urinate [18]. Moreover, the descending limb of the micturition reflex pathway may be mediated by α_1-adrenoreceptors [19]. Blockade of the α_{1A}-receptors reduces prostatic tone and is found, therefore, to improve the dynamic aspects of voiding [20].

α_{1B}-Receptors, on the other hand, populate the smooth muscle of arteries and veins, including the microvasculature of the prostate [21]. Blockade of these receptors in the cardiovascular system may result in dizziness and hypotension secondary to decreased total peripheral resistance via veno- and arterial dilation. This causes severe side effects, particularly among the many urologic patients with associated coexisting comorbidities.

Nonselective α-blockers

The first α-blocker that proved promising for the treatment of LUTS/BPH was phenoxybenzamine, an irreversibly binding, long-acting, nonselective α_1-/α_2-receptor blocker [22]. Its role in improving LUTS/BPH had in

Localization of α_1-Receptors

Bladder detrusor-α_{1D} > α_{1A}
Instability and irritative symptoms

Prostate/Urethra-α_{1A}
Smooth muscle contraction

Vasculature-α_{1A} [young patients]
α_{1B} > α_{1A} [older patients]
Smooth muscle contraction, vessel resistance

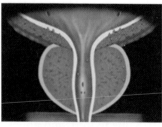

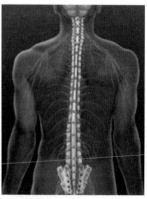

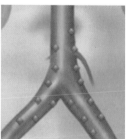

★ α_{1A}-Receptors
● α_{1B}-Receptors
▲ α_{1D}-Receptors

Spinal cord-α_{1D}
Lumbosacral cord innervation, control of urinary function

Figure 7.2 Localization of α_1 receptors. Images © Copyright Visible Health, Inc. Images © Copyright Visible Health, Inc. Created using drawMD Urology (www.drawmd.com) and reproduced with permission by Visible Health, Inc.

the past been applauded, but its significant adverse effects including dizziness, weakness, and palpitations limited the use of this drug for therapy [22]. The nonselective α-blocker was noted to exert its negative effect on the cardiovascular system with strong affinity, in addition to its effect on the prostate [23]. The effect on peripheral vascular α₁-receptors with resulting vasodilation and subsequent orthostatic hypotension, syncope, cardiac arrhythmias, nasal congestion, and pupillary dilation is less pronounced among the new, more selective α-blockers. Additionally, nonselective α-blockers affect histamine, serotonin, and acetylcholine receptors, with added malevolent effects [23]. Today, nonselective α-blockers are primarily used for the perioperative management of pheochromocytoma.

Selective α-blockers

α-Receptor blockers now used for the treatment of bothersome LUTS/BPH are primarily α₁-selective. These include terazosin (Hytrin®), doxazosin (Cardura®, Cardura® XL), tamsulosin (Flomax®), naftopidil (Flivas®), alfuzosin (Uroxatral®), and silodosin (Rapaflo®). Their targeted α₁-receptor blockade results in smooth muscle relaxation, notably within the cardiovascular system, urinary bladder, prostate, and urethra [24]. They are divided according to their ability to more specifically target the α_{1A}-AR subtype found primarily in prostatic tissue. Prazosin (Minipress®), indoramin (Doralese®), terazosin, alfuzosin, and doxazosin target the α_{1A}-receptor subtypes in the prostate gland with less binding affinity than do tamsulosin and silodosin [24].

In addition to their effects on α_{1A}-receptors, these agents may also decrease the expression of contractile proteins in prostate smooth muscle cells and minimally promote apoptosis [25]. Notably, doxazosin, a quinazoline-based α₁-blocker, was found in one study to increase the apoptotic activity in prostatic stromal cells within a 12-month period, a potential mechanism for the effect of α₁-blockade in improving bothersome LUTS [26]. This mechanism may be mediated by a decrease in TGF-β₁ [27]. Other quinazoline-based α₁-blockers such as prazosin and terazosin may act in a similar fashion, and not likely via α₁-receptor blockade but rather via inhibition of HERG-potassium channels [28]. However, the clinical impact of this prostatic apoptosis must be minimal, given that prostate-specific antigen (PSA) and prostate volume are not reduced by α-blockers in long-term randomized clinical trials [29].

Doxazosin

In regard to its efficacy, doxazosin, a long-acting α₁-blocker with once-daily dosing, was found in short-term clinical trials to demonstrate increases in urinary flow rate (Q_{max}) of about 1–4 mL/s and decreases in AUA-SI scores of up to 50% in men with symptomatic BPH (Figures 7.3 and 7.4). This clinical response to α₁-antagonism is noted to be dose dependent, as is the side-effect profile. Therefore, doxazosin is typically initiated at an oral dose of 1 mg daily, which is intended to minimize the frequency of side effects, notably postural hypotension and syncope. Depending on the patient response to therapy, the dose is titrated to 8 mg daily [30].

Terazosin

Terazosin is also a relatively long-acting α₁-blocker, with once-daily dosing. The Hytrin Community Assessment Trial (HCAT) is a multicenter study in which 2084 men aged ≥55 years, with moderate-to-severe LUTS as

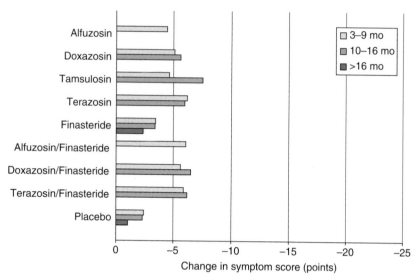

Figure 7.3 American Urological Association Symptom Index score improvements for medical therapies by duration of follow-up. Missing bars indicate that data were not available.

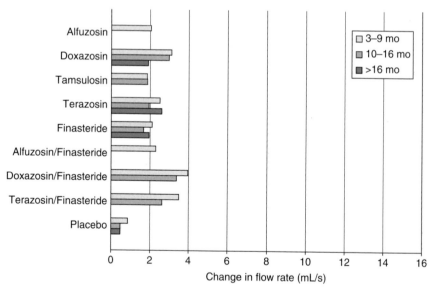

Figure 7.4 Peak urinary flow rate improvements for medical therapies by duration of follow-up. Missing bars indicate that data were not available.

defined by an AUA-SI score of 13 or more points, were randomized to treatment with terazosin (2, 5, or 10 mg) or placebo [31]. Terazosin was found to be significantly superior to placebo in all measurements of efficacy, particularly with regard to the improvement in reported symptoms with the AUA-SI score improvement from a baseline mean of 20.1 points, by 37.8% in the terazosin group, compared with only 18.4% in the placebo group. The mean change in Q_{max} from baseline was 2.2 mL/s for terazosin, compared with 0.8 mL/s for placebo (Figures 7.3 and 7.4). Treatment failure occurred in about 11% in the terazosin study group, compared with about 25% in the placebo group. Withdrawal from the study due to adverse effects of treatment occurred in 20% in the terazosin study group. Overall, terazosin given once daily is an effective medical therapy option for significantly reducing bothersome BPH/LUTS.

Alfuzosin

Alfuzosin is indicated for the management of moderate-to-severe urinary symptoms. It is an older medication, used in Europe in multiple dose-per-day formulations. In North America, alfuzosin is administered via an oral extended-release (ER) formulation (10 mg once daily), approved by the US Food and Drug Administration (FDA) in 2003 based on studies that showed improvements in irritative and obstructive urinary symptoms, as well as in Q_{max}, with alfuzosin ER compared with placebo [32] (Figures 7.3 and 7.4). There is evidence to suggest that pharmacotherapy with alfuzosin may even alter the natural history of BPH-related urinary symptoms and reduce certain complications (i.e. AUR) [33–36]. In a 2-year, open-label extension of a placebo-controlled study (N = 72), Jardin et al. found that patients who received alfuzosin therapy did not show any signs of BPH disease-related deterioration (i.e. bladder infection or AUR) [37]. A number of other long-term, open-label investigations have demonstrated a lower incidence of AUR with alfuzosin treatment, compared with the historical rates seen with watchful waiting. [33–36,38] For instance, in the 3-year prospective, open-label study of alfuzosin IR (2.5 mg three times daily) by Lukacs

et al., there was an extremely low incidence (0.3%) of AUR episodes overall, which is dramatically lower than the 2.9% overall rate seen in another investigation among patients with moderate BPH treated only with watchful waiting [36]. Admittedly, such cross-study comparison involves different patient cohorts, but the sharply lower incidence of AUR seen with alfuzosin between two similar groups of patients suggests that this difference is not spurious.

In one meta-analysis, the vasodilatory adverse-event profile experienced with alfuzosin ER 10 mg was similar to that experienced with placebo; other studies revealed that the incidence of ejaculatory dysfunction or erectile dysfunction (ED) was low at <1% [32]. Three studies were included in this meta-analysis, each with similar study design and inclusion/exclusion criteria, with enrollment of 984 patients with symptomatic BPH, randomized to receive either alfuzosin (N = 473) or placebo (N = 482) for 84 days. The number of study withdrawals was similar in both groups [alfuzosin 45 (9.5%) vs placebo 42 (8.7%)]. There were no significant changes in blood pressure observed with alfuzosin ER compared with placebo; hypotension and syncope were uncommon, and no first-dose vasodilatory effect was seen, which suggests no need to titrate the dose when initiating treatment with alfuzosin ER [32]. Findings from another meta-analysis revealed that alfuzosin ER helped to slow or prevent progression to more serious conditions as well; no patients treated with alfuzosin ER experienced AUR, compared with two patients who received placebo (0.4%) who did experience retention [32]. Data regarding the long-term efficacy and safety of the alfuzosin ER formulation have become available in the last decade [39]. In a long-term (i.e. 9 months), open-label extension of a 3-month double-blind, placebo-controlled trial in which all participants (N = 311) received alfuzosin ER 10 mg, the mean AUA-SI score improved significantly, from 17.1 at baseline to 9.3 at the study end ($p < 0.0001$); the mean Q_{max} rate improved from 9.1 to 11.3 mL/s ($p < 0.0001$). Twenty-nine (9.3%) patients discontinued treatment because of adverse events in 3.9% (12/311), and insufficient efficacy in 2.3% (7/311). Significant symptom relief was achieved rapidly with alfuzosin ER, and maintained at the study end. Bother scores also improved significantly, from 3.3 at baseline to 2.1 at the study end ($p < 0.0001$).

Tamsulosin

Tamsulosin is an α-blocker with greater specificity for the $α_{1A}$-AR compared with the $α_{1B}$-AR [40]. This drug is therefore expected to selectively target the smooth muscle cells contained within the prostate gland and exert minimal effects on the other α-AR subtypes that regulate blood pressure control and vasodilation. Some clinical trials suggest that tamsulosin provides relatively rapid-action onset based on symptom improvement and Q_{max}, with improvement noted within 24 h [41]. Initial short-term clinical trials suggest that tamsulosin increases Q_{max} by approximately 1.5 mL/s and decreases AUA-SI score by >35% [42] (Figures 7.3 and 7.4). Long-term studies (up to 60 weeks) also demonstrate that the beneficial effects of this $α_{1A}$-blocker are sustained over time, as measured by Q_{max} and AUA-SI scores [43]. Tamsulosin was tolerated during the study period, with side effects occurring in about 21% of patients. The most common side effects reported were dizziness (about 14.9%) and altered ejaculation (about 8.4%). Additional clinical studies have also demonstrated that tamsulosin can be coadministered with antihypertensive medications such as atenolol (Tenormin®), enalapril (Vasotec®), and nifedipine (Procardia®, Procardia® XL) without any increased risk of hypotensive or syncopal episodes [44]. Taken together, tamsulosin is a safe and efficacious drug for the treatment of BPH without any major vascular, or other, side effects.

Sildosin

Silodosin is an $α_{1A}$-AR antagonist, approved by the US FDA in 2008 for the treatment of LUTS associated with BPH. Shibata *et al.* examined the binding affinity of silodosin to cloned human $α_{1A}$-AR subtypes in an in vitro study using Chinese hamster ovary cells [45]. Silodosin was found to have a binding affinity for the $α_{1A}$-receptor subtype of almost 600 times that of the $α_{1B}$-AR, and approximately 60 times that of the $α_{1D}$-AR, confirming its selectivity for the $α_{1A}$-AR. On the other hand, tamsulosin demonstrated much less of an affinity, albeit still greater binding to the $α_{1A}$-AR compared with the $α_{1B}$- and $α_{1D}$-receptor subtypes, with a five- and threefold greater binding affinity for the $α_{1A}$-AR than for the $α_{1B}$- and the $α_{1A}$-AR, respectively. Silodosin is demonstrated, therefore, to be more selective than tamsulosin.

Several Japanese groups were the first to document the clinical efficacy of a 4 mg oral dosage of silodosin [46,47]. A few clinical studies performed in the US have since evaluated the efficacy and tolerability of an 8 mg oral daily dose of silodosin in men with BPH, with satisfactory results [48,49]. One 12-week, multicenter, randomized, double-blind, placebo-controlled trial enrolled men aged ≥50 years who had an AUA-SI score of ≥13 points, a Q_{max} between 4 and 15 mL/s, and a PVR volume of <250 mL [49]. Of the ~900 patients enrolled in the study, 466 received silodosin (8 mg daily), and 457 received a placebo drug. The mean improvements in AUA-SI score in the silodosin and placebo groups were −6.5 points and −3.6 points, respectively ($p < 0.001$). In addition, Q_{max} improved by +2.2 mL/s in the silodosin group, compared with +1.2 mL/s in the placebo group ($p = 0.006$). These profound clinical improvements have also been reported for other $α_{1A}$-blockers, with reported mean improvements of 2–2.5 points in AUA-SI scores compared with placebo [50].

Some studies have shown silodosin to be generally well tolerated. However, it has been associated with a higher incidence (>22%) of altered ejaculation [46,48,49]. Further studies are required to definitively establish the relative incidence of ejaculatory dysfunction, compared with other selective antagonists. As expected, given its higher affinity for the $α_{1A}$-receptor subtype, silodosin has been described as having a lower incidence of vascular effects, including orthostatic hypotension (<3%) [49]. In addition, the incidence of headache and dizziness is also reportedly low. Again, comparative data between silodosin and other selective antagonists are lacking.

Altogether, although the long-term efficacy and tolerability of silodosin require further study, this $α_{1A}$-selective antagonist appears nonetheless to significantly improve LUTS associated with BPH.

Naftopidil

Naftopidil is an $α_1$-blocker with high selectivity for the $α_{1A}$-receptor and also a notable affinity for the $α_{1D}$-receptor. The significance of this drug's affinity for the $α_{1D}$-receptor is represented by a study that demonstrated possible involvement of this receptor subtype in bladder storage and detrusor activity [51]. In an early study of the urodynamic effects of naftoptidil by Yasuda et al., Q_{max} rates increased and PVR decreased after 4–6 weeks of treatment on doses ranging from 25 to 75 mg/day [52]. Importantly, the authors also found that the bladder capacity at first desire to void increased significantly, which supports the understanding that naftopidil may do more to affect bladder filling and detrusor activity.

Naftopidil has shown a dose-dependent effect on objective measures of relief of the obstructive component in patients with BPH. For example, in one study in which 139 patients were randomized to treatment with 25 mg/day versus 75 mg/day, Yokoyoma et al. noted a dose-dependent improvement, as patients in the 75 mg/day group experienced improvements in voided volume, Q_{max}, and PVR, whereas those in the 25 mg/day group experienced an improvement in only their PVR volume [53]. On the other hand, Oh-oka found no difference in efficacy between patients taking 75 mg/day and those taking 50 mg/day, with similar improvements in Q_{max}, AUA-SI, and PVR volume among patients in either treatment arm [54]. Long-term studies on the efficacy of naftopidil are lacking.

Naftopidil has also shown benefits for irritative symptoms. For example, in a study of 81 men with complaints of urinary urgency at least once a day and AUA-SI scores of ≥8, Takahashi et al. reported reductions in AUA-SI from 19.1 to 6.5, with improvements in score from 4.6 to 3.2 noted after just 6 weeks of treatment [55]. Oh-oka studied the effect of naftopidil 75 mg/day in patients with symptomatic BPH and a primary complaint of nocturia, with a known reduced bladder capacity, over the course of 6 weeks of treatment. The patients reported a significant decrease in the frequency of nocturia from 3.1 to 1.2, as well as a decrease in daytime frequency. Furthermore, detrusor overactivity reported before treatment with naptopidil in 40 of the 122 patients studied was eliminated in 31 patients at the study end [56]. Symptoms of urinary urgency and the sensation of not adequately emptying the bladder improved significantly. Moreover, naftopidil seemed to have an effect on storage symptoms, as significant improvements were seen in bladder compliance and bladder capacity at the first desire to void.

α-Adrenergic antagonists and sexual dysfunction

Until recently, sexual dysfunction in older men has been perceived as of secondary importance. However, there is now clear evidence that most men remain sexually active into their seventies, and sexuality is an important component of quality of life in men with symptomatic BPH [57]. A concern for physicians when proceeding with medical treatment for BPH/LUTS has therefore been the negative impact of medical treatment on sexual function that may ensue. A recent study utilized Medical Treatment of Prostatic Symptoms (MTOPS) data to evaluate changes in sexual function related to finasteride, doxazosin, or combined therapy over 4 years [58]. A total of 2783 patients were included in this study, which required that they complete the Brief Male Sexual Function Inventory (BMSFI) at baseline and at least once during follow-up. Statistically significant differences in domains of the BMSFI including sexual drive, erectile function, ejaculatory function, and sexual problem assessment were demonstrated between the treatment arm and placebo, among patients in the finasteride and combined therapy groups. However, no changes in sexual function were seen across all domains of the

BMSFI in the doxazosin group. One finding that warrants further investigation is the possible synergism of combined therapy, in which worse ejaculatory function was noted when compared with finasteride alone.

Other studies have supported these findings, including a study by Rosen *et al.* that demonstrated better ejaculatory function in patients treated with the less selective α_1-blockers doxazosin, terazosin, and alfuzosin, compared with treatment with the α_{1A}-subtype selective tamsulosin, as well as compared with treatment with 5α-reductase inhibitors (5-ARIs) or combination therapy with α_1-blockers and 5-ARIs [38].

In an open-label study of 3076 men treated with alfuzosin 10 mg for 1 year, reduced stiffness of erection, reduced volume of ejaculate, and pain/discomfort on ejaculation were reported at baseline by 65.3%, 63.2%, and 20.2% of participants, respectively. At the study end-point, the mean Danish Prostate Symptom Score (DAN-PSS) including the sexual function domain (DAN-PSSsex) scores for each of these symptoms improved significantly (all $p < 0.001$) [35]. These improvements were apparent from the first assessment at 3 months and were maintained throughout the study, which also found alfuzosin to be effective in the improvement of LUTS as had previously been demonstrated in other studies. Alfuzosin may improve sexual function in those men with concomitant ED and ejaculatory dysfunction.

With long-term use of alfuzosin, lasting improvements in sexuality have consistently been observed [33–35]. For example, in their 3-year follow-up of patients, Lukacs and colleagues demonstrated improvements in patient sexuality using the UroLife BPH scale. Specifically, with up to 3 years of alfuzosin treatment, improvements in sexual-life subscores were seen among patients of all ages, with the greatest degree of sexual improvement occurring among those patients who reported severe symptoms at baseline, regardless of age [36]. Other studies [33–35,38] suggest that alfuzosin is not likely to give rise to unwanted sexual side effects, including ejaculatory dysfunction or ED. Clinical trials have shown, rather, that ejaculatory dysfunction and ED with alfuzosin are infrequent (0.0–0.6%), and in most cases these symptoms are judged by investigators not to be related to treatment [33–35]. These and other studies also indicate that long-term alfuzosin therapy tends to have a positive impact on patient BPH-related and bother-associated symptoms, again with the added benefit of fewer sexual side effects [33–36,38].

Tamsulosin, on the other hand, is associated with an increased incidence of ejaculatory dysfunction with symptoms among 8.4% of patients treated with the 0.4 mg dose to 18.1% of patients treated with the 0.8 mg dose [59]. In a phase III multicenter placebo-controlled study, Narayan and Tewari found a statistically significant difference in percentage of patients suffering from altered ejaculation in the tamsulosin arms versus placebo, with 11% dysfunction in the 0.4 mg group and 18% dysfunction in the 0.8 mg group [60]. It has also been theorized that ejaculatory dysfunction may also be linked to effects within the CNS, as tamsulosin shows a strong affinity for $5HT_{1A}$- and D_2-like receptors that are both involved with central regulation of ejaculation [61]. Ejaculatory dysfunction with tamsulosin has been reported to be as high as 26% [62]. Daily tamsulosin has been shown in one study to reduce ejaculate volume significantly in 90% of patients, and was associated with anejaculation in 35% of patients [39].

Silodosin has been shown to have even higher rates of ejaculatory dysfunction than are documented with tamsulosin. In a meta-analysis, Ding *et al.* reported consistently higher rates of ejaculatory dysfunction with silodosin compared with tamsulosin [63]. Overall, however, these effects on ejaculatory function may be less clinically concerning. A study performed by Hofner *et al.* comparing tamsulosin with alfuzosin and placebo revealed low discontinuation rates due to these symptoms, and revealed that patients did not report an overall negative impact on sexual function compared with the other groups [64].

$α_1$-blockers and intraoperative floppy iris syndrome

In 2005, a condition termed the intraoperative floppy iris syndrome (IFIS) was recognized [65], having initially been described as a group of intraoperative findings including iris billowing, miosis, and prolapse, observed in some patients undergoing routine phacoemulsification surgeries for cataract removal. An association between IFIS and the systemic use of $α_1$-AR antagonists, specifically tamsulosin, was suggested in the original report.

In its simplest form, the iris dilator smooth muscle, along with the sphincter muscle, was thought to produce pupil dilation through a balance of sympathetic adrenergic and parasympathetic muscarinic nerve activity [66]. $α_1$-AR antagonists seem to have a much greater effect on iris dilator muscle relaxation than $α_2$-AR antagonists, which suggests that $α_1$-ARs are the predominant subtype in the sympathetically mediated dilator muscle contraction. The specific $α_1$-AR subtype that appears to mediate contraction of the iris dilator smooth muscle has repeatedly been identified as the α_{1A}-AR. Therefore, since the α_{1A}-AR is the predominant subtype in both the prostatic stromal smooth muscle and the iris dilator muscle, a link between the use of α_1-antagonists for LUTS and iris dilator muscle relaxation associated with IFIS seems logical.

A recent review of the literature reveals the following salient points concerning IFIS and the use of α-blockers [67]. First, the risk of IFIS was substantial among men taking tamsulosin, ranging from about 43% to 90% in 10 retrospective and prospective studies (sometimes the denominator for these risks was patients, and sometimes the number of eyes at risk). Second, the risk of IFIS appears to be lower with older, generic α_1-blockers such as terazosin and doxazosin, with IFIS occurring in 0–6% of patients in four studies reporting on the risk of IFIS with these agents. Third, there are insufficient exposure data to estimate the risk of IFIS with alfuzosin and silodosin. Fourth, the dose, duration, or cessation of α_1-blocker treatment that influences the risk of IFIS is unclear. Fifth, if experienced ophthalmologists are aware of preoperative α_1-blocker use, pre- and intraoperative precautions can be taken to reduce the risk of IFIS complications and attain excellent visual outcomes, though it remains unclear if the residual risk and outcomes are any worse than among patients without IFIS. Recommendations concerning the use of α_1-blockers and IFIS noted in the 2010 AUA BPH Clinical Guidelines are as follows:

1 Recommendation: Men with LUTS secondary to BPH for whom alpha-blocker therapy is offered should be asked about planned cataract surgery. Men with planned cataract surgery should avoid the initiation of alpha-blockers until their cataract surgery is completed.

2 Recommendation: In men with no planned cataract surgery, there are insufficient data to recommend withholding or discontinuing alpha-blockers for bothersome LUTS secondary to BPH.

(Reference: 2010 AUA BPH Clinical Guidelines. http://www.auanet.org/education/guidelines/benign-prostatic-hyperplasia.cfm. Last accessed January 2014.)

Combination therapy

As mentioned earlier, both hormonal therapy and α-adrenergic therapy are effective treatments for symptomatic BPH. The hormonal therapy is generally believed to target the static component, while the α_1-adrenergic therapy is directed toward the dynamic component of BPH. Based on this assumption, it was believed that combination therapy could target both of these major components of BPH simultaneously.

The first randomized, double-blind, placebo-controlled study investigating combination therapy using α_1-adrenergic antagonists and 5-ARIs was the four-arm Veterans Administration Cooperative (VA COOP) study comparing placebo, finasteride alone, terazosin alone, and combination therapy with finasteride and terazosin [68]. After 1 year of treatment, the investigators concluded that short-term combination therapy was no more effective than a single agent in the treatment of BPH. Terazosin alone produced superior results in terms of improvements in AUA-SI scores and Q_{max}. Treatment with finasteride showed the most significant decrease in prostate size, but reports of bothersome symptoms did not correspond. A subsequent clinical trial, the Prospective European Doxazosin and Combined Therapy trial, also assessed whether combination therapy with

Table 7.1 Risk of benign prostatic hypertension progression as measured by American Urological Association-International Prostate Symptom Scores, rates of acute urinary retention, and requirement for surgical Intervention: tamsulosin versus dutasteride versus combination therapy

	Relative risk reduction (%) in increasing AUA-IPSS (>4 points)	Relative risk reduction (%) in AUR	Relative risk reduction (%) for requiring subsequent surgical treatment
Combination versus tamsulosin	41.3	69.6	70.6
Combination versus dutasteride	35.2	29.7	31.1

All values are presented as relative risk reduction compared to combination therapy group. Four-year incidences of AUR, BPH-related surgery, and BPH clinical progression and reduction in relative risk are with Combination therapy with dutasteride or tamsulosin therapy.
AUA-IPSS, American Urological Association-International Prostate Symptom Scores; AUR, acute urinary retention; BPH, benign prostatic hypertension.

α_1-adrenergic inhibitors and 5-ARIs could be used for the symptomatic treatment of BPH [69]. Study conclusions confirmed that doxazosin was a superior treatment for symptomatic BPH compared with finasteride alone or placebo. The addition of finasteride to doxazosin did not provide any increased benefit compared with doxazosin alone.

The applicability of the study's conclusion to the general population of men with symptomatic BPH was subsequently challenged due to the relatively small percentage of participants with larger prostates. It also failed to address whether combination therapy affected BPH progression or whether a longer duration of therapy affected the outcome.

The MTOPS study was a four-arm clinical trial (placebo, doxazosin, finasteride, and combination) that revisited the utility of combination therapy. The study leaders questioned whether combination therapy could prevent clinical disease progression by treatment with finasteride, doxazosin, or both [70]. The investigators followed a total of 3047 men for 4.5 years. The study participants all had relatively large prostate volumes

(average of 36.5 mL) at the beginning of the study. The clinical outcomes that were measured included the incidence of AUR, renal insufficiency, recurrent urinary tract infections (UTIs), and changes in AUA-SI score.

The MTOPS study clearly demonstrated that, compared with monotherapy, there was a significant risk reduction in the progression of BPH with combination therapy. This risk reduction included a sustained measurable decrease in AUA-SI score, a decreased risk of developing AUR, and a decreased incidence of surgical treatment for BPH (Table 7.1).

One way to assess BPH progression is by documenting an increase in AUA-SI score. The MTOPS study demonstrated that an increase in AUA-SI score of >4 points above baseline values was the most common individual adverse event in all groups at the end of the study. In fact, there was a 3.6/100 person-years risk of having this 4-point increase in the placebo arm of the study. In comparison, the risk of having a 4-point increase in AUA-SI was reduced to 1.9 person-years (45% reduction in risk) in the doxazosin group. Similarly, patients in the finasteride

Table 7.2 Drug-related adverse events occurring in ≥1% of subjects in any treatment group in the Medical Treatment of Prostatic Symptoms trial (McConnell et al. *N Engl J Med* 2003; 349:2387–2398.)

	Combination, % (N = 786)	Finasteride, % (N = 768)	Doxazosin, % (N = 756)
Erectile dysfunction	5.0*	4.5*	3.3
Abnormal ejaculation	3.0*	1.8*	1.1
Altered (decreased) libido	2.5*	2.4*	1.6
Dizziness	5.4*	2.3	4.4*
Postural hypotension	4.3*	4.0	2.6*
Dyspnea	1.2*	0.6	0.9
Peripheral edema	1.3*	0.9	0.7

*$P < 0.05$ compared with the placebo group.

group had a 30% reduction in risk. Patients enrolled in the combination therapy arm of the study experienced a 66% reduction in the risk of higher AUA-SI. In fact, this risk reduction was larger than any of the medical therapies used alone.

The MTOPS study also analyzed the contribution of monotherapy and combination therapy to the incidence of AUR [70]. Doxazosin did not significantly reduce the rate of AUR compared with the placebo group (0.4/100 person-years). However, both the finasteride monotherapy (0.4/100 person-years) and combination therapy (0.1/100 person-years) groups significantly lowered the rate of development of urinary retention compared with the placebo group (0.6/100 person-years). Table 7.2 reveals an insignificant decrease of 35% in the doxazosin group, and a significant decrease of 68% and 81% in the finasteride mono-therapy and combination therapy groups, respectively.

The MTOPS study also demonstrated a significant reduction in the rate of invasive surgical treatment over a 5-year period when either finasteride monotherapy or combination therapy with finasteride and doxazosin is used [70]. Men enrolled in the placebo group had a 1.3/100 person-years risk of having invasive surgery for BPH (such as TURP or transurethral microwave thermotherapy). The risk of requiring these invasive treatments for progression of BPH was reduced by 64% and 67% in the finasteride and combination therapy groups, respectively. Doxazosin did not significantly reduce the incidence of invasive treatments.

As previously stated, the MTOPS trial demonstrated a decrease in the progression of BPH associated with combination therapy with finasteride and doxazosin. Since the initiation of MTOPS, studies have shown that patients with larger prostates and higher PSA levels are at increased risk for BPH progression, and are therefore arguably more likely to benefit from combination therapy. Kaplan *et al.* utilized data from the MTOPS trial and found that patients with prostate volumes greater than 25 mL would indeed benefit from combination therapy [71]. However, the number needed to treat (NNT) when comparing combination therapy versus placebo is approximately 58 for a <25 mL gland, 39 for a 25–40 mL gland, and 18 for a

>40 mL gland. For the more clinically relevant question of the marginal value of adding finasteride to doxazosin monotherapy, the NNT is 172 for glands <25 mL, 79 for glands 25–40 mL, and 52 for glands >40 mL. Thus, combination therapy should be considered when a prostate volume of >40 mL is suspected. To successfully predict prostate volume size, a study carried out in 2007 by Bohnen *et al.* investigated PSA ranges that would be most useful in determining PSA volumes less than 30 mL, greater than 30 mL, greater than 40 mL, and greater than 50 mL. They showed that PSA was predictive of prostate volumes of >30 mL and with even more accuracy for prostate volumes greater than 40 or 50 mL. The area under the curve was 0.79, 0.86, and 0.92 to predict a prostate volume of >30 mL, >40 mL, and PV >50 mL, respectively [72]. They found that PSA ranges from 0 to 2 and from 2.1 to 4.0 favor prostate volumes of 30 mL. PSA values greater than 4 favor prostate volumes of >40 or 50 mL. Thus, clinicians can utilize PSA values and begin combination therapies when estimated prostate volumes exceed 40 mL.

The Combination of Avodart and Tamsulosin (CombAT) trial was a 4-year, multicenter, randomized, double-blind study designed to investigate the benefits of combination therapy with dutasteride and tamsulosin, compared with each monotherapy in improving symptoms and long-term outcomes in men with moderate-to-severe LUTS due to BPH [73]. The study involved more than 4800 men, and of the men studied, 1492 were treated with a combination of dutasteride and tamsulosin, 1502 were prescribed dutasteride alone, and 1519 were prescribed tamsulosin alone. Eligible patients were 50 years with an estimated prostate volume of 30 mL and PSA level of 1.5 ng/mL. In pivotal 2-year phase 3 trials, oral dutas-

teride 0.5 mg once daily improved urinary symptoms, decreased total prostate volume (TPV), and reduced the risk of AUR and BPH-related surgery in men with moderate-to-severe symptoms of BPH and prostate enlargement [73]. The efficacy and tolerability of dutasteride were maintained for up to 4 years in open-label extension studies. Results of the preplanned, 2-year interim analysis of the CombAT trial showed that the combination of dutasteride and tamsulosin was superior to either drug as monotherapy in improving BPH-related symptoms, Q_{max}, and BPH-related health status. In another analysis of CombAT trial data, Roehrborn *et al.* concluded that in men with moderate-to-severe LUTS and prostate enlargement (i.e. ≥30 mL) combination therapy provides a significantly greater degree of benefit than tamsulosin or dutasteride monotherapy [74]. In terms of the long-term progression events, combination therapy was significantly superior to tamsulosin monotherapy, but not dutasteride monotherapy, at reducing the relative risk of AUR or BPH-related surgery [74]. Combination therapy was also significantly superior to both monotherapies at reducing the relative risk of BPH clinical progression. Combination therapy provided significantly greater symptom benefit than either monotherapy at 4 years.

In comparing naftopidil with the well-known and more commonly used $α_1$-blocker, tamsulosin, Kawachi *et al.* retrospectively compared patients taking tamsulosin or naftopidil over 2 years and found that failure rates due to overactive bladder symptoms were more common with patients taking tamsulosin [75]. Ukimura *et al.* performed a multicenter prospective randomized-controlled study to determine the clinical efficacy between naftopidil and tamsulosin. Groups were divided into 0.2 mg of

tamsulosin daily (*N* = 28) or 50 mg of naftopidil daily (*N* = 31) for 6–8 weeks. After 2
weeks, the naftopidil group demonstrated
significant improvements in daytime frequency and nocturia, while patients on tamsulosin showed no significant improvements
in either symptom. Importantly, the effects
of the two α_1-blockers were similar in regard
to obstructive LUTS at the end of the treatment period [76]. Though naftopidil administration shows promise, especially for
patients with severe symptoms of urgency
and nocturia, long-term randomized placebo-controlled trials are necessary to make
definitive decisions regarding the use of this
pharmacologic agent.

Adverse effects of combination therapy for benign prostatic hyperplasia

Combination therapy for the treatment of
BPH is also associated with drug-related
adverse events. For example, as mentioned
in prior sections, patients assigned to the
doxazosin group in the MTOPS trial had an
increased rate of dizziness and postural hypotension compared with patients enrolled in
the placebo group. Similarly, ED, decreased
libido, and abnormal ejaculation occurred
with increased frequency in the combination
group compared with placebo. The adverse
events experienced by patients on combination therapy were similar to those for each
drug alone. However, the rates of altered
ejaculation, peripheral edema, and dyspnea
were increased in this group [77] (Table 7.2).
Similarly, drug-related adverse events were
also reported for men enrolled in the CombAT
trial (Table 7.3). Although there was a significantly higher overall frequency of adverse
events in the combination group, there was
a low and nonsignificant increase in the
incidence of any individual adverse related
events using combination therapy compared
with either monotherapy.

Summary

Selective α-AR blockers, including alfuzosin,
doxazosin, tamsulosin, and terazosin, are
regarded in the 2010 AUA Clinical Guidelines

Table 7.3 Drug-related adverse events occurring in ≥1% of subjects in any treatment group in the Combination of Avodart and Tamsulosin trial

	Combination, % (*N* = 1610)	Dutasteride, % (*N* = 1623)	Tamsulosin, % (*N* = 1611)
Erectile dysfunction	9	7	5
Retrograde ejaculation	4	<1	1
Altered (decreased) libido	4	3	2
Ejaculation failure	3	<1	<1
Semen volume decreased	2	<1	<1
Loss of libido	2	1	1
Dizziness	2	<1	2
Gynecomastia	2	2	<1
Nipple pain	1	<1	<1
Breast tenderness	1	1	<1

Dos and don'ts

- Patient education is paramount in the decision to treat LUTS/BPH with α-blockers or combination therapy.
- Side effects of α-blockers should be clearly explained to the patients, particularly given the inherent increased risk of falls in the elderly that are likely to be treated with this medication.
- Patients should be asked about any history of cataracts or planned cataracts extraction procedure, for appropriate planning regarding the use of α-blockers.

for BPH and elsewhere as an option for the treatment of bothersome moderate-to-severe LUTS (AUA-SI score ≥8) due to BPH, with each agent demonstrating about equal clinical efficacy, although with varying side effects as discussed in the text. Silodosin appears to function equivalent to the other α-AR blockers. Dizziness was the most common unfavorable event, with doxazosin and terazosin notable for requiring dose titration and close blood-pressure monitoring; abnormalities in ejaculation and hypotension are also among the adverse effects of these treatments. Although there are slight differences in the adverse-events profiles of these agents, all five appear to have equal clinical effectiveness. The effectiveness and efficacy of the five α-AR blockers under consideration appear to be similar. There is a paucity of head-to-head comparative effectiveness data, but available data support this contention.

IFIS is also an entity of concern, and the guidelines recommend patient education to protect from the development of this condition, and withholding or discontinuing the α-blockers about the time of planned cataract surgery. The nonselective α-blockers prazosin and phenoxybenzamine are not recommended.

Combination therapy with α-AR blockers and a 5-ARI has also proven to be effective, particularly in patients with known prostatic enlargement. The MTOPS trial did well to demonstrate the benefit of this combination therapy versus monotherapy with α-AR blockers, with reduced incidence of AUR and with fewer patients progressing to surgical treatments for symptomatic relief. The CombAT study also supports this positive effect of combination therapy.

Bibliography

1 McVary, KT. A review of combination therapy in patients with benign prostatic hyperplasia. *Clin Ther.* 2007;29:387.

2 Rhodes T, Girman CJ, Jacobsen SJ, Roberts RO, Guess HA, Lieber MM. Longitudinal prostate growth rates during 5 years in randomly selected community men 40 to 79 years old. *J Urol.* 1999;161(4):1174–9.

3 Roehrborn CG, Mcconnell J, Bonilla J, Rosenblatt S, Hudson PB, Malek GH, *et al.* Serum prostate specific antigen is a strong predictor of future prostate growth in men with benign prostatic hyperplasia. PROSCAR long-term efficacy and safety study. *J Urol.* 2000;163(1):13–20.

4 Berry SJ, Coffey DS, Walsh PC, Ewing LL. The development of human benign prostatic hyperplasia with age. *J Urol.* 1984;132(3):474–9.

5 Fawzy A, Braun K, Lewis GP, Gaffney M, Ice K, Dias N. Benign prostatic hypertrophy and the role of alpha-adrenergic blockade J Urol. 1995; 154(1):105–9.

6 Furuya S, Kumamoto Y, Yokoyama E, Tsukamoto T, Izumi T, Abiko Y. Alpha-adrenergic activity and urethral pressure in prostatic zone in benign prostatic hypertrophy. *J Urol.* 1982;128(4):836–9.

7 Schwinn DA, Roehrborn CG. Alpha1-adrenoceptor subtypes and lower urinary tract symptoms. *Int J Urol.* 2008;15(3):193–9.

8 Kobayashi S, Tang R, Shapiro E, Lepor H. Characterization and localization of prostatic alpha 1 adrenoceptors using radioligand receptor binding on slide-mounted tissue section. *J Urol.* 1993;150:2002–6.

9 Lepor H, Laddu A. Terazosin in the treatment of benign prostatic hyperplasia: the United States experience. *Br J Urol.* 1992;70(Suppl 1):2–9.

10 Yokoyama E, Furuya S, Kumamoto Y. [Quantitation of alpha-1 and beta adrenergic receptor densities in the human normal and hypertrophied prostate]. *Nippon Hinyokika Gakkai Zasshi.* 1985;76:325–7.

11 Sugaya K, Nishijima S, Miyazato M, Ashitomi K, Hatano T, Ogawa Y. Effects of intrathecal injection of tamsulosin and naftopidil, alpha-1A and -1D adrenergic receptor antagonists, on bladder activity in rats. *Neurosci Lett.* 2002;328(1):74–6.

12 van der Vaart CH, Roovers JP, de Leuw JR, Heintz AP. Associated between urogenital symptoms and depression in community-dwelling women aged 20 to 70 years. *Urology.* 2007;69(4):691.

13 Asplund R, Henriksson S, Johannson S, Isacsson G. Nocturia and depression. *BJU Int.* 2004;93(9):1253.

14 Fitzgerald MP, Litman HJ, Link CL, McKinlay JB. The association of nocturia with cardiac disease, diabetes, body mass index, age, and diuretic use: results of the BACH survey. *J Urol.* 2007;177(4):1385.

15 Vaughan CP, Brown CJ, Goode PS, Burgio KL, Allman RM, Johnson TM 2nd. The association of nocturia wit incident falls in an elderly community-based cohort. *Int J Clin Pract.* 2010;64(5):577.

16 Lepor H. Managing and preventing acute urinary retention. *Rev Urol.* 2005;7(Suppl 8):S26–33.

17 Arrighi N, Bodei S, Zani D, Peroni A, Simeone C, Mirabella G, *et al.* [Alpha1 adrenoceptors in human urinary tract:expression, distribution and clinical implications.] *Urologia.* 2007;74(2):53–60.

18 De groat WC, Yoshiyama M, Ramage AG, Yamamoto T, Somogyi GT. Modulation of voiding and storage reflexes by activation of alpha1-adrenoceptors. *Eur Urol.* 1999;36(Suppl 1): 68–73.

19 Yamaguchi O. Latest treatment for lower urinary tract dysfunction: therapeutic agents and mechanism of action. *Int J Urol.* 2013;20(1):28–39.

20 Caine M. Alpha-adrenergic mechanisms in dynamics of benign prostatic hypertrophy. *Urology.* 1988;32(6 Suppl):16–20.

21 Piascik MT, Hrometz SL, Edelmann SE, Guarino RD, Hadley RW, Brown RD. Immunocytochemical localization of the alpha-1B adrenergic receptor and the contribution of this and the other subtypes to vascular smooth muscle contraction: analysis with selective ligands and antisense oligonucleotides. *J Pharmacol Exp Ther.* 1997;283(2):854–68.

22 DIBENZYLINE® *(phenoxybenzamine hydrochloride)* package insert. Colts Neck, NJ: WellSpring Pharmaceutical Corporation; 1999.

23 Robertson D, Biaggioni I. Chapter 10. Adrenoceptor Antagonist Drugs. In: Katzung BG, Masters SB, Trevor AJ, eds. *Basic & clinical pharmacology.* 12th ed. New York, NY: McGraw-Hill; 2012.

24 Bultitude, MF. (2012), *Campbell-Walsh urology.* 10th ed. *BJU Int.* 109: E10. doi:10.1111/j.1464-410X.2011.10907.x.

25 Lin VK, Benaim EA, McConnell JD. Alpha-blockade downregulates myosin heavy chain gene expression in human benign prostatic hyperplasia. *Urology.* 2001;57(1):170–5.

26 Kyprianou N, Litvak JP, Borkowski A, Alexander R, Jacobs SC. Induction of prostate apoptosis by doxazosin in benign prostatic hyperplasia. *J Urol.* 1998;159(6):1810–5.

27 Ilio KY, Park II, Pins MR, Kozlowski JM, Lee C. Apoptotic activity of doxazosin on prostate stroma in vitro is mediated through an autocrine expression of TGF-beta1. *Prostate.* 2001;48(3):131–5.

28 Thomas D, Wimmer AB, Wu K, Hammerling BC, Ficker EK, Kuryshev YA, *et al.* Inhibition of human ether-a-go-go-related gene potassium channels by alpha 1-adrenoceptor antagonists prazosin, doxazosin, and terazosin. *Naunyn Schmiedebergs Arch Pharmacol.* 2004;369(5):462–72.

29 Kaplan SA, Roehrborn CG, McConnell JD, Meehan AG, Surynawanshi S, Lee JY, *et al.* Long-term treatment with finasteride results in a clinically significant reduction in total prostate volume compared to placebo over the full range of baseline prostate sizes in men enrolled in the MTOPS trial. *J Urol.* 2008;180(3):1030–2.

30 Macdonald R, Wilt TJ, Howe RW. Doxazosin for treating lower urinary tract symptoms compatible with benign prostatic obstruction: a systematic review of efficacy and adverse effects. *BJU Int.* 2004;94(9):1263–70.

31 Roehrborn CG, Oesterling JE, Auerbach S, Kaplan SA, Lloyd LK, Milam DE, *et al.* The Hytrin Community Assessment Trial study: a one-year

study of terazosin versus placebo in the treatment of men with symptomatic benign prostatic hyperplasia. HYCAT Investigator Group. *Urology.* 1996;47(2):159–68.

32 Roehrborn CG, Van kerrebroeck P, Nordling J. Safety and efficacy of alfuzosin 10 mg once-daily in the treatment of lower urinary tract symptoms and clinical benign prostatic hyperplasia: a pooled analysis of three double-blind, placebo-controlled studies. *BJU Int.* 2003;92(3):257–61.

33 Leungwattanakij S, Watanachote D, Noppakulsatit P, Petchpaibuol T, Choeypunt N, Tongbai T, *et al.* Sexuality and management of benign prostatic hyperplasia with alfuzosin: SAMBA Thailand. *J Sex Med.* 2010;7(9):3115–26.

34 Rosen R, Seftel A, Roehrborn CG. Effects of alfuzosin 10 mg once daily on sexual function in men treated for symptomatic benign prostatic hyperplasia. *Int J Impot Res.* 2007;19(5):480–5.

35 Van Moorselaar RJ, Hartung R, Emberton M, Harving N, Matzkin H, Elhilali M, *et al.* Alfuzosin 10 mg once daily improves sexual function in men with lower urinary tract symptoms and concomitant sexual dysfunction. *BJU Int.* 2005;95(4):603–8.

36 Lukacs B, Grange JC, McCarthy C, Comet D. Clinical uroselectivity: a 3-year follow-up in general practice. BPH Group in General Practice. *Eur Urol.* 1998;33(Suppl 2):28–33.

37 Jardin A, Bensadoun H, Delauche-Cavallier MC, Stalla-Bourdillon A, Attali P. Long-term treatment of benign prostatic hyperplasia with alfuzosin: a 24–30 month survey. BPHALF Group. *Br J Urol.* 1994;74(5):579–84.

38 Rosen RC, Wei JT, Althof SE, Seftel AD, Miner M, Perelman MA. Association of sexual dysfunction with lower urinary tract symptoms of BPH and BPH medical therapies: results from the BPH Registry. *Urology* 2009; 73:562–6.

39 Hellstrom WJ, Sikka SC. Effects of acute treatment with tamsulosin versus alfuzosin on ejaculatory function in normal volunteers. *J Urol.* 2006;176:1529–33.

40 Elhilali M, Emberton M, Matzkin H, van Moorselaar RJ, Hartung R, Harving N, *et al.* Long-term efficacy and safety of alfuzosin 10 mg once daily: a 2-year experience in "real-life" practice. *BJU Int.* 2006;97(3):513–9.

41 Roehrborn CG, Schwinn DA. Alpha1-adrenergic receptors and their inhibitors in lower urinary tract symptoms and benign prostatic hyperplasia. *J Urol.* 2004;171(3):1029–35.

42 Lepor H. Phase III multicenter placebo-controlled study of tamsulosin in benign prostatic hyperplasia. Tamsulosin Investigator Group. *Urology.* 1998;51(6):892–900.

43 Arnold EP. Tamsulosin in men with confirmed bladder outlet obstruction: a clinical and urodynamic analysis from a single centre in New Zealand. *BJU Int.* 2001;87(1):24–30.

44 Ichioka K, Ohara H, Terada N, Matsui Y, Yoshimura K, Terai A, *et al.* Long-term treatment outcome of tamsulosin for benign prostatic hyperplasia. *Int J Urol.* 2004;11(10):870–5.

45 Lowe FC. Coadministration of tamsulosin and three antihypertensive agents in patients with benign prostatic hyperplasia: pharmacodynamic effect. *Clin Ther.* 1997;19(4):730–42.

46 Shibata K, Foglar R, Horie K, Obika K, Sakamoto A, Ogawa S, *et al.* KMD-3213, a novel, potent, alpha 1a-adrenoceptor-selective antagonist: Characterization using recombinant human alpha 1-adrenoceptors and native tissues. *Mol Pharmacol.* 1995;48:250–8.

47 Kawabe K, Yoshida M, Homma Y, for the Silodosin Clinical Study Group. Silodosin, a new alpha1A-adrenoceptor-selective antagonist for treating benign prostatic hyperplasia: Results of a phase III randomized, placebo-controlled, double- blind study in Japanese men. *BJU Int.* 2006; 98:1019–24.

48 Takao T, Tsujimura A, Kiuchi H, Matsuoka Y, Miyagawa Y, Nonomura N, *et al.* Early efficacy of silodosin in patients with lower urinary tract symptoms suggestive of benign prostatic hyperplasia. *Int J Urol.* 2008;15:992–6.

49 *Rapaflo (silodosin) package insert.* Corona, CA: Watson Pharmaceuticals; 2013.

50 Marks LS, Gittelman MC, Hill LA, Volinn W, Hoel G. Rapid efficacy of the highly selective alpha-1A-adrenoceptor antagonist silodosin in men with signs and symptoms of benign prostatic hyperplasia: Pooled results of 2 phase 3 studies. *J Urol.* 2009;181:2634–40.

51 American Urological Association. Guideline on the management of benign prostatic hyperplasia (BPH). Chapter 3: Results of the treatment outcomes analyses [updated 2010]. Available from: http://www.auanet.org/common/pdf/education/clinical-guidance/Benign-Prostatic-Hyperplasia.pdf

52 Malloy B, Price D, Price R, Bienstock A, Dole M, Funk B, et al. Alpha1-adrenergic receptor subtypes in human detrusor. *J Urol.* 1998;160(3 Pt 1): 937–43.

53 Yasuda K, Yamanishi T, Tojo M, Nagashima K, Akimoto S, Shimazaki J. Effect of naftopidil on urethral obstruction in benign prostatic hyperplasia: assessment by urodynamic studies. *Prostate.* 1994;25(1):46–52.

54 Yokoyama T, Kumon H, Nasu Y, Takamoto H, Watanabe T. Comparison of 25 and 75 mg/day naftopidil for lower urinary tract symptoms associated with benign prostatic hyperplasia: a prospective, randomized controlled study. *Int J Urol.* 2006;13:932–8.

55 Oh-oka H. Usefulness of naftopidil for dysuria in benign prostatic hyperplasia and its optimal dose–comparison between 75 and 50 mg. *Urol Int.* 2009;82:136–42.

56 Takahashi S, Tajima A, Matsushima H, Kawamura T, Tominaga T, Kitamura T. Clinical efficacy of an alpha1A/D-adrenoceptor blocker (naftopidil) on overactive bladder symptoms in patients with benign prostatic hyperplasia. *Int J Urol.* 2006;13:15–20.

57 Oh-oka H. Effect of naftopidil on nocturia after failure of tamsulosin. *Urology.* 2008;72:1051–5.

58 Rosen R, Altwein J, Boyle P, Kirby RS, Lukacs B, Meuleman E, et al. Lower urinary tract symptoms and male sexual dysfunction: the multinational survey of the aging male (MSAM-7). *Eur Urol.* 2003;44(6):637–49.

59 Fwu CW, Eggers PW, Kirkali Z, McVary KT, Burrows PK, Kusek JW. Change in sexual function in men with lower urinary tract symptoms (LUTS)/ benign prostatic hyperplasia (BPH) associated with long-term treatment with doxazosin, finasteride, and combined therapy. *J Urol.* 2013. doi: 10.1016/j.juro.2013.12.014. (Epub ahead of print)

60 Narayan P, Tewari A. US 93–01 Study Group, authors. A second phase III multicenter placebo controlled study of 2 dosages of modified release tamsulosin in patients with symptoms of benign prostatic hyperplasia. *J Urol.* 1998;160:1701–6.

61 Giuliano F. Impact of medical treatments for benign prostatic hyperplasia on sexual function. *BJU Int* 2006;97(Suppl 2):34–8.

62 Lepor H, for the Tamsulosin Investigator Group. Long-term evaluation of tamsulosin in benign prostatic hyperplasia: placebo-controlled, double-blind extension of phase III trial. *Urology.* 1998;51:901–6.

63 Ding H, Du W, Hou ZZ, Wang HZ, Wang ZP. Silodosin is effective for treatment of LUTS in men with BPH: a systematic review. *Asian J Androl.* 2013;15(1):121–8.

64 Hofner K, Claes H, De Reijke TM, Folkestad B, Speakman MJ, for the European Tamsulosin Study Group. Tamsulosin 0.4 mg once daily: effect on sexual function in patients with lower urinary tract symptoms suggestive of benign prostatic obstruction. *Eur Urol.* 1999;36:335–41.

65 Chang, DF, Campbell JR. Intraoperative floppy iris syndrome associated with tamsulosin. *J Cataract Refract Surg.* 2005;31(4):664–73.

66 Schwinn, DA, Afshari NA. Alpha(1)-Adrenergic receptor antagonists and the iris: new mechanistic insights into floppy iris syndrome. *Surv Ophthalmol.* 2006;51(5):501–12.

67 AlHussaini Z, McVary KT. Alpha-blockers and intraoperative floppy iris syndrome: ophthalmic adverse events following cataract surgery. *Curr Urol Rep.* 2010;11(4):242–8.

68 Lepor H, Williford WO, Barry MJ, Brawer MK, Dixon CM, Gormley G, et al. The efficacy of terazosin, finasteride, or both in benign prostatic hyperplasia. *Veterans Affairs Cooperative Studies Benign Prostatic Hyperplasia Study Group. N Engl J Med.* 1996;335(8):533–9.

69 Kirby RS, Roehrborn C, Boyle P, Bartsch G, Jardin A, Cary MM, et al. Efficacy and tolerability of doxazosin and finasteride, alone or in combination, in treatment of symptomatic benign prostatic hyperplasia: the Prospective European Doxazosin and Combination Therapy (PREDICT) trial. *Urology.* 2003;61(1):119–26.

70 McConnell JD, Roehrborn CG, Bautista OM, Andriole GL Jr, Dixon CM, Kusek JW, et al. The long-term effect of doxazosin, finasteride, and combination therapy on the clinical progression of benign prostatic hyperplasia. *N Engl J Med.* 2003;349(25):2387–98.

71 Kaplan SA, McConnell JD, Roehrborn CG, Meehan AG, Lee MW, Noble WR, et al. Medical Therapy of Prostatic Symptoms (MTOPS) Research Group. Combination therapy with doxazosin and finasteride for benign prostatic hyperplasia in patients with lower urinary tract symptoms and a baseline total prostate volume of 25 mL or greater. *J Urol.* 2006;175:217–20.

72 Bohnen AM, Groeneveld FP, Bosch JL. Serum prostate-specific antigen as a predictor of prostate volume in the community: the Krimpen study *Eur Urol.* 2007;511645–52.52; discussion 1652–3.

73 Roehrborn CG, Barkin J, Siami P, Tubaro A, Wilson TH, Morrill BB, *et al.* Clinical outcomes after combined therapy with dutasteride plus tamsulosin or either monotherapy in men with benign prostatic hyperplasia (BPH) by baseline characteristics: 4-year results from the randomized, double-blind Combination of Avodart and Tamsulosin (CombAT) trial. *BJU Int.* 2011;107(6):946–54.

74 Roehrborn CG, Siami P, Barkin J, Damião R, Major-Walker K, Nandy I, *et al.* The effects of combination therapy with dutasteride and tamsulosin on clinical outcomes in men with symptomatic benign prostatic hyperplasia: 4-year results from the CombAT study. *Eur Urol.* 2010; 57(1):123–31.

75 Kawachi Y, Sakurai T, Sugimura S, Iwata S, Noto K, Honda S, *et al.* Long-term treatment and prognostic factors of alpha 1-blockers for lower urinary tract symptoms associated with benign prostatic hyperplasia: a pilot study comparing naftopidil and tamsulosin hydrochloride. *Scand J Urol Nephrol.* 2010;44:38–45.

76 Ukimura O, Kanazawa M, Fujihara A, Kamoi K, Okihara K, Miki T, *et al.* Naftopidil versus tamsulosin hydrochloride for lower urinary tract symptoms associated with benign prostatic hyperplasia with special reference to the storage symptom: a prospective randomized controlled study. *Int J Urol.* 2008;15(12):1049–54.

77 McConnell JD, Roehrborn CG, Bautista OM, Andriole GL Jr, Dixon CM, Kusek JW, *et al.* The long-term effect of doxazosin, finasteride, and combination therapy on the clinical progression of benign prostatic hyperplasia. *N Engl J Med.* 2003;349(25):2387–98.

CHAPTER 8

5α-Reductase Inhibitors

Claudius Füllhase[1] & Roberto Soler[2]

[1]Department of Urology, Großhadern Hospital, Ludwig-Maximilians-University, Munich, Germany
[2]Division of Urology, Federal University of São Paulo, São Paulo, Brazil

Key points

- Testosterone is converted into dihydrotestosterone (DHT) by 5α-reductases.
- DHT is involved in prostate growth.
- 5α-Reductase inhibitors (5ARIs) reduce the levels of prostatic DHT and reduce prostate volume.
- Finasteride and dutasteride improve urinary symptoms associated with benign prostatic hyperplasia (BPH), improve urinary flow rate, and reduce prostate volume.
- Finasteride and dutasteride reduce the risk of acute urinary retention and BPH-related surgery.
- Finasteride and dutasteride lead to sexual adverse effects (AEs), such as decreased libido, erectile dysfunction, and ejaculation dysfunction. The likelihood of new sexual AEs with 5ARI treatment seems to decrease with longer duration of therapy.
- Similar efficacy and tolerability were reported when finasteride and dutasteride were directly compared.
- The effect of 5ARIs on prostate cancer is still a matter of debate.

Introduction and history of 5α-reductase inhibitors

5α-Reductases (5ARs) are a group of enzymes (isozymes) involved in steroid hormone metabolism [1]. One of their most-known reactions is the conversion from the steroid hormone testosterone into DHT. DHT is one of the most important androgens responsible for the development and activity of male sex organs and characteristics, and prostate growth [2]. Among others, "responsibility for the development and activity of male sex organs" includes the growth of the prostate. Inhibition of 5ARs by 5α-reductase inhibitors (5ARIs) reduces the levels of DHT, and consequently the effects of DHT, such as the growth of the prostate.

In 1940, the relationship between the testes hormone and BPH was reported [3], but it was not until decades later that the therapeutic possibilities to target the BPH–testosterone relationship to hinder benign prostate growth were realized on a full scale [4]. Jean Wilson found in 1968 that DHT, not testosterone, is the main androgen in the prostate [5–7]. His discovery also had no therapeutic implications at first. It was in the 1970s that a group of endocrinologists from Cornell University, New York, reported in a series of publications their findings on a hereditary form of pseudo-hermaphroditism in several families in the

Male Lower Urinary Tract Symptoms and Benign Prostatic Hyperplasia, First Edition.
Edited by Steven A. Kaplan and Kevin T. McVary.
© 2014 John Wiley & Sons, Ltd. Published 2014 by John Wiley & Sons, Ltd.

Dominican Republic [8,9], which brought about the "breakthrough." Julianne Imperato-McGinley and colleagues [9] were able to link this form of pseudohermaphroditism, a female phenotype, with the presence of XY chromosomes, to a lack of DHT, which in turn is due to an insufficient conversion from testosterone to DHT based on a deficiency of 5ARs. Testosterone is needed for the formation of the prostate, but only DHT is responsible for the growth of the prostate. The seminal role of 5ARs in this scenario became first evident through the description of the Dominican pseudohermaphrodites [4].

5ARs had already been discovered years earlier, in 1951, in slices of rat liver [10]. However, their crucial role for testosterone–DHT transformation within the prostate was first established in the seminal work by Jean Wilson from Texas University in the 1970s [11,12]. Following these scientific achievements, the pharmaceutical industry started to search for inhibitors of 5ARs to tackle DHT-related BPH. In 1992, the US Food and Drug Administration (FDA) approved the first 5-ARI, finasteride, for the treatment of symptomatic BPH, and later on for treatment of alopecia [4,13–15]. Whereas finasteride inhibits just one isoform of 5AR, another 5-ARI, dutasteride, inhibits two isoforms of 5AR (dual inhibitor) [16]. Dutasteride was approved for the treatment of BPH in 2002 [4,17].

Hypothetical rationale, preclinical, and early clinical (phase I–II) evidence for the use of 5α-reductase inhibitors in benign prostatic hyperplasia

Testosterone is the main circulating androgen. Within the cells, testosterone is, among others (depending on the cell type), reduced to DHT by 5ARs of the nuclear membrane. In some cells, testosterone can be converted by other enzymes into estrogen, for example. DHT binds to the androgen receptor (AR; a binding protein) to form the DHT-AR complex, which then translocates from the cytosol to the nucleus. The binding affinity of DHT to the AR is 10 times higher than the affinity of testosterone towards AR, thus explaining, in part, the higher androgenic potency of DHT compared with testosterone. In the nucleus, the DHT–AR complex binds to the chromatin and influences DNA transcription and, as such, ultimately, the metabolism of androgenic action [5,12].

Whereas the content of testosterone and androstenedione, another androgen, was the same, the content of DHT was significantly higher in tissue of hypertrophic prostate glands than in normal, not-hypertrophied prostate gland tissue [6]. DHT and testosterone were given to dogs that had been castrated at a young age; thereby, only DHT caused accelerated growth of the prostate with histological signs of hypertrophy [18]. Interestingly, the accumulation of DHT in hypertrophic prostate tissue is related to neither an increased formation by 5ARs nor a decreased degradation of DHT [6,18]. Accumulation of DHT might be explained by an altered AR expression with increasing age [19,20].

Biochemical-wise, several substances can be used to inhibit 5ARs competitively or uncompetitively [1]. For example, zinc, a cation, is known to inhibit 5AR1, which is why it is used in dermatological ointments to treat acne, another DHT-related condition [21]. However, for oral human use, so far only two pharmaceutical compounds have been approved as 5ARIs by the FDA and the European Medicines Agency: finasteride (Proscar®), formerly known as MK-906, which mainly inhibits 5AR2; and dutasteride

(Avodart®), formerly known as GK745, which is a dual inhibitor of 5AR1 and 5AR2. On the quest for the first specific 5ARI, several compounds were tested preclinically, but most of them had androgenic or antiandrogenic effects by themselves. Derivatives from the 4-Azasteroid group, such as 17β-(N,N-diethyl)carbamoyl-4-methyl-4-aza-5α-androstan-3-one (4-MA) and 17β-(N-t-butyl)carbamoyl-4-aza-5α-androst-1-en-3-one (MK-906, finasteride), which were developed in the Laboratories of Merck Sharp & Dohme, had the most promising preclinical results as specific 5AR2-inhibitors and showed no genuine androgenic or antiandrogenic action [22].

In vitro, both of those compounds showed a high potency to inhibit the conversion of ^{3}H-radiolabeled testosterone into [^{3}H]-DHT [23]. 4-MA, administered subcutaneously, was shown in vivo to reduce the DHT levels in rat prostatic tissue [23]. In dogs, treated for more than 40 days with 4-MA orally, the compound dose-dependently reduced the levels of prostatic DHT, reduced prostate volumes, and caused histological changes, such as atrophy of the epithelium, in the prostate (but not in the testes) [13]. The same results were found in dogs treated with MK-906 for 16 weeks [24]. A reduction in rat prostate volume following administration of 4-azasteroid-5ARIs is also mainly due to an atrophy of epithelial cells, with a concomitant reduction in secretory capacity up to 50% (dose-dependently) [25]. The effects on prostatic apoptosis of MK-906 are less pronounced than following castration, most likely due to increased levels of testosterone (not DHT) in the prostate following 5ARI treatment compared with castration [26]. Despite the increase in prostatic testosterone following MK-906 administration, prostates have remained small (atrophic) throughout a 2-year treatment period, as tested in long-term rat experiments, thus indicating that DHT

alone (and not testosterone) has a trophic effect on the prostate [27]. Following the "successful" animal experiments, MK-906 was tested for its biochemical activity, safety, and tolerability in 350 volunteers in 1986 [28]. In healthy men, a single dose of 10–100 mg of finasteride (MK-906) reduced serum DHT levels dose-dependently by 70–82% but had no influence on serum testosterone levels [14], thus suggesting that it affects only DHT-related androgenic effects (such as prostatic growth) but does not influence testosterone-dependent functions, such as libido. In another phase I clinical study, it was shown that in healthy men, 5 mg of finasteride reduces DHT by up to 65% [29]. Other hormone levels, such as FH, FSH, cortisol, or estradiol, were not affected by finasteride intake [28]. In men with confirmed BPH, awaiting surgery, treatment with finasteride over 7 days decreased prostatic DHT levels by 92% [30]. Six months of treatment with 5 mg of finasteride reduced serum DHT levels by 80% but had no influence on serum testosterone levels [28]. Successful phase I and phase II clinical trials led to the first phase III clinical trial, the results of which were reported in the New England Journal of Medicine in 1992, and finally led to the approval of finasteride for the treatment of BPH by the FDA in the same year [4,15].

Clinical evidence (phase III or higher) for the use of 5α-reductase inhibitors in benign prostatic hyperplasia

Finasteride

The safety and efficacy of finasteride in men with BPH were evaluated in a large randomized, multicenter, double-blind, placebo-controlled study. A total of 895 men with BPH were enrolled in the study and were equally randomized to receive placebo, 1 mg of finasteride, or 5 mg of finasteride for 12 months. Decreases in symptom scores were significantly higher in men using 5 mg of finasteride compared with placebo, while this difference was not significant in those taking 1 mg of finasteride. Maximal urinary flow rate increased significantly at 6 and 12 months in both finasteride-treated groups compared with both baseline and placebo group values. From 5 to 12 months, the maximal flow rate was slightly but significantly higher in the group using 5 mg of finasteride than in the group using 1 mg. During the first 6 months the median size of the prostate decreased progressively in both finasteride-treated groups and was significantly smaller than in the placebo group. After 12 months, the prostate had shrunk by 19% and by 18% from baseline in the groups given 5 mg and 1 mg of finasteride, respectively [31].

Following two studies of similar methodology, including that mentioned above, patients were invited to take part in an open extension to the study in which all patients received 5 mg of finasteride to evaluate its long-term safety and efficacy for 36 months. Prostate volume was reduced from baseline by approximately 27%, the maximum urinary flow rate improved by approximately 2.3 mL/s, and symptom scores improved by 3.6 points [32].

The effect of the use finasteride on the risk of acute urinary retention (AUR) and the need for surgical treatment were evaluated in men with BPH, moderate to severe urinary symptoms, and an enlarged prostate on digital rectal examination. A total of 3040 men were randomized to receive either 5 mg of finasteride or placebo and were followed for 4 years. Differences in the rates of surgery and AUR were evident within 4 months, with continued divergence throughout the 4-year period. The 4-year incidence of surgery

for BPH was 10% in the placebo group and 5% in the finasteride group (risk reduction: 55%). The 4-year incidence of AUR was 7% in the placebo group and 3% in the finasteride group (risk reduction: 57%). On the basis of these results, 15 men would need to be treated for 4 years to prevent one event (either surgery or AUR) [33].

A secondary analysis of the Prostate Cancer Prevention Trial (PCPT) was undertaken to determine if 5 mg of finasteride prevents incident clinical BPH in healthy older men. From the whole study population of the PCPT, participants who at baseline reported BPH medical treatment, BPH surgery, or International Prostate Symptom Score of ≥8 were excluded. Incident clinical BPH was defined as the first event of report of medical treatment, surgery, or sustained, clinically significant BPH symptoms. In both unadjusted and adjusted proportional hazards models, finasteride decreased the risk of incident clinical BPH by 40%. The number needed to treat (NNT) to prevent one case of clinical BPH over 7 years was 58 for men 55–59 years of age, 42 for men 60–64 years of age, and 31 for men ≥65 years of age. In addition, for men aged ≥65, the 5- and 6-year NNT values were 54 and 40, respectively [34].

Dutasteride

Three identical clinical trials were designed to evaluate the effect of 0.5 mg of dutasteride daily on the treatment of men with lower urinary tract symptoms due to an enlarged prostate and BPH compared with placebo. These three studies set inclusion criteria that were not used in the first studies with finasteride: prostate-specific antigen (PSA) of >1.5 ng/mL, prostate volumes of >30 mL, and AUA-SI score of ≥12 points. Previous studies with finasteride suggested that 5ARIs are most effective in men with these particularities.

Statistically significant differences (dutasteride vs placebo) were noted during the earliest post-treatment prostate volume measurement in each study (month 1, 3, or 6) and continued throughout month 24. The mean percentage change from baseline for the total prostate volume was −25.7%. At 24 months, the AUA-SI was reduced by 2.3 points in the placebo-treated patients and by 4.5 points in the dutasteride-treated patients. The change from baseline was demonstrated as early as 3 months in one study but reached significance in the pooled results from 6 months. In the pooled analysis, Q_{max} increased by 0.6 mL/s in the placebo groups and 2.2 mL/s in the dutasteride groups at 24 months. In the three individual studies, the differences in Q_{max} between placebo and dutasteride were significantly different statistically from baseline in all studies by month 3. At 24 months, serum PSA increased from baseline in the placebo groups by 15.8% compared with a 52.4% decrease in the dutasteride group. The relative risk of AUR with dutasteride compared with placebo was 0.43, and the risk reduction was 57%. The relative risk for BPH-related surgical interventions was 0.52 with dutasteride compared with placebo, and the risk reduction was 48% [17].

The long-term efficacy and safety of the use of 0.5 mg of dutasteride were evaluated in a 2-year open-label extension of the above-mentioned double-blind studies. The study analyzed two groups: men previously receiving 0.5 mg of dutasteride [dutasteride/dutasteride (D/D) group] and previously receiving placebo [placebo/dutasteride (P/D) group]. Both groups had significant improvements in AUA-SI scores and Q_{max} from month 24 to 48, but the D/D group exhibited significantly greater improvements compared with the P/D group. Likewise, the reduction in prostate volume was higher in the D/D group. Therefore, long-term treatment with dutasteride resulted in continuing improvements in urinary symptoms and flow rate, and further reductions in prostate volume, in men with symptomatic BPH. The reduction in risk of AUR and BPH-related surgery, seen in the double-blind phase, was durable over the 4-year term of the studies [35].

Finasteride versus dutasteride

The Enlarged Prostate International Comparator Study (EPICS) was designed to assess the efficacy and safety of dutasteride 0.5 mg compared with finasteride 5 mg for 12 months in treating men with BPH. A total of 1630 men were randomized to receive either finasteride 5 mg or dutasteride 0.5 mg. The change in prostate volume, which was the primary end-point, was similar in both groups. At month 3, there was an adjusted mean percentage reduction in prostate volume of 18.5% for men in the finasteride group versus 18.3% in the dutasteride group. At month 12, the reduction was 26.7% in the finasteride group versus 26.3% in the dutasteride group. There was also no significant difference between the groups regarding the secondary outcomes. At month 12, improvements in AUA-SI scores and Q_{max} were similar in both treatment groups. Also, PSA levels consistently decreased from baseline to months 3 and 12 in both groups. From baseline, PSA levels in the finasteride group decreased by a mean of 38.9% at month 3 and 47.7% at month 12, while there was a mean decrease of 40.3% at month 3 and 49.5% at month 12 in the dutasteride group [36].

Side effects of 5α-reductase inhibitor treatment

Side effects of 5ARI are related to sexual function and include decreased libido, erectile dysfunction (ED), and ejaculatory dysfunction

(EjD). Gynecomastia is also more frequent than with placebo. Evidence from a number of studies suggests that the likelihood of new sexual AEs with 5ARI treatment decreases with longer duration of therapy. Analysis of 4-year data from the Proscar® Long-term Efficacy and Safety Study (PLESS) demonstrated that, compared with placebo, men treated with finasteride experienced new drug-related sexual AEs with an increased frequency only during the first year of therapy [37]. Similarly, the incidence of drug-related sexual AEs decreased with longer duration of therapy in an analysis of the 4-year safety and tolerability of dutasteride [38]. In different studies, with durations from 6 months to 4.5 years, the use of 5 mg of finasteride versus placebo led to an interval of incidence of decreased libido of 2.4–18% versus 1.0–6.3%, ED of 3.0–15.8% versus 1.7–6.3%, and EjD of 0.2 to 7.7% versus 0.1–1.7%. Likewise the use of 0.5 mg of dutasteride versus placebo led to an interval of incidence of decreased libido of 0.5–6.0% versus 0.3–3.0%, ED of 1.3–11.0% versus 1.2 to 6.0%, and EjD of 0.3–3.0% versus 0.0–0.1% [39]. The head-to-head comparison of finasteride and dutasteride in EPICS showed similar rates of sexual adverse events in 12 months [36]. Recently, prolonged AEs on sexual function such as ED and diminished libido in a subset of men have been reported [39].

5α-Reductase inhibitors and prostate cancer

Prostate cancer (PCa) is known to grow androgen-dependently [40]. In logical consequence, 5ARIs, reducing DHT levels, and having as such an indirect antiandrogenic effect might be a treatment option in an already-diagnosed PCa. A very recent study, the Reduction by Dutasteride of Clinical Progression Events in Expectant Management trial, assessed whether dutasteride could inhibit PCa progression in low-risk cancer patients, who would otherwise undergo active surveillance [41]. Another trial, the Avodart® After Radical Therapy for Prostate Cancer Study, assessed whether dutasteride delays biochemical progression in patients with biochemical failure following a radical therapy [42]. However, currently scientific data on new or innovative indications of 5ARIs in PCa are too scarce, and it can be deduced that 5ARIs do not have a primary role as first-line PCa therapy.

Regardless of their active therapeutic value, 5ARIs are of relevance in two aspects regarding PCa: diagnosis and prevention. Regardless of which standard or serum PSA threshold is used, 5ARIs are known to reduce serum PSA levels. According to the "finasteride PSA study group," the measured serum PSA level should be doubled in BPH patients taking a 5ARI not to mask a PCa diagnosis [43]. The same recommendation was made by the PLESS study group [44] and others [45].

The role of 5ARIs in PCa prevention has been passionately discussed in the recent past. Initially, it was a post hoc finding of the Combination of Avodart and Tamsulosin trial that patients who were receiving dutasteride had numerically a lower rate of prostate biopsies. The results suggested that dutasteride might reduce the risk of PCa, and the findings resulted in the initiation of two large randomized controlled trials: PCPT and Reduction by Dutasteride of Prostate Cancer Events (REDUCE), which evaluated the role of finasteride, and dutasteride, respectively, in PCa prevention [46,47]. A daily dose of 5 mg of finasteride, in men without BPH [as assessed by normal digital rectal examination, low serum PSA levels, and low American Urological Association (AUA) symptom score], reduced PCa prevalence by almost 25% over a 7-year period. However, a lower PCa detection rate was counterweighted by a significantly increased rate of high-risk PCa diagnosis in the finasteride group [46]. Similarly, REDUCE reported a risk reduction of 22.8% over a 4-year period with 0.5 mg of dutasteride once daily but at the same time also an increased occurrence of high-grade PCa [47].

The findings from PCPT, REDUCE, and several other clinical trials led to a consensus paper from an expert panel in 2008, which stated that an asymptomatic man, undergoing an annual PSA screening, "might benefit from a discussion of benefits and risks (including the possibility of high-grade PCa) of preventive 5ARI intake." However, at the time, several panel members believed that the higher detection rate of high-grade PCa following preventive 5ARI intake might be due to confounding factors. For example, as a confounding factor, a biopsy in a volume-reduced prostate might uncover more high-grade PCa due to an increased sampling density. In the

mean time, however, the FDA performed an extensive work-up (including a histological re-examination of the REDUCE specimen and various statistical estimation calculations) to address this topic. Their final conclusion, published in 2011 in the *New England Journal of Medicine*, was that 5ARIs indeed increase the risk of high-grade PCa (and this is not due to any bias or confounding factor) [48]. Consequently, the FDA issued a safety announcement, not approving 5ARIs for the use of PCa prevention, and obliged pharmaceutical companies to print a warning label on 5ARI package inserts. This decision has been criticized by others again, because the FDA would overestimate the risks in comparison with the benefits; particularly because, so far, the higher rate of high-grade PCa in the trials could not be linked to an increased mortality [49]. So far, there is no clear statement of the big international urological associations (and their guidelines) whether or not 5ARIs should or should not be used off-label (or at least be offered in an informed consent manner) to healthy ageing or aged men for the purpose of PCa prevention. Currently, the use of 5ARI for PCa prevention cannot be recommended.

Dos and don'ts

- 5ARIs do not have a rapid onset of action. Thus, for men with baseline severe symptoms, the use of 5ARIs alone may not be the best alternative.

- 5ARIs are more effective in men with large prostates, reduce the risk of AUR and BPH-related surgeries, and reduce disease progression. Thus, 5ARIs are a good treatment choice for men at risk of BPH-related complications and BPH progression, especially with large prostates.

- Sexual adverse events may occur with the use of 5ARI. Therefore, sexually active men should be warned of the risk.

- The benefits versus the risks of 5ARIs (particularly the risk of high-grade prostate cancer) should be discussed with the patient. Currently, 5ARI cannot be recommended for PCa prevention.

Bibliography

1 Azzouni F, Godoy A, Li Y, Mohler J. The 5 alpha-reductase isozyme family: a review of basic biology and their role in human diseases. *Adv Urol.* 2012;2012:530121.

2 Wilson JD. Role of dihydrotestosterone in androgen action. *Prostate Suppl.* 1996;6:88–92.

3 Huggins C, Steven R. The effect of castration on benign hypertrophy of the prostate in man. *J Urol.* 1940;43:705–14.

4 Marks LS. 5alpha-reductase: history and clinical importance. *Rev Urol.* 2004;6 Suppl 9:S11–21.

5 Bruchovsky N, Wilson JD. The intranuclear binding of testosterone and 5-alpha-androstan-17-beta-ol-3-one by rat prostate. *J Biol Chem.* 1968;243(22):5953–60.

6 Siiteri PK, Wilson JD. Dihydrotestosterone in prostatic hypertrophy. I. The formation and content of dihydrotestosterone in the hypertrophic prostate of man. *J Clin Invest.* 1970;49(9):1737–45.

7 Bruchovsky N, Wilson JD. Discovery of the role of dihydrotestosterone in androgen action. *Steroids.* 1999;64(11):753–9.

8 Peterson RE, Imperato-McGinley J, Gautier T, Sturla E. Male pseudohermaphroditism due to steroid 5-alpha-reductase deficiency. *Am J Med.* 1977;62(2):170–91.

9 Imperato-McGinley J, Peterson RE, Gautier T, Sturla E. Androgens and the evolution of male-gender identity among male pseudohermaphrodites with 5alpha-reductase deficiency. *N Engl J Med.* 1979;300(22):1233–7.

10 Schneider JJ, Horstmann PM. Effects of incubating desoxycorticosterone with various rat tissues. *J Biol Chem.* 1951;191(1):327–38.

11 Wilson JD, Lasnitzki I. Dihydrotestosterone formation in fetal tissues of the rabbit and rat. *Endocrinology.* 1971;89(3):659–68.

12 Wilson JD. Recent studies on the mechanism of action of testosterone. *N Engl J Med.* 1972;287(25):1284–91.

13 Brooks JR, Berman D, Glitzer MS, Gordon LR, Primka RL, Reynolds GF, et al. Effect of a new 5 alpha-reductase inhibitor on size, histologic characteristics, and androgen concentrations of the canine prostate. *Prostate.* 1982;3(1):35–44.

14 Rittmaster RS, Stoner E, Thompson DL, Nance D, Lasseter KC. Effect of MK-906, a specific 5 alpha-reductase inhibitor, on serum androgens and androgen conjugates in normal men. *J Androl.* 1989;10(4):259–62.

15 Gormley GJ, Stoner E, Bruskewitz RC, Imperato-McGinley J, Walsh PC, McConnell JD, et al. The effect of finasteride in men with benign prostatic hyperplasia. The Finasteride Study Group. *N Engl J Med.* 1992;327(17):1185–91.

16 Gisleskog PO, Hermann D, Hammarlund-Udenaes M, Karlsson MO. A model for the turnover of dihydrotestosterone in the presence of the irreversible 5 alpha-reductase inhibitors GI198745 and finasteride. *Clin Pharmacol Ther.* 1998;64(6):636–47.

17 Roehrborn CG, Boyle P, Nickel JC, Hoefner K, Andriole G. Efficacy and safety of a dual inhibitor of 5-alpha-reductase types 1 and 2 (dutasteride) in men with benign prostatic hyperplasia. *Urology.* 2002;60(3):434–41.

18 Gloyna RE, Siiteri PK, Wilson JD. Dihydrotestosterone in prostatic hypertrophy. II. The formation and content of dihydrotestosterone in the hypertrophic canine prostate and the effect of dihydrotestosterone on prostate growth in the dog. *J Clin Invest.* 1970;49(9):1746–53.

19 Banerjee PP, Banerjee S, Brown TR. Increased androgen receptor expression correlates with development of age-dependent, lobe-specific spontaneous hyperplasia of the brown Norway rat prostate. *Endocrinology.* 2001;142(9):4066–75.

20 Bethel CR, Chaudhary J, Anway MD, Brown TR. Gene expression changes are age-dependent and lobe-specific in the brown Norway rat model of prostatic hyperplasia. *Prostate.* 2009;69(8):838–50.

21 Pierard GE, Pierard-Franchimont C. Effect of a topical erythromycin-zinc formulation on sebum delivery. Evaluation by combined photometric-multi-step samplings with Sebutape. *Clin Exp Dermatol.* 1993;18(5):410–3.

22 Li X, Singh SM, Labrie F. Synthesis and in vitro activity of 17 beta-(N-alkyl/arylformamido)- and 17 beta-[(N-alkyl/aryl)alkyl/arylamido]-4-methyl-4-aza-3-oxo-5 alpha-androstan-3-ones as inhibitors of human 5 alpha-reductases and antagonists of the androgen receptor. *J Med Chem.* 1995;38(7):1158–73.

23 Brooks JR, Baptista EM, Berman C, Ham EA, Hichens M, Johnston DB, et al. Response of rat ventral prostate to a new and novel 5 alpha-reductase inhibitor. *Endocrinology.* 1981;109(3):830–6.

24 Juniewicz PE, Hoekstra SJ, Lemp BM, Barbolt TA, Devin JA, Gauthier E, et al. Effect of combination treatment with zanoterone (WIN 49596), a steroidal androgen receptor antagonist, and finasteride (MK-906), a steroidal 5 alpha-reductase inhibitor, on the prostate and testes of beagle dogs. *Endocrinology*. 1993;133(2):904–13.

25 Ghusn HF, Shao TC, Klima M, Cunningham GR. 4-MAPC, a 5 alpha-reductase inhibitor, reduces rat ventral prostate weight, DNA, and prostatein concentrations. *J Androl*. 1991;12(5):315–22.

26 Rittmaster RS, Manning AP, Wright AS, Thomas LN, Whitefield S, Norman RW, et al. Evidence for atrophy and apoptosis in the ventral prostate of rats given the 5 alpha-reductase inhibitor finasteride. *Endocrinology*. 1995;136(2):741–8.

27 Prahalada S, Rhodes L, Grossman SJ, Heggan D, Keenan KP, Cukierski MA, et al. Morphological and hormonal changes in the ventral and dorsolateral prostatic lobes of rats treated with finasteride, a 5-alpha reductase inhibitor. *Prostate*. 1998;35(3):157–64.

28 Stoner E. The clinical development of a 5 alpha-reductase inhibitor, finasteride. *J Steroid Biochem Mol Biol*. 1990 ;37(3):375–8.

29 Vermeulen A, Giagulli VA, De Schepper P, Buntinx A, Stoner E. Hormonal effects of an orally active 4-azasteroid inhibitor of 5 alpha-reductase in humans. *Prostate*. 1989;14(1):45–53.

30 McConnell JD, Wilson JD, George FW, Geller J, Pappas F, Stoner E. Finasteride, an inhibitor of 5 alpha-reductase, suppresses prostatic dihydrotestosterone in men with benign prostatic hyperplasia. *J Clin Endocrinol Metab*. 1992;74(3):505–8.

31 Gormley GJ, Stoner E, Bruskewitz RC, Imperato-McGinley J, Walsh PC, McConnell JD, et al. The effect of finasteride in men with benign prostatic hyperplasia. The Finasteride Study Group. *N Engl J Med*. 1992;327(17):1185–91.

32 Stoner E. Three-year safety and efficacy data on the use of finasteride in the treatment of benign prostatic hyperplasia. *Urology*. 1994;43(3):284–92; discussion 92–4.

33 McConnell JD, Bruskewitz R, Walsh P, Andriole G, Lieber M, Holtgrewe HL, et al. The effect of finasteride on the risk of acute urinary retention and the need for surgical treatment among men with benign prostatic hyperplasia. *N Engl J Med*. 1998;338(9):557–63.

34 Parsons JK, Schenk JM, Arnold KB, Messer K, Till C, Thompson IM, et al. Finasteride reduces the risk of incident clinical benign prostatic hyperplasia. *Eur Urol*. 2012;62(2).

35 Debruyne F, Barkin J, van Erps P, Reis M, Tammela TL, Roehrborn C. Efficacy and safety of long-term treatment with the dual 5 alpha-reductase inhibitor dutasteride in men with symptomatic benign prostatic hyperplasia. *Eur Urol*. 2004;46(4): 488–94; discussion 95.

36 Nickel JC, Gilling P, Tammela TL, Morrill B, Wilson TH, Rittmaster RS. Comparison of dutasteride and finasteride for treating benign prostatic hyperplasia: the Enlarged Prostate International Comparator Study (EPICS). *BJU Int*. 2011;108(3).

37 Wessells H, Roy J, Bannow J, Grayhack J, Matsumoto AM, Tenover L, et al. Incidence and severity of sexual adverse experiences in finasteride and placebo-treated men with benign prostatic hyperplasia. *Urology*. 2003;61(3):579–84.

38 Schulman C, Pommerville P, Hofner K, Wachs B. Long-term therapy with the dual 5alpha-reductase inhibitor dutasteride is well tolerated in men with symptomatic benign prostatic hyperplasia. *BJU Int*. 2006;97(1):73–9; discussion 9–80.

39 Traish AM, Hassani J, Guay AT, Zitzmann M, Hansen ML. Adverse side effects of 5alpha-reductase inhibitors therapy: persistent diminished libido and erectile dysfunction and depression in a subset of patients. *J Sex Med*. 2011;8(3):872–84.

40 Huggins C, Hodges CV. Studies on prostatic cancer: I. The effect of castration, of estrogen and of androgen injection on serum phosphatases in metastatic carcinoma of the prostate. 1941. *J Urol*. 2002;168(1):9–12.

41 Fleshner NE, Lucia MS, Egerdie B, Aaron L, Eure G, Nandy I, et al. Dutasteride in localised prostate cancer management: the REDEEM randomised, double-blind, placebo-controlled trial. *Lancet*. 2012;379(9821):1103–11.

42 Schröder F, Bangma C, Angulo JC, Alcaraz A, Colombel M, McNicholas T, et al. Dutasteride treatment over 2 years delays prostate-specific antigen progression in patients with biochemical failure after radical therapy for prostate cancer: Results from the randomised, placebo-controlled Avodart After Radical Therapy for Prostate Cancer Study (ARTS). *Eur Urol*. 2013;63(5):779–87.

43 Oesterling JE, Roy J, Agha A, Shown T, Krarup T, Johansen T, et al. Biologic variability of prostate-specific antigen and its usefulness as a marker for prostate cancer: effects of finasteride. The Finasteride PSA Study Group. *Urology.* 1997; 50(1):13–8.

44 Andriole GL, Guess HA, Epstein JI, Wise H, Kadmon D, Crawford ED, et al. Treatment with finasteride preserves usefulness of prostate-specific antigen in the detection of prostate cancer: results of a randomized, double-blind, placebo-controlled clinical trial. PLESS Study Group. Proscar Long-Term Efficacy and Safety Study. *Urology.* 1998;52(2):195–201; discussion 201–2.

45 Andriole GL, Marberger M, Roehrborn CG. Clinical usefulness of serum prostate specific antigen for the detection of prostate cancer is preserved in men receiving the dual 5alpha-reductase inhibitor dutasteride. *J Urol.* 2006;175(5):1657–62.

46 Thompson IM, Goodman PJ, Tangen CM, Lucia MS, Miller GJ, Ford LG, et al. The influence of finasteride on the development of prostate cancer. *N Engl J Med.* 2003;349(3):215–24.

47 Andriole GL, Bostwick DG, Brawley OW, Gomella LG, Marberger M, Montorsi F, et al. Effect of dutasteride on the risk of prostate cancer. *N Engl J Med.* 2010;362(13):1192–202.

48 Theoret MR, Ning YM, Zhang JJ, Justice R, Keegan P, Pazdur R. The risks and benefits of 5alpha-reductase inhibitors for prostate-cancer prevention. *N Engl J Med.* 2011;365(2):97–9.

49 Kim J, Amos CI, Logothetis C. 5alpha-Reductase inhibitors for prostate-cancer prevention. *N Engl J Med.* 2011;365(24):2340.

CHAPTER 9

Antimuscarinics

Nadir I. Osman & Christopher R. Chapple

Department of Urology, Royal Hallamshire Hospital, Sheffield, UK

Key points

- Storage lower urinary tract symptoms (LUTS) are typically more bothersome than voiding LUTS.
- The bladder is an important contributor to storage LUTS in a significant proportion of men.
- Antimuscarinics (anti-M) may work through urothelial/suburothelial mechanisms or through the afferent system rather than simply blocking efferent signals.
- Anti-M are considered safe and efficacious as a monotherapy in men with predominant overactive bladder (OAB) or in combination with an alpha-blocker provided the postvoid residual is <200 mL.
- Caution is advised when treating those at greater risk of urinary retention such as men with a postvoid residual of >200 mL, men with large prostates, men with confirmed bladder outlet obstruction (BOO) and the elderly.

Introduction

LUTS are a prevalent problem in ageing men [1] and often adversely affect quality of life due to their bothersome nature [2]. For most men, there is an overlap between voiding and storage LUTS [3] (Figure 9.1), yet it is the storage LUTS that are characteristically more troublesome and have a greater impact on quality of life [4]. Paradoxically, most medical and surgical therapies have been aimed at improving voiding LUTS, which are commonly prostate targeted, as traditionally benign prostatic hyperplasia (BPH) has been assumed to be the originator of LUTS in men. In the past decade, the role of the bladder in the pathogenesis of storage LUTS has become widely recognized and has led to a paradigm shift in the management of male LUTS with the emergence of bladder-targeted therapies [5].

Overactive bladder (OAB) is a highly bothersome symptom syndrome that comprises an important subset of storage LUTS and is defined as "urinary urgency with or without urgency incontinence usually accompanied by frequency and nocturia" [6]. Urgency is the essential component of the syndrome and has been defined as "the sudden and compelling desire to void that is difficult to defer" usually for fear of leakage [6]. The urodynamic abnormality most commonly associated with OAB is detrusor overactivity (DO), the nonvolitional contraction of the detrusor muscle during bladder filling. In men, this association is stronger than in women, occurring in 69% and 90% of individuals with OAB without incontinence

Male Lower Urinary Tract Symptoms and Benign Prostatic Hyperplasia, First Edition.
Edited by Steven A. Kaplan and Kevin T. McVary.
© 2014 John Wiley & Sons, Ltd. Published 2014 by John Wiley & Sons, Ltd.

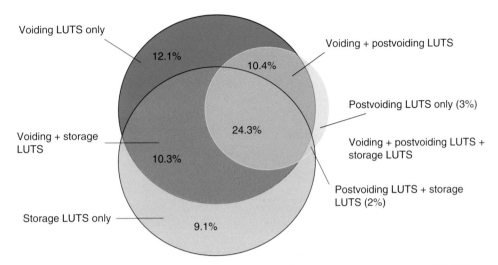

Figure 9.1 Overlap between voiding, storage and post-voiding lower urinary tract symptoms (LUTS) in men: most men have both voiding and storage LUTS. Adapted from Coyne KS, Sexton CC, Kopp ZS, Ebel-Bitoun C, Milsom I, Chapple C. The impact of overactive bladder on mental health, work productivity and health-related quality of life in the UK and Sweden: results from EpiLUTS. BJU international. 2011;108(9):1459–71.

(OAB-dry) and OAB with incontinence (OAB wet), respectively [7].

Anti-M have for many years been the mainstay of pharmacotherapy for women with OAB, while in men these agents have been avoided due to the fear of precipitating voiding problems and urinary retention. There is now a growing evidence base to support the efficacy and safety of anti-M in men with storage LUTS/OAB. This chapter discusses the mechanism of action of anti-M in the context of the pathophysiology of storage LUTS/OAB in men before focusing on the evidence relating to their safety and efficacy with an emphasis on the key aspects of prescribing these agents in clinical practice

Mechanism of action

The etiology of storage LUTS/OAB in men is complex and incompletely understood (Figure 9.2). In some men, it appears that symptoms are secondary to BOO due to BPH, as evidenced by the resolution of symptoms after bladder outlet surgery in approximately two-thirds of men [8] and the resolution of DO in a similar proportion of patients [9]. In such patients, a suggested mechanism of DO is hypersensitivity of cholinergic receptors based on the histological finding of denervation in obstructed bladders ("denervation hypersensitivity") [10]. In other men, symptoms and/or DO occur in the absence of BOO or continue after relief of obstruction. OAB itself may or may not be associated with DO. Several pathophysiological hypotheses have been proposed to explain OAB encompassing dysfunctions of the efferent system, the urothelium and suburothelium, the detrusor muscle, the afferent nerves, and the central control mechanism of lower urinary tract function. The putative mechanisms remain the subject of discussion and have been discussed in detail elsewhere [11].

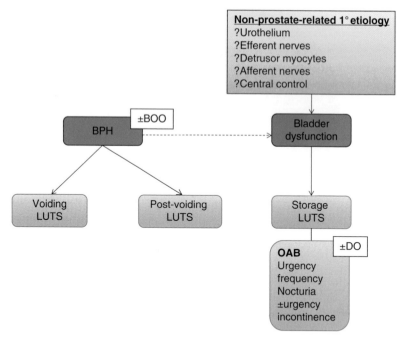

Figure 9.2 Relationship between benign prostatic hyperplasia (BPH), bladder outlet obstruction (BOO) and Storage lower urinary tract symptoms (LUTS)/overactive bladder (OAB). Storage LUTS/OAB may occur due etiologies affecting bladder function not related to BPH. OAB is commonly associated with detrusor overactivity (DO) in men.

The longstanding view of the mechanism by which anti-M exert their effect in OAB is antagonism of the postjunctional muscarinic M_3 receptors resulting in the prevention of excitation–contraction coupling and detrusor contraction (Figure 9.3) [12]. This view is problematic, as clinical evidence suggests that in usual doses, anti-M do not affect bladder emptying in OAB patients while improving storage LUTS, while with higher doses, impairment of voiding contraction occurs (Figure 9.4). An alternative mechanism on the afferent system was suggested with the finding of muscarinic receptors in the urothelium, suburothelium, and afferent nerves. This may explain why OAB patients without DO experience symptom relief with anti-M therapy, and it is suggested that such patients may represent one end of the OAB spectrum. A further suggested mechanism is inhibition of smooth muscle "micromotion," a phenomenon that is postulated to occur due to a leak of acetylcholine from the postganglionic parasympathetic nerve during the storage phase of micturition leading to activation of sensory afferent fibers and the sensation of urgency [13]. Alternatively, anti-M may exert their effect through a direct action on the prostate. The prostate has cholinergic innervation of the stromal and glandular components [14], and muscarinic receptors have been found mainly associated with epithelial cells, which, along with the relatively little muscarinic mediated prostatic contraction, suggests a role in glandular growth or function [15].

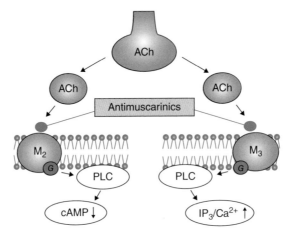

Figure 9.3 Traditional explanation for mechanism of action of antimuscarinics in patients with storage lower urinary tract symptoms (LUTS)/overactive bladder presumed secondary to detrusor overactivity. Antimuscarinics act on both the M_2 and M_3 receptors that are present in the detrusor. M_3 receptors are thought to be most important for detrusor contraction. Acetylcholine (Ach) is released from parasympathetic nerve endings then act on M_2 and M_3 receptors. Activation of M_2 receptors inhibits adenylyl cyclase which causes a reduction in intracellular cyclic AMP which is a mediator of bladder relaxation. M_3 receptor stimulation leads to activation of phospholipase C (PLC) and inositol triphosphate (IP_3) generation which leads to intracellular Ca^{2+} release and activation of the cell contractile apparatus. Reproduced from Karl-Eric Anderesson. Antimuscarinics for the treatment of overactive bladder. The Lancet Neurology. Jan 2004 with permission from Elsevier.

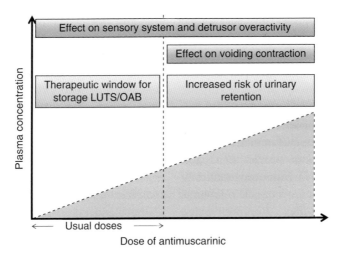

Figure 9.4 At usual doses antimuscarinics have a low plasma concentration allowing anatgonism of the effects of acetylcholine (ACh) in the urothelial and myocyte signaling pathways during bladder filling ("therapeutic window") whilst not affecting detrsuor voiding contraction. When doses are increased voiding contraction may become impaired resulting in urinary retention. LUTS, lower urinary tract symptoms; OAB, overactive bladder. Adapted from Karl-Erik Andersson. Antimuscarinic Mechanisms and the Overactive Detrusor: An Update. *European Urology*, Volume 59, Issue 3, 2011, 377–386.

Muscarinic receptors comprise five sub-types and are present throughout the body (e.g. salivary gland M_1/M_3, gut M_2/M_3, brain M_1, and cardiovascular system M_2). In the bladder, although M_2 receptors predominate (75%), M3 receptors (25%) are mainly responsible for the normal voluntary voiding contraction, whereas the role of M2 receptors in detrusor function is not yet established.

Clinical studies

Many randomized placebo controlled trails have demonstrated the efficacy and safety of several anti-M agents in men as monotherapy or in combination with alpha-blockers (AB). The aim of combining an anti-M with an AB is to achieve a synergy of the effects of both agents in men with concomitant BPH and OAB where both storage and voiding LUTS are present [16]. AB work by antagonizing the alpha-1a adrenoreceptor that predomi-nates in prostatic smooth muscle thereby ameliorating the dynamic component of BPH. Combination therapy consists of commencing both agents either simultaneously or sequen-tially, that is adding on an anti-M in patients with residual storage LUTS/OAB despite being on AB. The available studies can be cat-egorized as those conducted in men with stor-age LUTS/OAB without proven BOO and those conducted in men with urodynamically confirmed BOO. We discuss the main findings of the pivotal studies. Comprehensive reviews of existing studies have been pub-lished elsewhere [17–19] (Table 9.1).

Evidence in men with storage lower urinary tract symptoms

The Tolterodine and Tamsulosin in Men with LUTS Including OAB: Evaluation and Efficacy Study (TIMES) was a 12-week randomized placebo controlled trial in men greater than age 40 years meeting both the criteria for LUTS/BPH and OAB trials [20]. Patients were randomized to receive tolterodine extended release (ER; 4 mg) monotherapy, tamsulosin (0.4 mg) monotherapy or combination ther-apy with both tamsulosin (0.4 mg) and tolterodine ER (4 mg) or placebo. Those with evidence of benign prostatic obstruction ($Q_{max} < 5$ mL/s and/or postvoid residual (PVR) > 200 mL and/or history of retention) were excluded. Of the combination therapy 80% of patients reported treatment benefit at 12 weeks while in the tamsulosin, toltero-dine and placebo groups this was 71%, 65% and 62% respectively. By 12 weeks toltero-dine monotherapy significantly reduced urgency urinary incontinence episodes versus placebo but no other parameters. By comparison combination therapy led to significant reductions in OAB symptom out-comes in including bladder diary variables, International Prostate Symptom Score (IPSS) total and storage subscores including reduc-tion in each of the individual storage symp-tom scores. The occurrence of acute urinary retention (AUR) was low and comparable between groups; 0.5%, 0%, 0.4% and 0% for the tolterodine, tamsulosin, combination and placebo groups respectively. There was no significant difference in PVR or Q_{max} between placebo and tolterodine monother-apy or combination therapy. In post-hoc analyses, tolterodine monotherapy improved several bladder diary measures and IPSS stor-age subscores in men with smaller prostates [vol < 30 mL and prostate-specific antigen (PSA) < 1.3 ng/mL] not seen in men with larger prostates (vol > 30 mL and PSA > 1.3 ng/mL) [21,22].

That tolterodine ER monotherapy was not particularly effective in the TIMES study is at odds with multiple other reports describing

Table 9.1 Pivotal 12-week randomized placebo controlled studies investigating antimuscarinics for male lower urinary tract symptoms

Reference	Patients (n)	Length (weeks)	End points	Study groups	AUR needing catheterization (%)
Kaplan et al. (TIMES) [20]	879	12	PPTB Bladder diary IPSS	Tolterodine Tamsulosin Tolterodine + tamsulosin Placebo	0 0 <1
Chapple et al. (ADAM) [27]	652	12	IPSS Symptom bother Bladder diary Flow rate PVR	Tolterodine ER + AB Placebo + AB	<1 <1
MacDiarmid et al. [26]	420	12	IPSS QoL Flow rate PVR	Oxybutynin + Tamsulosin Placebo + tamsulosin	0 0
Kaplan et al. (VICTOR) [28]	398	12	Bladder diary IPSS Flow rate PVR	Solifenacin + tamsulosin Placebo + tamsulosin	1.5 0
Abrams et al. [30]	221	12	Urodynamics	Tolterodine Placebo	0 1.2
Kaplan et al. [31]	222	12	Urodynamics	Solifenaciin + tamsulosin Placebo + tamsulosin	<1 0

AB, alpha-blockers; ADAM, ADd-on to an Alpa-blocker in Men; AUR, acute urinary retention; ER, extended release; IPSS, International Prognostic Scoring System; PPTB, patient perception of treatment benefit; PVR, postvoid residual; QoL, quality of life; TIMES, Tolterodine and Tamsulosin in Men with Lower Urinary Tract Symptoms Including Overactive Bladder: Evaluation and Efficacy Study; VICTOR, VESIcare® In Combination With Tamsulosin in OAB Residual Symptoms.

efficacy for anti-M monotherapy in men with storage LUTS/OAB [23–25]. This is probably a product of the characteristics of study participants who had a relatively high IPSS scores at baseline [19.5–20.6] compared with other studies. Also, patients in the TIMES were required to have features for entry into both OAB and LUTS/BPH trials and so a greater proportion of this group may have had symptoms as a consequence of prostate dysfunction and may not have responded as well to anti-M.

The ER formulation of oxybutynin was studied in a 12-week double-blinded rand-omized controlled trial including a total of 420 men [26]. Men included were >45 years with IPSS score ≥13 and storage subscore ≥8 while those with a Q_{max} of <8 mL/s with a voided volume of ≥125 mL and PVR > 150 mL on two separate occasions were excluded. Participants were randomized to receive tamsulosin (0.4 mg) with oxybutynin ER 10 mg or tamsulosin (0.4 mg) with placebo. There was a significant advantage in terms of improvement in IPSS and storage sub-score for combination of tamsulosin/Oxybutinin versus tamsulosin monotherapy in addition to greater improvement in IPSS QoL scores. An increase PVR of >300 mL was seen in 2.9% of those receiving tamsulosin/oxybutynin versus 0.5% in tamsulosin/placebo group.

The tolterodine XL ADd-on to an Alpablocker in Men (ADAM) study was a further 12 week randomized placebo controlled study that studied the effect of sequential tolterodine XL (4 mg) in men already taking AB (for >1 month) compared with placebo [27]. Men included were >40 years with symptoms of urgency, frequency and at least moderate symptom on the patient perception of bladder condition questionnaire (PPBC) after at least 1-month treatment with alpha-blocker monotherapy. A significant advantage over of placebo was found in total number of voids, OAB-q symptoms scores and IPSS storage subscore. In terms of total urgency episodes, there was a significant improvement in the add-on antimuscarinic group compared with placebo (−2.9 vs −1.8; $p = 0.0010$). Daytime and night-time urgency episodes were similarly significantly improved. An improvement in the PPBC occurred in 63.6% of the combination group and 61.6% of AB + placebo group, though the difference was not statistically significant. AUR requiring catheterization occurred in <1% of patients in each group. No statistically significant change in Q_{max} was observed in either group, although a statistically significant increase in PVR occurred in the add-on anti-M group this was not deemed clinically significant. When subjects were stratified by baseline PSA values, those with a PSA above the mean had a statistically significant decrease in Q_{max} and increase in PVR, although these changes were also not deemed clinically significant.

Sequential therapy with solifenacin after failure of tamsulosin to alleviate storage LUTS was assessed in the 12-week double-randomized VESIcare® In Combination With Tamsulosin in OAB Residual Symptoms study [28]. A total of 398 men with persistent storage LUTS after monotherapy with tamsulosin (0.4 mg) were randomized to therapy with solifenacin (5 mg) or placebo. Men included were aged >45 years with a frequency of ≥8/day, ≥1 urgency episode/day, total IPSS ≥ 13, PPBC ≥ 3, PVR ≤ 200 mL, and Q_{max} ≥ 5 mL/s. A significant reduction in the total number of urgency episodes for solifenacin/tamsulosin versus solifenacin/placebo was observed (−2.18 vs −1.10, p <0.001), although there was no statistically significant difference between the groups in terms of the total number of voids. Around 1.5% of the tamsulosin/solifenacin group developed AUR requiring catheterization, compared with none of the tamsulosin/placebo group.

Flexible dose fesoterodine in patients with persistent OAB symptoms despite treatment with AB was recently evaluated in a 12-week study randomized study that included a total of 943 subjects [29]. Patients were randomized into two groups: fesoterodine (4 mg) with the option to increase to the dose to 8 mg at week 4 and go down to 4 mg again at week 8 and placebo. There was no significant difference between the two groups in terms of the primary end-point of urgency episodes with both groups showing no significant improvement from baseline. However, there were improvements in the total number of micturitions and the OAB-q bother score that were significantly greater for fesoterodine over placebo. Only one patient in each group developed AUR requiring catheterization.

Evidence in men with confirmed bladder outlet obstruction

Given the frequent coexistence of voiding and storage LUTS, it is important to ascertain whether obstruction is a contraindication to the use of anti-M. Several studies have now addressed this question. The safety of tolterodine 2 mg BD was assessed in a small randomized trial in men aged >40 years with urodynamically confirmed BOO and DO [30]. A total of 149 and 72 subjects were randomized to toletrodine or placebo respectively. Patients underwent urodynamic studies at baseline and at 12 weeks. There was no statistically significant difference in terms of Q_{max} and pdet@Q_{max} between both groups. Tolterodine resulted in an increase in PVR compared with placebo (25 mL vs 0 mL, $p \leq .004$) and a reduction in the bladder contractility index (BCI; −5 vs +5, $p = .0045$). Overall, AUR was reported in one patient who was in the placebo group. The incidence of adverse events was similar between the groups.

A recent 12-week randomized study evaluated the safety of combination of tamsulosin oral controlled absorption system (OCAS) with solifenacin at a dose of 6 mg or 9 mg in men aged >45 years with an IPSS score of >8 and reduced flow ($Q_{max} \leq 12$ mL/s), and urodynamic evidence of BOO (BOO index >20) [31]. In total, 222 men were randomized into three groups: tamsulosin 0.4 mg/solifenacin 6 mg, tamsulosin 0.4 mg/solifenacin 9 mg, or tamsulosin 0.4 mg/placebo. At 12 weeks, there were no significant differences in terms of Q_{max}, Pdet@Q_{max}, and BCI between the treatment groups and placebo. Overall AUR occurred in only one patient who was in the tamsulosin/solifenacin 6 mg group.

Comparison between agents

While a number of anti-M have been studied in clinical trials, there is a lack of trials performing a head-to-head comparison of different agents. A small randomized study including 107 men compared tolterodine, solifenacin, or darifenacin [32]. All three agents showed efficacy in reducing the total number of voids and IPSS. In terms of improvement in IPSS and urgency, tolterodine and solifenacin had an advantage in comparison with darifenacin. There was a greater increase in PVR (+16.2 mL, $p < 0.001$) and rates of AUR (56%) with darifenacin in addition to a greater incidence of constipation, leading the authors to conclude that darifenacin was not an optimal agent to use in men with LUTS/BPH. Further larger studies are needed to establish definitively whether there is differential efficacy across agents in this patient group

Antimuscarinic safety in men with lower urinary tract symptoms/benign prostatic hyperplasia

Although there is a strong body of evidence to support the safety of anti-M in men with LUTS/BPH, there is the limitation that most studies excluded men with larger PVRs (usually >200 mL) who would represent a greater risk of AUR due to a presumed reduction in the detrusor contractile function. Furthermore, in the studies that measured prostate size, volumes were generally low. Additionally, studies were generally of 12 weeks' duration which is arguably not long enough to accurately determine the true risk of AUR, which may increase with length of follow-up. As such, anti-M are generally not recommended in men with a PVR of >200 mL, who have low peak flow rates, or who have larger prostates or a previous history of AUR. Age also appears to be an important factor, and a retrospective survey from the UK showed that the risk of AUR increased from 0.1 per 1000 person-years in men aged 20–49 years to 6.9 per 1000 person-years in men aged 80–84 years [33]. AUR was most likely to occur during the initial 30 days, especially during the first 2 weeks, but reduced significantly thereafter. These data need to be interpreted with a degree of caution, as the participant characteristics are unclear. There remains a need for longer-term studies to better assess the risk of AUR and determine the safe upper limit in terms of baseline PVR.

Other important treatment issues

Two common issues with anti-M use are poor adherence and persistence. In a year-long study in 45,576 receiving anti-M for OAB, an average of only 32% of the total number of days were covered by medication use [34]. Common reasons for low adherence are a lack of perceived efficacy or poor tolerability to treatment side effects. For similar reasons, persistence rates are also low, and a recent analysis of UK prescription data found that the proportion of patients still on their originally prescribed agent at 12 months ranged from 14 to 35% for different agents in common use [35]. While the efficacy of anti-M is often dose-dependent, the occurrence of side effects related to the wide distribution of muscarinic receptors may limit dose escalation. Side effects are similarly dependent on dosage, with common complaints being dry mouth, constipation, tiredness, blurred vision, and cognitive impairment, which the elderly are at particular risk from. Less commonly, anti-M are contraindicated for usage including patients with gastroparesis, severe liver impairment, and narrow-angle glaucoma. In clinical practice, if a patient has failed to gain symptomatic relief or has been unable to tolerate side effects, an alternative anti-M agent is commonly tried, although there is no evidence for differential efficacy across agents, and it remains unclear why an alternative agent in such cases is successful.

Practical aspects of antimuscarinic use

Anti-M as monotherapy or in combination with AB are currently recommended for use in men with LUTS/BPH with predominant storage LUTS in both the American urology association (AUA) [36] and European Association of Urology (EAU) guidelines [37] (Figure 9.5). The AUA guidelines recommend that PVR be checked before the initiation of therapy and that anti-M be used with caution in men with a PVR of >250–300 mL, while the EAU guideline recommends caution when used in men with BOO. The EAU treatment algorithm provides the option of anti-M monotherapy in men with storage LUTS/OAB only, while in those coexistent voiding LUTS, an AB is recommended initially, typically for a period of 4–6 weeks, after which an anti-M is an option in men with residual storage LUTS/OAB. Monitoring of PVR within the first month of treatment using bladder ultrasound is advisable.

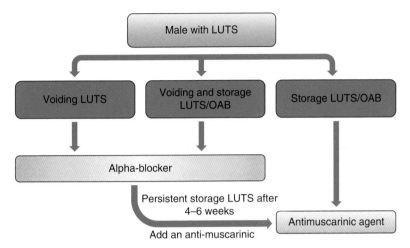

Figure 9.5 Simplified male lower urinary tract symptoms (LUTS) pharmacotherapy treatment algorithm.

Dos and don'ts

- Assess whether patients suffer from bothersome storage LUTS/OAB.
- Estimate or measure prostate volume.
- In men with only storage LUTS/OAB, consider anti-M monotherapy after suitable lifestyle interventions have failed to improve symptoms sufficiently.
- In men with both voiding and storage LUTS/OAB, consider a sequential anti-M after an initial trial with AB if residual storage LUTS/OAB persist.
- Check PVR at baseline and within the first month of treatment with an anti-M.
- Use caution when prescribing anti-M in men with confirmed BOO, low flow rate, and elevated PVR (>200 mL), and in elderly men.

Conclusion

The available evidence supports the use of anti-M alone in men with only storage LUTS/OAB where a primary bladder dysfunction is suspected. In men who have concomitant voiding and storage LUTS/OAB, the combination of an AB with an anti-M allows the synergistically alleviation of both components. Men with smaller prostates based on prostate volume measurement/estimation or serum PSA may benefit more from anti-M therapy, while those with larger glands or suspected BOO may be more at risk of problems such as raised PVR, reduced flow or AUR; in such patients caution is recommended. Future studies are required to ascertain the risk of AUR beyond 12 weeks and delineate the safe upper limit for baseline PVR. Additionally, the characteristics of men who are most likely to benefit from anti-M treatment need to be better defined.

Conflict of interest

Christopher Chapple is a consultant and researcher for Allergan, Astellas, Pfizer, and Recordati. Nadir Osman has no conflict of interest.

Bibliography

1 Kupelian V, Wei JT, O'Leary MP, Kusek JW, Litman HJ, Link CL, *et al.* Prevalence of lower urinary tract symptoms and effect on quality of life in a racially and ethnically diverse random sample: the Boston Area Community Health (BACH) Survey. *Arch Intern Med.* 2006;166(21):2381–7. Epub 2006/11/30.

2 Coyne KS, Sexton CC, Kopp ZS, Ebel-Bitoun C, Milsom I, Chapple C. The impact of overactive bladder on mental health, work productivity and health-related quality of life in the UK and Sweden: results from EpiLUTS. BJU Int. 2011;108(9): 1459–71. Epub 2011/03/05.

3 Sexton CC, Coyne KS, Kopp ZS, Irwin DE, Milsom I, Aiyer LP, et al. The overlap of storage, voiding and postmicturition symptoms and implications for treatment seeking in the USA, UK and Sweden: EpiLUTS. BJU Int. 2009;103 Suppl 3:12–23. Epub 2009/04/02.

4 Coyne KS, Wein AJ, Tubaro A, Sexton CC, Thompson CL, Kopp ZS, et al. The burden of lower urinary tract symptoms: evaluating the effect of LUTS on health-related quality of life, anxiety and depression: EpiLUTS. BJU Int. 2009;103 Suppl 3: 4–11. Epub 2009/04/02.

5 Chapple CR, Roehrborn CG. A shifted paradigm for the further understanding, evaluation, and treatment of lower urinary tract symptoms in men: focus on the bladder. Eur. Urol. 2006;49(4):651–8. Epub 2006/03/15.

6 Abrams P, Cardozo L, Fall M, Griffiths D, Rosier P, Ulmsten U, et al. The standardisation of terminology in lower urinary tract function: report from the standardisation sub-committee of the International Continence Society. *Urology.* 2003;61(1):37–49. Epub 2003/02/01.

7 Hashim H, Abrams P. Is the bladder a reliable witness for predicting detrusor overactivity?

J Urol. 2006;175(1):191–4; discussion 4–5. Epub 2006/01/13.

8 Abrams PH, Farrar DJ, Turner-Warwick RT, Whiteside CG, Feneley RC. The results of prostatectomy: a symptomatic and urodynamic analysis of 152 patients. *J Urol.* 1979;121(5):640–2. Epub 1979/05/01.

9 Machino R, Kakizaki H, Ameda K, Shibata T, Tanaka H, Matsuura S, *et al.* Detrusor instability with equivocal obstruction: A predictor of unfavorable symptomatic outcomes after transurethral prostatectomy. *Neurourol Urodyn.* 2002;21(5):444–9. Epub 2002/09/17.

10 Speakman MJ, Brading AF, Gilpin CJ, Dixon JS, Gilpin SA, Gosling JA. Bladder outflow obstruction—a cause of denervation supersensitivity. *J Urol.* 1987;138(6):1461–6. Epub 1987/12/01.

11 Roosen A, Chapple CR, Dmochowski RR, Fowler CJ, Gratzke C, Roehrborn CG, *et al.* A refocus on the bladder as the originator of storage lower urinary tract symptoms: a systematic review of the latest literature. *Eur Urol.* 2009;56(5):810–9. Epub 2009/08/18.

12 Andersson KE, Yoshida M. Antimuscarinics and the overactive detrusor—which is the main mechanism of action? *Eur Urol.* 2003;43(1):1–5. Epub 2003/01/01.

13 Drake MJ, Mills IW, Gillespie JI. Model of peripheral autonomous modules and a myovesical plexus in normal and overactive bladder function. *Lancet.* 2001;358(9279):401–3. Epub 2001/08/15.

14 Ventura S, Pennefather J, Mitchelson F. Cholinergic innervation and function in the prostate gland. *Pharmacol. Ther.* 2002;94(1–2):93–112. Epub 2002/08/23.

15 Witte LP, Chapple CR, de la Rosette JJ, Michel MC. Cholinergic innervation and muscarinic receptors in the human prostate. *Eur Urol.* 2008; 54(2):326–34. Epub 2007/12/28.

16 Chapple CR, Smith D. The pathophysiological changes in the bladder obstructed by benign prostatic hyperplasia. *Br J Urol.* 1994;73(2):117–23. Epub 1994/02/01.

17 Kaplan SA, Roehrborn CG, Abrams P, Chapple CR, Bavendam T, Guan Z. Antimuscarinics for treatment of storage lower urinary tract symptoms in men: a systematic review. *Int J Clin Pract.* 2011;65(4):487–507. Epub 2011/01/08.

18 Athanasopoulos A, Chapple C, Fowler C, Gratzke C, Kaplan S, Stief C, *et al.* The role of antimuscarinics in the management of men with symptoms of overactive bladder associated with concomitant bladder outlet obstruction: an update. *Eur Urol.* 2011;60(1):94–105. Epub 2011/04/19.

19 Blake-James BT, Rashidian A, Ikeda Y, Emberton M. The role of anticholinergics in men with lower urinary tract symptoms suggestive of benign prostatic hyperplasia: a systematic review and meta-analysis. *BJU Int.* 2007;99(1):85–96. Epub 2006/10/10.

20 Kaplan SA, Roehrborn CG, Rovner ES, Carlsson M, Bavendam T, Guan Z. Tolterodine and tamsulosin for treatment of men with lower urinary tract symptoms and overactive bladder: a randomized controlled trial. *J Am Med Assoc.* 2006;296(19): 2319–28. Epub 2006/11/16.

21 Roehrborn CG, Kaplan SA, Jones JS, Wang JT, Bavendam T, Guan Z. Tolterodine extended release with or without tamsulosin in men with lower urinary tract symptoms including overactive bladder symptoms: effects of prostate size. *Eur Urol.* 2009;55(2):472–9. Epub 2008/06/28.

22 Roehrborn CG, Kaplan SA, Kraus SR, Wang JT, Bavendam T, Guan Z. Effects of serum PSA on efficacy of tolterodine extended release with or without tamsulosin in men with LUTS, including OAB. *Urology.* 2008;72(5):1061–7; discussion 7. Epub 2008/09/27.

23 Kaplan SA, Roehrborn CG, Dmochowski R, Rovner ES, Wang JT, Guan Z. Tolterodine extended release improves overactive bladder symptoms in men with overactive bladder and nocturia. *Urology.* 2006;68(2):328–32. Epub 2006/08/15.

24 Kaplan SA, Goldfischer ER, Steers WD, Gittelman M, Andoh M, Forero-Schwanhaeuser S. Solifenacin treatment in men with overactive bladder: effects on symptoms and patient-reported outcomes. *The Aging Male.* 2010;13(2):100–7. Epub 2009/12/17.

25 Roehrborn CG, Abrams P, Rovner ES, Kaplan SA, Herschorn S, Guan Z. Efficacy and tolerability of tolterodine extended-release in men with overactive bladder and urgency urinary incontinence. *BJU Int.* 2006;97(5):1003–6. Epub 2006/04/29.

26 MacDiarmid SA, Peters KM, Chen A, Armstrong RB, Orman C, Aquilina JW, *et al.* Efficacy and safety of extended-release oxybutynin in combination with tamsulosin for treatment of lower urinary tract symptoms in men: randomized, double-blind, placebo-controlled study. *Mayo Clin. Proc.* 2008;83(9):1002–10. Epub 2008/09/09.

27 Chapple C, Herschorn S, Abrams P, Sun F, Brodsky M, Guan Z. Tolterodine treatment improves storage symptoms suggestive of overactive bladder in men treated with alpha-blockers. *Eur. Urol.* 2009;56(3): 534–41. Epub 2008/12/17.

28 Kaplan SA, McCammon K, Fincher R, Fakhoury A, He W. Safety and tolerability of solifenacin add-on therapy to alpha-blocker treated men with residual urgency and frequency. *J Urol.* 2009;182(6):2825–30. Epub 2009/10/20.

29 Kaplan SA, Roehrborn CG, Gong J, Sun F, Guan Z. Add-on fesoterodine for residual storage symptoms suggestive of overactive bladder in men receiving alpha-blocker treatment for lower urinary tract symptoms. *BJU Int.* 2012;109(12):1831–40. Epub 2011/10/05.

30 Abrams P, Kaplan S, De Koning Gans HJ, Millard R. Safety and tolerability of tolterodine for the treatment of overactive bladder in men with bladder outlet obstruction. *J Urol.* 2006;175(3 Pt 1): 999–1004; discussion Epub 2006/02/14.

31 Kaplan SA, He W, Koltun WD, Cummings J, Schneider T, Fakhoury A. Solifenacin plus tamsulosin combination treatment in men with lower urinary tract symptoms and bladder outlet obstruction: a randomized controlled trial. *Eur Urol.* 2012. Epub 2012/07/27.

32 Kaplan SA, Zoltan E, Te AE. Safety and efficacy of tolterodine, solifenacin, and darifenacin in men with lower urinary tract symptoms (LUTS) on alpha-blockers with persistent overactive bladder symptoms (OAB)Abstract 2036. *J Urol.* 2008; 179:701.

33 Martin-Merino E, Garcia-Rodriguez LA, Masso-Gonzalez EL, Roehrborn CG. Do oral antimuscarinic drugs carry an increased risk of acute urinary retention? *J Urol.* 2009;182(4):1442–8. Epub 2009/08/18.

34 Pelletier EM, Vats V, Clemens JQ. Pharmacotherapy adherence and costs versus nonpharmacologic management in overactive bladder. *Am J Manag Care.* 2009;15(4 Suppl):S108–14. Epub 2009/04/16.

35 Wagg A, Compion G, Fahey A, Siddiqui E. Persistence with prescribed antimuscarinic

therapy for overactive bladder: a UK experience. *BJU Int*. 2012;110(11):1767–74. Epub 2012/03/14.

36 McVary KT, Roehrborn CG, Avins AL, Barry MJ, Bruskewitz RC, Donnell RF, *et al*. Update on AUA guideline on the management of benign prostatic hyperplasia. *J Urol*. 2011;185(5):1793–803. Epub 2011/03/23.

37 Oelke M, Bachmann, A., Descazeaud, A., Emberton, M., Gravas, S., Michel, MC, *et al. European Association of Urology guidelines on male lower urinary tract symptoms*; 2012 [updated February 2012; cited March 2013]. Available from: http://www.uroweb.org/gls/pdf/12_Male_LUTS_LR May 9th 2012.pdf.

CHAPTER 10

The Use of Phosphodiesterase Type 5 Inhibitors in the Treatment of Lower Urinary Tract Symptoms Due to Benign Prostatic Hyperplasia

Casey Lythgoe & Kevin T. McVary

Division of Urology, Southern Illinois University School of Medicine, Springfield, IL, USA

Key points

- Phosphodiesterase type 5 inhibitors (PDE5-Is) are a safe and effective treatment for men over the age of 45 with lower urinary tract symptoms (LUTS) due to benign prostatic hyperplasia (BPH) alone or in combination with alpha-blockers.
- PDE5-Is consistently improve International Prostate Symptom Score (IPSS) scores, but Q_{max} and postvoid residual (PVR) are unlikely to be affected by this medication.
- Side effects most commonly include flushing, gastroesophageal reflux, headache, and dyspepsia.
- Further research into long-term effectiveness of PDE5-Is is warranted, along with cost-effectiveness studies.

Introduction

The relationship between LUTS secondary to BPH and erectile dysfunction (ED) has been frequently investigated for the high prevalence of both conditions in older men. This large body of epidemiologic data supports a causal relationship between LUTS and ED [1]. This association between LUTS and sexual dysfunction has been emerging in the level of concern by patients, government agencies, investigators, and the healthcare providers who treat such men. It is well established that both LUTS and ED independently reduce the quality of life (QoL). In combination, these two clinical entities logically compound life distress. The association between these two diseases has also garnered attention, as investigators have hypothesized a common pathophysiology to explain the idea that they are causally linked. This common-theme hypothesis has taken on a life of its own as pharmaceutical companies have expanded the indications for their drugs for both diseases.

Male Lower Urinary Tract Symptoms and Benign Prostatic Hyperplasia, First Edition.

Edited by Steven A. Kaplan and Kevin T. McVary.

© 2014 John Wiley & Sons, Ltd. Published 2014 by John Wiley & Sons, Ltd.

Epidemiology

The first large-scale study reporting on an age-independent association between LUTS and male sexual dysfunction was presented by Lukacs *et al.* [2]. Based on data from a study of 5849 men who underwent a 1-year observational trial with alfuzosin, baseline LUTS were strongly correlated with different aspects of sexual dysfunction. Additional studies have been published in the last decade, of which more than 35,000 men have contributed data on ED and LUTS. Based on these results, there is on average an increase of approximately 100% in ED rates in men with concomitant moderate or severe LUTS. The results are consistent overall across studies [1].

The largest and most widely cited study to date is the Multinational Survey of the Aging Male by Rosen *et al.* [3], in which the relationship between LUTS and both ED and ejaculatory dysfunction (EjD) is measured by the International Index of Erectile Function, IPSS, and Danish Prostate Symptom Score, a validated measure of ejaculation, low desire, and ejaculation-related bother in aging men [4]. Data from 12,815 men aged 50–80 years from the United States and six European countries were analyzed. Thirty-one percent of respondents had moderate to severe LUTS, and 48.7% reported on difficulties achieving an erection, with 10% on a complete absence of erection. Within each age category, the frequency of ED was strongly related to the severity of LUTS with a relative risk (RR) increasing from 3.1 (moderate LUTS) to 5.9 (severe LUTS) regardless of the coexistence of comorbid conditions, such as diabetes, hypertension, cardiac disease, or hyperlipidemia (Figure 10.1).

The impact of LUTS on men's sexual health was evaluated as part of a cross-sectional epidemiological study (the Epidemiology of Lower Urinary Tract Symptoms Study) to assess the prevalence LUTS among men and

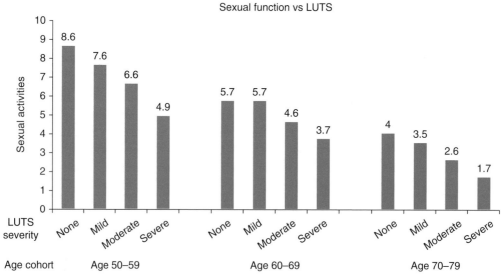

Figure 10.1 Graph showing how sexual function declines as the severity of lower urinary tract symptoms (LUTS) increases and with age. Severity of LUTS assessed by International Prognostic Scoring System: none, 0; mild, 1–7; moderate, 8–19; severe, 20–35. Rosen 2003 [3]. Reproduced with permission of Elsevier.

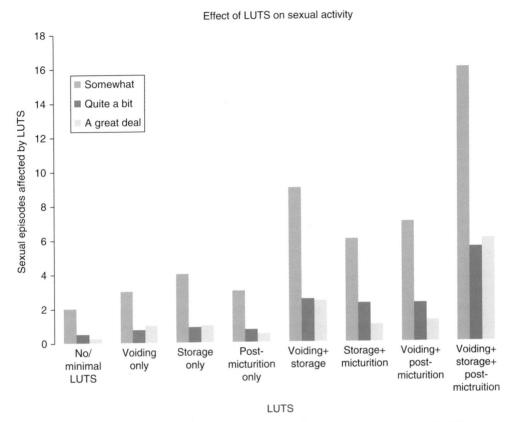

Figure 10.2 Decreased enjoyment of sexual activity due to lower urinary tract symptoms (LUTS): Epidemiology of Lower Urinary Tract Symptoms Study. Wein 2009 [5]. Reproduced with permission of John Wiley & Sons Ltd.

women aged 40 years or older in the USA, the UK, and Sweden [5]. The analysis included 11,834 men with a mean age of 56.1 years, 71% of whom reported being currently sexually active. Twenty-six percent had mild to severe ED, 7% had EjD, and 16% had premature ejaculation. This problem (premature ejaculation) had not previously been assessed. However, a strong, dose-related relationship between LUTS and male sexual dysfunction was again observed (Figure 10.2).

Men with multiple LUTS had more severe ED, and more frequent EjD and premature ejaculation. In the logistic regression analysis, older age, hypertension, diabetes, depression, urgency with fear of leaking,

and leaking during sexual activity were significantly associated with ED. More frequent LUTS were associated with most of the common sexual dysfunctions in men, highlighting again the importance of assessing the sexual health of all men presenting with LUTS.

In summary, the major epidemiologic findings to date include: (1) a consistent dose response association between increased frequency of LUTS and ED, (2) a significantly higher prevalence of LUTS in men suffering from ED as compared with men with normal erections, and (3) a statistically significant increase in the risk of ED for increasing urinary complaints in logistic regression models after controlling for age and comorbidities. According to these reproducible and robust data, considering strength of association, internal consistency, and dose–response effects, a causal link between LUTS and ED is strongly supported [6]. Moreover, the association between ED and LUTS has biologic plausibility, given the interrelationships of the known pathophysiological mechanisms of these disease states.

Lower urinary tract symptoms treatment

The treatment of LUTS secondary to BPH underwent a major paradigm shift with the advent of alpha-blockers in the 1990s. Used alone or in combination with 5-alpha-reductase inhibitors (5ARIs), medical treatment soon became the standard of care for LUTS/BPH. Unfortunately, these medications can be associated with bothersome sexual side effects that vary between different classes of medications, different medications within the same classes, and different combinations of drugs.

The primary purpose of treating LUTS is to improve symptoms and reduce bother while at the same time causing as few side effects as possible, while there should ideally be few adverse events including on sexual function. In fact, almost all therapies for BPH-related LUTS are associated with some sexual side effects, although they differ in type, frequency, and severity.

Surprisingly, even in active surveillance of LUTS, there is some alteration on sexual function. The impact on ED in men with LUTS undergoing active surveillance is variable during a short period, with some men finding that their sexual function improves and others finding that it deteriorates.

However, in the long run, sexual function tends to deteriorate. The effect of alpha-blockers (AB) on ED in men with LUTS is variable during a short period, with men reporting either no change or a modest improvement of unknown significance. However, the effect of AB on EjD in men with LUTS is significantly affected by two agents (tamsulosin and silodosin). The other AB have little or no impact on EjD. The effect of 5ARIs on sexual function in men with LUTS is modest but global with effects on penile erection, ejaculation, and sexual desire. It was originally thought that the effects were fully reversible, and there have been reports of persistence of the sexual side effects following cessation of therapy when these drugs have been used to treat male pattern baldness. The veracity of this finding is unclear at present.

Pathophysiology of lower urinary tract symptoms and the phosphodiesterase-5 signal pathway

Although the mechanisms underlying the relationship between LUTS and ED have not been fully elucidated, several pathophysiological theories have been currently proposed in the literature, while the possible common links between these pathways are still under investigation. Sexual dysfunction is frequently found in aging men with LUTS secondary to BPH and is linked to LUTS/BPH via the nitric oxide synthase (NOS)/cyclic guanosine monophosphate (cGMP) pathway, Ras homolog gene family, member A (RhoA)/Ras homolog (Rho)-kinase signaling, pelvic atherosclerosis associated with chronic hypoxia, and autonomic adrenergic hyperactivity.

Nitric oxide synthase/cyclic guanosine monophosphate pathway

The NOS/cGMP pathway in erectile function has been well characterized, but investigations have recently focused on the link between BPH/LUTS and ED using the NOS pathway as a common link between the two entities [7] (Figure 10.3).

Investigators have suggested that BPH may result from proliferation of prostatic stroma and epithelium and/or from increased prostatic smooth muscle tone. A critical regulator of prostate innervation and smooth muscle tone is nitric oxide (NO), derived from NOS. Since NO is a key regulator of proliferation and smooth muscle relaxation, and NOS signaling is altered in patients with BPH, investigators have proposed that decreased NO in patients leads to increased severity of LUTS [8]. NOS is found in endothelial and neuronal forms in nerves within the prostate as well as in the basal cells of the glandular epithelium [9]. Also, NOS expression of both forms is reduced in the transition zone of the prostate in BPH [10]. The subsequent reduction in bioavailable NO results in increased smooth muscle cell contraction at the bladder neck and smooth muscle cell proliferation within the stroma of the prostate, resulting in worsening of bladder outlet obstruction (BOO) [11]. Further, in vitro models have demonstrated an antiproliferative effect on prostatic smooth muscle cells by NO donors, such as sodium nitroprusside, via a negative effect on the proliferation of the protein kinase C signal transduction pathway [12]. Phosphodiesterase (PDE) mRNA and protein have been localized across the whole human urogenital tract, with different patterns of expression and concentrations [13]. The hypothesis that impaired NO/cGMP signaling contributes to the pathophysiology of BPH provided further background for a potential role of NO donor drugs and PDE5-i in the management of BPH-associated LUTS [7]. In this respect, PDE5-i increased the levels of cAMP and cGMP in the human prostate and plasma, and the distribution of PDE5-i was found to be higher in the prostate than in the plasma of treated men [11]. In addition, PDE5-i have shown antiproliferative effects in the prostatic stroma [14].

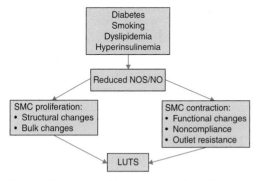

Figure 10.3 Nitric oxide synthase/nitric oxide (NOS/NO) theory of erectile dysfunction and lower urinary tract symptoms (LUTS). SMC, smooth muscle cell. McVary 2005 [27]. Reprinted with permission of MedReviews®, LLC.

Ras homolog gene family, member A/Ras homolog-kinase signaling

It is theorized that smooth muscle relaxation in the penis and prostate, and the NO pathway may be mitigated by pathways that circumvent the relaxing effects of NO. The Rho kinase pathway is one such pathway in which RhoA is activated by guanosine-5′-triphosphate (GTP), translocated to the cell membrane where it acts as a kinase to maintain the phosphorylated state of myosin light chain by inhibition of myosin phosphatase. Actin and myosin cross-bridging and contraction then ensue independent of intracellular calcium levels [15]. Upregulation of RhoA/ROCK has been established in diabetes-related ED [16–18] and may provide further insight into the multifactorial nature of BPH/LUTS and ED. Despite the seemingly independent mechanism of ROCK signaling, some evidence suggests that the Rho kinase pathway is also involved in the inhibition of eNOS, which may lead to decreased smooth muscle relaxation, thus providing a way for PDE5 inhibitors (PDE5-Is) to overcome smooth muscle contraction and BOO resulting from the ROCK pathway [19].

Pelvic atherosclerosis and chronic hypoxia

Pelvic atherosclerosis is thought to affect the voiding function through fibrosis and contraction of smooth muscle cells in the prostate and bladder through alterations in the NOS pathway and inhibitory effects on vascular endothelial growth factor (VEGF), inducing a state of chronic hypoxia in the bladder and prostate that is associated with ED and LUTS [20]. Investigators have demonstrated in rabbits that chronic hypoxia due to pelvic arterial disease resulted in significant detrusor fibrosis and increased bladder pressures. This fibrosis was also associated with significantly higher levels of transforming growth factor beta 1 (TGF-β1) in the bladder tissue [21,22] (Figure 10.4).

Increased levels of TGF-β1 are inhibitory to NOS function and NO production [23], which results in impaired prostatic smooth muscle relaxation [24], potentially contributing to BOO. Prostate smooth muscle isolated from rabbits with pelvic atherosclerosis showed significant contraction on isometric tension measurements as well as structural damage [25]. Chronic pelvic ischemia secondary to atherosclerosis is also associated with prostatic glandular atrophy, resulting in decreased levels of VEGF. VEGF is also an important regulator of the NOS pathway [26] and therefore associated with the PDE5 mechanism.

Autonomic hyperactivity

Autonomic hyperactivity (AH), a component of the metabolic syndrome, refers to a dysregulation of sympathetic and parasympathetic tone. While the relationship between AH and the PDE5 pathway is unclear, animal models have shown clearly that prostatic hyperplasia and ED are induced by AH [27]. Increased sympathetic tone results in penile flaccidity and antagonizes penile erection. Several epidemiologic studies that did not account for confounding showed an increased risk of LUTS with components of metabolic syndrome and AH including type II diabetes, beta blocker requirements, sedentary lifestyle, hypertension, and obesity [28,29].

AH has been shown to lead to LUTS and subjective dysfunctional voiding [30]. In this study, increased American Urological Association symptom scores, BPH Impact Index Scores, and even prostate size significantly correlated with markers for AH such as increased serum norepinephrine levels or abnormal hypertensive response to tilt table testing. This relation remained significant after controlling for confounders [body mass index (BMI), insulin level, physical inactivity, and age].

Rat models have demonstrated an effect on prostatic growth and differentiation through manipulation of autonomic activity. The spontaneously hypertensive rats (SHRs) that develop increased autonomic activity, prostate hyperplasia and ED show an improvement in their ED after brief

Control

Moderate ischemia

Hypercholesterolemia

Severe ischemia

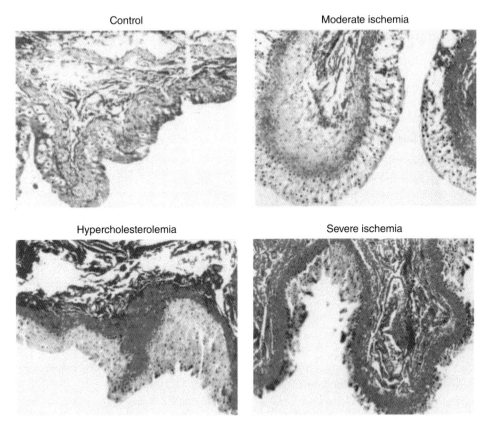

Figure 10.4 Masson's trichrome stain of urothelium in bladder tissues from control, hypercholesterolemia, moderate bladder ischemia, and severe bladder ischemia groups. Chronic moderate bladder ischemia produces marked structural damage in urothelium, causing thickening, disruption of mucosa, vacuolization, and dense fibrosis of the suburothelial layer. Severe bladder ischemia produced more extensive changes causing thickening of urothelium, distortion of mucosa, and more extensive fibrosis in the suburothelial layer. Hypercholesterolemia produced only mild regional thickening of the urothelium but did not produce any destructive changes or fibrosis of the suburothelial layer. Azadozoi 1999 [22]. Reproduced with permission of Elsevier.

aggressive treatment of their hypertension [31]. In a different model, hyperlipidemic rats developed simultaneous prostatic enlargement, bladder overactivity, and ED after being fed a high-fat diet. It remains unclear whether the increase in LUTS or ED is a consequence of an alteration in the function of the bladder/penis itself that generates increased central activation or is the result of a central increase in sensitivity to peripheral signals.

Studies using SHRs, which were shown to develop increased autonomic activity, prostatic hyperplasia, LUTS, and ED, further support a significant role of the autonomic nervous system in promoting the common pathophysiology of these disorders. SHRs had an overabundance of sympathetic fibers innervating the bladder, prostate, and penis, and showed an improvement in erectile function after antihypertensive therapy.

Mechanism of action of phosphodiesterase-5 inhibitors in benign prostatic hyperplasia/lower urinary tract symptoms

Bladder

PDE5 is widely expressed in human bladder tissue and modulates proliferative and smooth muscle relaxant effects through cGMP. A PDE-resistant cGMP analog demonstrated consistent antiproliferative and relaxant effects in human bladder cells. All PDE5-Is showed similar activities, but vardenafil had activity levels similar to that of the cGMP analog. Also, vardenafil significantly reduced nonvoiding contractions of smooth muscle at a level comparable with that of tamsulosin [14].

The RhoA/Rho kinase (ROCK) pathway has been shown to have an important role in the regulation of human bladder muscle tone [7]. As emerging data demonstrated a link between bladder dysfunction and the PDE5 pathway, it seemed plausible that a link existed between PDE5 and the RhoA/Rho kinase pathway. Morelli *et al.* investigated the relationship between the PDE5 pathway and RhoA/Rho kinase, and the effect of vardenafil-induced cGMP accumulation on RhoA/ROCK signaling in the bladder. In this study, vardenafil prevented RhoA membrane translocation and activation, which decreased ROCK activity in rats genetically prone to overactive bladder. Vardenafil dosing led to an accumulation of cGMP, which interrupted the RhoA/ROCK signaling pathway. These results suggested that an improvement in overactive bladder symptoms in rats may be at least partially due to cGMP-dependent RhoA/ROCK inhibition [15].

Prostate

While PDE5-Is have demonstrable effects on bladder musculature, the effect of PDE5-Is locally in prostatic smooth muscle tissue has also proven to be an important part of the physiologic activity of these medications in the treatment of LUTS. Zhao *et al.* found that PDE5-Is increased plasma levels of cyclic nucleotides as well as in prostatic tissue. The elevated ratio of cyclic nucleotides in prostatic tissue to plasma levels indicated a longer duration of action in the prostate [11]. The cyclic nucleotide cGMP has also been implicated in the function of the prostate via the NO-cGMP signal pathway. NOS that exists in the prostate in its neuronal and endothelial forms has been found in prostatic basal cells as well [32], and its expression is reduced in the transition zone of the prostate in BPH. In rat models, reduced expression of NOS resulted in increased smooth muscle cell proliferation and contraction of the prostatic urethra contributing to BOO [11].

Vasculature

Morelli *et al.* found that PDE5 is highly expressed in human vesicular-deferential artery, and investigated the effect of PDE5-Is on prostatic blood flow. PDE5 activity in the arteries, as measured by cGMP breakdown, was significantly reduced by tadalafil, resulting in increased relaxation response to NO donors, as well as improving prostate tissue oxygenation comparable with controls [33]. Similarly, Morelli's study of PDE5-Is' effects on bladder hypoxia showed significant reductions in hypoxia-related induction of smooth muscle specific genes by administration of vardenafil. Together, these data provide strong support for a common link between pelvic vasculature dysfunction and LUTS as well as objective data regarding the usefulness of PDE5-Is in the bladder and prostate via improved blood flow and reduced hypoxia to these organs [15].

Spinal cord

Recently, investigators demonstrated the presence of PDE5 in the lumbosacral spinal cord in a rat model [34]. In addition, the authors showed that sildenafil had no urodynamic effects in normal rats, but pronounced effects in rats obstructed at the bladder outlet. The obstructed rats also had changes in afferent neurons primarily residing in the dorsal root ganglia, suggesting that the PDE5-I might affect their sensitivity to cGMP and thus towards PDE5-I. Sildenafil administered in a small dose (1 µg) directly to the sacral spinal cord had urodynamic effects that could not be explained by a peripheral site of action. The urodynamic effects of PDE5-I in bladder-obstructed rats may thus be mediated at least in part via effects on the sacral spinal cord.

Summary of randomized controlled trials of phosphodiesterase-5 inhibitors versus placebo

LUTS associated with BPH are a common condition of middle-aged and older men. Interestingly, sexual dysfunction is also highly prevalent among this group of men, yet current therapies for the treatment of LUTS/BPH (i.e. AB, 5ARIs, and phytotherapies) are associated with bothersome sexual side effects. This combination of disease and treatment associated side effects set the stage for the discovery for a treatment modality that could help both LUTS and ED. It was suggested for the first time in 2002 that PDE5-Is could improve urinary symptom scores in men [35]. In 2006, Mulhall *et al.* demonstrated in a cohort of men with IPSS scores of >10 and ED that PDE5-Is can improve LUTS [36]. After these uncontrolled studies, several clinical trials have investigated the use of PDE5-Is in LUTS/BPH men. McVary *et al.* performed a systematic review and meta-analysis to determine the relative efficacy and safety of PDE5-Is alone or in combination with AB, and to define the best candidates for this treatment based on clinical features and LUTS severity. In this review, 107 publications were reviewed, but only seven met criteria as randomized controlled trials of PDE5-Is versus placebo for the study. Ultimately, data from 2749 patients were included in the studies that were reviewed in this analysis. The following is a summary of these trials.

Gacci *et al.* examined the treatment response to sildenafil in men with moderate to severe LUTS associated with BPH in a double-blind placebo controlled trial [37]. The sildenafil group ($n = 189$) showed an improvement in IPSS scores of 8.6 points, while the placebo groups IPSS scores improved by only 2.4 points. No change in Q_{max} was observed in either group. This study also examined the effect of BMI with regards to treatment and improvement of LUTS with PDE5 inhibitor and found improvements in IPSS scores regardless of BMI with no change in Q_{max} regardless of BMI [38].

McVary *et al.* studied the efficacy of tadalafil once daily for LUTS/BPH. This study was a single-blind placebo controlled trial with 281 men taking 5 mg of tadalafil for 6 weeks followed by dose escalation to 20 mg for 6 weeks or 12 weeks of placebo. IPSS scores at 6 weeks showed significant improvements for the tadalafil group versus placebo (−2.8 vs −1.2). At 12 weeks, the improvements in the IPSS scores persevered (−3.8 vs −1.7). Notably, when postvoid residual was measured, no significant change was seen. Similarly, there were no changes in uroflometry across groups [39].

Stief *et al.* studied vardenafil dosed twice daily at 10 mg for the treatment of BPH/LUTS in a randomized double-blind placebo-controlled study. Men with IPSS scores of ≥12 were assessed with IPSS, Q_{max}, and PVR after 8 weeks of treatment. Vardenafil showed significant improvements in the mean IPSS score compared with placebo (−5.9 vs 3.6), although only nominal improvements were seen in irritative and obstructive IPSS subscores, erectile function, and Urolife QoL-9 scores. Q_{max} and PVR did not change significantly [40].

In an effort to delineate the dose of PDE5 inhibitor needed to treat BPH/LUTS, Roehrborn *et al.* assigned patients to 12-week treatments of placebo or tadalafil at doses of 2.3, 5, 10, or 20 mg. Mean IPSS scores showed improvements at all dosages compared with placebo. Interestingly, improvements in IPSS scores were documented at 4, 8, and 12 weeks for patients taking tadalafil. Tadalafil showed significant improvements in IPSS obstructive subscore for the 2.5 mg dose, while the 5, 10, and 20 mg dosages showed improvements in both IPSS obstructive and irritative subscores. Q_{max} did not improve at any tadalafil dose. The authors concluded that the 5 mg dosage appeared to provide a positive risk–benefit profile [41].

In a similar study evaluating the effect of once-daily tadalafil on BPH/LUTS, Porst *et al.* evaluated 581 men in a multinational randomized, double-blind, placebo-controlled study. Statistically significant improvements in patient IPSS scores were noted at each dose: −5.4 (2.5 mg), 6.8 (5 mg), 7.9 (10 mg), and 8.2 (20 mg) versus 2.0 for placebo. All *p*-values were <0.05. There were no significant changes in Q_{max} or PVR [42].

Tamimi *et al.* evaluated the PDE5 inhibitor UK-369,003 in a multicenter, double-blind, placebo- and active-controlled study with 418 men over the age of 40 and IPSS scores of 13 or higher. The initial Q_{max} rate was 5–15 mL/s. Patients were given doses of 10, 25, 50, or 100 mg in a modified release (MR) formulation, and 40 mg in an immediate-release formulation for 12 weeks. They found an increasing efficacy with increasing dose of the MR medication. The 100 mg MR and 4 mg immediate release dose IPSS improvements were −2.91 and −2.50 better than placebo respectively. Interestingly, in contrast to the other studies reviewed in this chapter, UK-369,003 improved Q_{max} significantly by 2.1 mL/s compared with 0.84 for placebo [43].

In a continued analysis of tadalafil, Porst *et al.* investigated the efficacy and onset of tadalafil on BPH/LUTS as well as patient and clinician perceptions of changes in urinary symptoms. Once again, tadalafil improved the IPSS results compared with placebo (−5.6 vs −3.6), and IPSS results were apparent after 1 week and statistically significant at 4 weeks. As with many of the other studies investigating the effect of PDE5-Is on Q_{max} and PVR, no significant change was seen in this study [44].

In another randomized controlled trial (RCT), there were no differences from baseline in men randomized to placebo versus tadalafil 20 mg daily for 12 weeks in either noninvasive or invasive urodynamics. This study was conducted to demonstrate the safety of tadalafil daily in terms of negative impact on bladder contractility and found no such effect. Notably, it also did not find any positive effect on contractility or the bladder outlet condition [45].

A systematic review of published material regarding the use of PDE5-Is for LUTS due to BPH was recently published that synthesized the results of several articles totaling 3214 patients enrolled in trials of PDE inhibitors [37]. In this review, 107 publications were reviewed, but only seven met the criteria as RCTs of PDE5-Is versus placebo. It is clear from this analysis that the relationship between ED and LUTS and the effect of PDE5-Is on these conditions has been well studied. Almost 2,800 patients have been studied in RCT comparing PDE5-Is against a placebo. IPSS scores were significantly improved for all treatment groups compared with placebo with a mean difference of almost 3 points on the IPSS. This is an improvement that is clinically relevant for symptomatic men and perceived by patients. The efficacy seems to be quite similar across the different classes of PDE5-Is and the different dosages.

provide a platform from which we may study and compare the effect of treatment for BPH/LUTS, they do not provide empiric data for analysis. Urodynamics is currently the best method for obtaining data that are not influenced by patient perception. The previously mentioned RCTs included several urodynamic parameters, such as Q_{max}, PVR, and uroflowmetry (Table 10.1).

Despite significant symptomatic improvement in the PDE5 inhibitor arms, no urodynamic changes were found in these studies, suggesting that PDE5-Is alone must exert their clinical activity differently than AB. AB are acting mainly to relieve prostatic obstruction, while PDE5-Is may be relieving LUTS via a relaxation effect on the bladder smooth muscle tone [37].

Summary of randomized controlled trials of phosphodiesterase-5 inhibitors and urodynamics

Measurement of improvement in symptoms secondary to BPH and BOO after treatment can be difficult, given that the main tools to do so are validated questionnaires such as the IPSS score. While these questionnaires

Safety

The overall rate of adverse events was calculated to be 16% in the treatment group, whereas that for the placebo group was only 6%. Common side effects of the medications included flushing, gastroesophageal reflux, headache, and dyspepsia, and these are consistent with the side effects noted in the RCT of PDE5-I for ED [37].

Table 10.1 Comparison of urodynamic parameters measured in placebo versus phosphodiesterase type 5 inhibitor randomized controlled trials [37]

Trial	Postvoid residual	Q_{max}	Q_{ave}	V_{comp}
McVary et al. [38]	–	No change	–	–
McVary et al. [39]	No change	No change	No change	No change
Stief et al. [40]	No change	No change	–	–
Roehrborn et al. [41]	No change	No change	No change	–
Porst et al. [42]	No change	No change	–	–
Tamimi et al. [43]	–	No change	–	–
Porst et al. [44]	No change	No change	–	–

Gacci 2012 [37]. Reproduced with permission of Elsevier.

Evidence-based outcomes
of alpha blocker/
phosphodiesterase-5 inhibitor
combination on lower urinary
tract symptoms

Given the association between BPH/LUTS and ED, current evidence regarding the functional outcomes of combination therapy is still modest: A meta-analysis regarding combination therapy concluded that combination therapy results in a reduction in the IPSS score of 1.8 [37]. Interestingly, it was noted in this review that combination PDE5-I and alpha blocker therapy can improve the maximum urinary flow rate significantly compared with α-adrenergic blockers alone, whereas PDE5-Is alone cannot increase Q_{max} compared with placebo. An examination of the various trials involved in this analysis may provide some further insight into the efficacy of certain PDE5-I/alpha blocker combinations.

One large study with 203 subjects treated with combination doxazosin and sildenafil or either drug alone showed significantly decreased IPSS scores, with consistent QoL improvements [46]. When alfuzosin and sildenafil are compared and contrasted, the combination of the two drugs reduced IPSS scores by 24.1%, alfuzosin alone by 15.6%, and sildenafil alone by 11.8%. Voiding diaries were used to assess frequency and showed a reduction of 34.4% for combination therapy and reductions of 26.4% and 14.3% for alfuzosin and sildenafil alone, the latter of which was not statistically significant. Q_{max} was also observed to improve by 21.1% for combination therapy versus 11.7% for alfuzosin, although sildenafil improved Q_{max} by only 6.2%, which did not reach statistical significance [47]. The combination of alfuzosin and tadalafil was compared during a 12-week study that showed reduced IPSS scores (41.6%), along with QoL improvement (49.5%), both of which were statistically superior to either drug used alone: alfuzosin – IPSS, 27.2%; Q_{max}, 21.7%; QoL, 27.2%; tadalafil – IPSS, 8.4%; Q_{max}, 9.5%; QoL, 28.8% [48]. Another trial compared tamsulosin with sildenafil with Q_{max} and QoL parameters measured that, notably, included a 4-day-per-week administration and showed no significant difference in IPSS or QoL, but Q_{max} was increased [49]. Finally, a study comparing combination therapy of tamsulosin and tadalafil also showed a significant reduction in IPSS scores [50].

In 2011, tadalafil (Cialis once a day) was approved by the Food and Drug Administration for the treatment of ED and LUTS secondary to BPH based on three phase III clinical trials that demonstrated significant improvements in IPSS scores in men over the age of 45 with bothersome LUTS. In addition, it was approved for simultaneous treatment of ED and BPH/LUTS. Tadalafil is contraindicated for concomitant use of organic nitrates such as nitroglycerin and isosorbide dinitrate, as it may potentiate the hypotensive effect of these medications. Caution is warranted in the use of tadalafil in patients with unstable angina, New York Heart Association (NYHA) Class 2 or greater heart disease, hypotension, or cerebrovascular accident (CVA) in the last 6 months. Concurrent consumption of alcohol is discouraged, as it may lead to orthostatic hypotension.

While properly powered data on the safety, use, and efficacy of AB with PDE5-Is are limited, there are several studies that have examined the combined/synergistic effects of these two medications, and their results warrant examination. Given that the target mechanisms for both of these medications may potentially interact with vascular organs resulting in symptomatic hemodynamic events, several studies have been performed to examine the safety of combination therapy of AB and PDE5-Is. In middle-aged men, the combination of sildenafil with alfuzosin did not show any significant hemodynamic changes [47]. Similarly, another study examining hemodynamic changes in patients receiving tamsulosin and tadalafil failed to find any significant resultant hypotension [50]. When doxazosin, at a dose of 8 mg, was combined with tadalafil, however, a significant decrease in systolic blood pressure was observed of 9.8 mmHg. The other arm of that same trial used tamsulosin instead of doxazosin, and no significant hypotension was observed, though the dose of tamsulosin was 0.4 mg [51]. A study of patients receiving doxazosin and vardenafil also failed to show any hypotensive events [52]. One study did show that sildenafil alone at a dose of 100 mg decreased systolic blood pressure by 11 mmHg, but when tamsulosin was added, no further alteration in blood pressure was observed [49].

Limitations

The information provided by the studies involving PDE5-Is contributes to a growing database of information from which clinicians can draw recommendations with regard to PDE5-Is in the treatment of BPH/LUTS. The nature of these studies, however, lessens the overall value due to the small size populations, inconsistent recording of safety data, and short duration. One recent long-term study showed that patients randomized to placebo that were switched to 5 mg of tadalafil also showed an improvement. Patients switched to higher dosages of medication (i.e. 2.5–5 mg) had improved IPSS scores, while those maintained on one dose did not show any additional improvement at 1 year but did not deteriorate either [53]. Unfortunately, no data exist so far with regard to ejaculation or global sexuality improvement that would be useful in the context of the treatment of BPH/LUTS and ED with PDE5-Is. Also, there are no randomized control trials comparing different classes of PDE5-Is, nor are there any studies reporting side-effect profiles such as sexual outcomes for combination therapy of PDE5-Is and 5ARIs. Finally, the cost-effectiveness of PDE5-I therapy has not been addressed satisfactorily.

Dos and don'ts

- PDE5-Is can be a useful therapy in treating men with LUTS secondary to BPH.
- PDE5-I/alpha blocker combination therapy can significantly improve symptoms related to BPH.
- Do not use PDE5-Is in combination with other drugs that may induce vasodilation such as nitroprusside, nitroglycerine, or isosorbide.
- Do not use PDE5-Is in patients with NYHA class 2 (or worse) heart disease, history of CVA in the last 6 months, unstable angina, or hypotension.
- Caution patients against the concurrent use of PDE5-Is and alcohol.

Bibliography

1 Nicolosi A, Moreira ED Jr, Shirai M, Bin Mohd Tambi MI, Glasser DB. Epidemiology of erectile dysfunction in four countries: cross-national study of the prevalence and correlates of erectile dysfunction. *Urology*. 2003;61:201–6.

2 Lukacs B, Leplège A, Thibault P, Jardin A. Prospective study of men with clinical benign prostatic hyperplasia treated with alfuzosin by general practitioners: 1-year results. *Urology*. 1996; 48(5):731–40.

3 Rosen R, Altwein J, Boyle P, Kirby RS, Lukacs B, Meuleman E, *et al*. Lower urinary tract symptoms and male sexual dysfunction: the multinational survey of the aging male (MSAM-7). *Eur Urol*. 2003;44(6):637–49.

4 Hansen BJ, Flyger H, Brasso K, Schou J, Nordling J, Thorup Andersen J, *et al*. Validation of the self-administered Danish Prostatic Symptom Score (DAN-PSS-1) system for use in benign prostatic hyperplasia. *Br J Urol*. 1995;76(4):451–8.

5 Wein AJ, Coyne KS, Tubaro A, Sexton CC, Kopp ZS, Aiyer LP. The impact of lower urinary tract symptoms on male sexual health: EpiLUTS. *BJU Int*. 2009;103(Suppl 3):33–41. doi:10.1111/j.1464-410X.2009.08447.x.19.

6 Gacci M1, Eardley I, Giuliano F, Hatzichristou D, Kaplan SA, Maggi M, *et al*. Critical analysis of the relationship between sexual dysfunctions and lower urinary tract symptoms due to benign prostatic hyperplasia. *Eur Urol*. 2011;60(4):809–25. doi:10.1016/j.eururo.2011.06.037. Epub 2011 Jun 29.

7 Kedia GT, Uckert S, Jonas U, Kuczyk MA, Burchardt M. The nitric oxide pathway in the human prostate: clinical implications in men with lower urinary tract symptoms. *World J Urol* 2008;26:603–9.

8 Podlasek CA, Zelner DJ, Bervig TR, Gonzalez CM, McKenna KE, McVary KT. Characterization and localization of nitric oxide synthase isoforms in the BB/WOR diabetic rat. *J Urol*. 2001;166(2): 746–55.

9 Richter K, Heuer O, Uckert S, Stief CG, Jonas U, Wolf G. Immunocytochemical distribution of nitric oxide synthases in the human prostate [Abstract 347]. *J Urol*. 2004;171(Suppl):262–6.

10 Bloch W, Klotz T, Loch C, Schmidt G, Engelmann U, Addicks K. Distribution of nitric oxide synthase implies a regulation of circulation, smooth muscle

tone, and secretory function in the human prostate by nitric oxide. *Prostate*. 1997;33:1–8.

11 Zhao C, Kim SH, Lee SW, Jeon JH, Kang KK, Choi SB, *et al*. Activity of phosphodiesterase type 5 inhibitors in patients with lower urinary tract symptoms due to benign prostatic hyperplasia. *BJU Int*. 2011;107(12):1943–7.

12 Guh JH, Hwang TL, Ko FN, Chueh SC, Lai MK, Teng CM. Antiproliferative effect in human prostatic smooth muscle cells by nitric oxide donor. *Mol Pharmacol*. 1998;53:467–74.

13 Montorsi F, Corbin J, Phillips S. Review of phosphodiesterases in the urogenital system: new directions for therapeutic intervention. *J Sex Med*. 2004;1(3):322–36.

14 Filippi S, Morelli A, Sandner P, Fibbi B, Mancina R, Marini M, *et al*. Characterization and functional role of androgen-dependent PDE5 activity in the bladder. *Endocrinology*. 148(3):1019–29.

15 Morelli A, Filippi S, Sandner P, Fibbi B, Chavalmane AK, Silvestrini E, *et al*. Vardenafil modulates bladder contractility through cGMP-mediated inhibition of RhoA/Rho kinase signaling pathway in spontaneously hypertensive rats. *J Sex Med*. 2009;6(6):1594–608.

16 Chang S, Hypolite JA, Changolkar A, Wein AJ, Chacko S, DiSanto ME. Increased contractility of diabetic rabbit corpora smooth muscle in response to endothelin is mediated via Rho-kinase beta. *Int J Impot Res*. 2003;15(1):53–62.

17 Bivalacqua TJ, Champion HC, Usta MF, Cellek S, Chitaley K, Webb RC, *et al*. RhoA/Rho-kinase suppresses endothelial nitric oxide synthase in the penis: A mechanism for diabetes-associated erectile dysfunction. *Proc Natl Acad Sci USA*. 2004;101: 9121–6.7.

18 Vignozzi L, Morelli A, Filippi S, Ambrosini S, Mancina R, Luconi M, *et al*. Testosterone regulates RhoA/Rho-kinase signaling in two distinctanimal models of chemical diabetes. *J Sex Med*. 2007; 4:620–32.

19 Mouli S, McVary KT. PDE5 inhibitors for LUTS. *Prostate Cancer Prostatic Dis*. 2009;12(4):316–24. doi:10.1038/pcan.2009.27. Epub 2009 Aug 18.

20 Tarcan T, Azadzoi KM, Siroky MB, Goldstein I, Krane RJ. Age related erectile and voiding dysfunction: the role of arterial insufficiency. *Br J Urol*. 1998;82(Suppl 1):26–33.

21 Azadzoi KM, Tarcan T, Siroky MB, Krane RJ. Atherosclerosis induced chronic ischemia causes

bladder fibrosis and noncompliance in the rabbit. *J Urol.* 1999;161:1626–35.

22 Azadozoi K, Tarcan T, Kozlowski R, Krane R, Siroky M. Overactivity and structural changes in the chronically ischemic bladder. *J Urol.* 1999:162 (5) 1768–78.

23 Zhang HY, Phan SH. Inhibition of myofibroblast apoptosis by transforming growth factor β1. *Am J Respir Cell Mol Biol.* 1999;21:658–5.

24 Kozlowski R, Kershen RT, Siroky MB, Krane RJ, Azadzoi KM. Chronic ischemia alters prostate structure and reactivity in rabbits. *J Urol.* 2001;165:1019–26.

25 Azadozoi KM *et al.* Chronic ischemia increases prostatic smooth muscle contraction in the rabbit. *J Urol.* 2003;170:659–63.

26 Papapetropoulos A, García-Cardeña G, Madri JA, Sessa WC. Nitric oxide production contributes to the angiogenic properties of vascular endothelial growth factor in human endothelial cells. *J Clin Invest.* 1997;100(12):3131–9.

27 McVary KT. Sexual function and alpha-blockers. *Rev Urol.* 2005;7(Suppl 8):S3–11.

28 Hammarsten J, Hogstedt B. Clinical, anthropometric, metabolic and insulin profile of men with fast annual growth rates of benign prostatic hyperplasia. *Blood Press.* 1999;8:29.

29 Meigs JB, Mohr B, Barry MJ, Collins MM, McKinlay JB. Risk factors for clinical benign prostatic hyperplasia in a community-based population of healthy aging men. *J Clin Epidemiol.* 2001;54:935.

30 McVary KT, Rademaker A, Lloyd GL, *et al.* Autonomic nervous system overactivity in men with lower urinary tract symptoms secondary to benign prostatic hyperplasia. *J Urol.* 2005;174: 1327–433.

31 Hale TM, Okabe H, Bushfield TL, *et al.* Recovery of erectile function after brief aggressive antihypertensive therapy. *J Urol.* 2002;168:348–54.

32 Richter K, Heuer O, Uckert S, Stief CG, Jonas U, Wolf G. Immunocytochemical distribution of nitric oxide synthases in the human prostate [Abstract 347]. *J Urol.* 2004;171(Suppl):262–6.

33 Morelli A, Sarchielli E, Comeglio P, Filippi S, Mancina R, Gacci M, *et al.* Phosphodiesterase type 5 expression in human and rat lower urinary tract tissues and the effect of tadalafil on prostate gland oxygenation in spontaneously hypertensive rats. *J Sex Med.* 2011;8(10):2746–60.

34 Füllhase C, Hennenberg M, Giese A, Schmidt M, Strittmatter F, Soler R, *et al.* Presence of phosphodiesterase type 5 (PDE5) in the spinal cord and its involvement in bladder outflow obstruction related bladder overactivity. *J Urol.* 190(4):1430–5.

35 Sairam K, Kulinskaya E, McNicholas TA, Boustead GB, Hanbury DC. Sildenafil influences lower urinary tract symptoms. *BJU Int.* 2002;90(9):836–9.

36 Mulhall JP, Guhring P, Parker M, Hopps C. Assessment of the impact of sildenafil citrate on lower urinary tract symptoms in men with erectile dysfunction. *J Sex Med.* 2006;3(4):662–7.

37 Gacci M, Corona G, Salvi M, Vignozzi L, McVary KT, Kaplan SA, *et al.* A systematic review and meta-analysis on the use of phosphodiesterase 5 inhibitors alone or in combination with α-blockers for lower urinary tract symptoms due to benign prostatic hyperplasia. *Eur Urol.* 2012;61(5): 994–1003

38 McVary KT, Monnig W, Camps JL Jr, Young JM, Tseng LJ, van den Ende G. Sildenafil citrate improves erectile function and urinary symptoms in men with erectile dysfunction and lower urinary tract symptoms associated with benign prostatic hyperplasia: a randomized, double-blind trial. *J Urol.* 2007;177:1071–7.

39 McVary KT, Roehrborn CG, Kaminetsky JC, Auerbach SM, Wachs B, Young JM, *et al.* Tadalafil relieves lower urinary tract symptoms secondary to benign prostatic hyperplasia. *J Urol.* 2007; 177:1401–7.

40 Stief CG, Porst H, Neuser D, Beneke M, Ulbrich E. A randomised, placebo-controlled study to assess the efficacy of twice daily vardenafil in the treatment of lower urinary tract symptoms secondary to benign prostatic hyperplasia. *Eur Urol.* 53; 2008:1236–44.

41 Roehrborn CG, McVary KT, Elion-Mboussa A, Viktrup L. Tadalafil administered once daily for lower urinary tract symptoms secondary to benign prostatic hyperplasia: a dose finding study. *J Urol.* 2008;180:1228–1234.

42 Porst H, McVary KT, Montorsi F, Sutherland P, Elion-Mboussa A, Wolka AM, *et al.* Effects of once-daily tadalafil on erectile function in men with erectile dysfunction and signs and symptoms of benign prostatic hyperplasia. *Eur Urol.* 2009; 56(4):727–35.

43 Tamimi NA, Mincik I, Haughie S, Lamb J, Crossland A, Ellis P. A placebo-controlled study

investigating the efficacy and safety of the phosphodiesterase type 5 inhibitor UK-369,003 for the treatment of men with lower urinary tract symptoms associated with clinical benign prostatic hyperplasia. *BJU Int.* 2010;106(5):674–80.

44 Porst H, Kim ED, Casabé AR, Mirone V, Secrest RJ, Xu L, *et al.* Efficacy and safety of tadalafil once daily in the treatment of men with lower urinary tract symptoms suggestive of benign prostatic hyperplasia: results of an international randomized, double-blind, placebo-controlled trial. *Eur Urol.* 2011;60:1105–13.

45 Dmochowski R, Roehrborn C, Klise S, Xu L, Kaminetsky J, Kraus S. Urodynamic effects of once daily tadalafil in men with lower urinary tract symptoms secondary to clinical benign prostatic hyperplasia: a randomized, placebo controlled 12-week clinical trial. *J Urol.* 2010; 183(3):1092–7.

46 Jin Z, Zhang ZC, Liu JH, Lu J, Tang YX, Sun XZ, *et al.* An open, comparative, multicentre clinical study of combined oral therapy with sildenafil and doxazosin GITS for treating Chinese patients with erectile dysfunction and lower urinary tract symptoms secondary to benign prostatic hyperplasia. *Asian J Androl.* 2011;13:630.

47 Kaplan SA, Gonzalez RR, Te AE. Combination of alfuzosin and sildenafil is superior to monotherapy in treating lower urinary tract symptoms and erectile dysfunction. *Eur Urol.* 2007;51:1717.

48 Liguori G, Trombetta C, De Giorgi G, Pomara G, Maio G, Vecchio D, *et al.* Efficacy and safety of combined oral therapy with tadalafil and alfuzosin: an integrated approach to the management of patients with lower urinary tract symptoms and erectile dysfunction. Preliminary report. *J Sex Med.* 2009;6:544.

49 Tuncel A, Nalcacioglu V, Ener K, Aslan Y, Aydin O, Atan A. Sildenafil citrate and tamsulosin combination is not superior to monotherapy in treating lower urinary tract symptoms and erectile dysfunction. *World J Urol.* 2010;28:17.

50 Bechara A1, Romano S, Casabé A, Haime S, Dedola P, Hernández C, *et al.* Comparative efficacy assessment of tamsulosin vs. tamsulosin plus tadalafil in the treatment of LUTS/BPH. Pilot study. *J Sex Med.* 2008;5:2170.

51 Kloner RA, Jackson G, Emmick JT, Mitchell MI, Bedding A, Warner MR, *et al.* Interaction between the phosphodiesterase 5 inhibitor, tadalafil and 2 alpha-blockers, doxazosin and tamsulosin in healthy normotensive men. *J Urol.* 2004;172:1935.

52 Ng CF, Wong A, Cheng CW, Chan ES, Wong HM, Hou SM. Effect of vardenafil on blood pressure profile of patients with erectile dysfunction concomitantly treated with doxazosin gastrointestinal therapeutic system for benign prostatic hyperplasia. *J Urol.* 2008;180:1042.

53 Donatucci CF, Brock GB, Goldfischer ER, Pommerville PJ, Elion-Mboussa A, Kissel JD, *et al.* Tadalafil administered once daily for lower urinary tract symptoms secondary to benign prostatic hyperplasia: a 1-year, open-label extension study. *BJU Int.* 2011;107:1110–6.

CHAPTER 11

Combination Medical Therapy for Male Lower Urinary Tract Symptoms

Claus G. Roehrborn
Department of Urology, UT Southwestern Medical Center, Dallas, TX, USA

Key points

- There are clearly defined mechanisms of action for alpha adrenergic receptor blockers (AARBs), 5α-reductase inhibitors (5ARIs), antimuscarinics, and, to a lesser degree, phosphodiesterase type 5 inhibitors (PDE5-Is) in the management of men with lower urinary tract symptoms (LUTS) suggestive of benign prostatic hyperplasia (BPH).
- There are currently five AARBs approved for the treatment of LUTS/BPH, two 5ARIs, and one PDE5-I, while antimuscarinics are used based mostly on a post hoc analysis of male subsets of large-scale trials in patients with overactive bladder (OAB).
- Combinations of AARB + 5ARI, AARB + antimuscarinics, and AARB + PDE5-I have all been studied in uncontrolled and controlled clinical trials.
- In properly chosen patients, the various combinations have been found to be effective in symptom relief and often superior to monotherapy.
- Adverse events associated with these combination therapies have been generally tolerable, self-limited, and reversible.
- There are intriguing possibilities for other combination therapies such as 5ARIs + PDE5-I that have to date not been properly explored.

Combination medical therapy: alpha receptor blocker + 5α-reductase inhibitor

Introduction and mechanisms of action

A recent systematic review and associated tables (Tables 11.1–11.3) serve as the basis for this section [1]. AARBs presumably work by relaxation of the smooth muscle at the bladder neck, the prostate, and its capsule, and perhaps in the central nervous system and spinal cord where there are also alpha receptors [2–5]. 5ARIs work by actually addressing the underlying condition of BPH, by preferentially shrinking the glandular epithelial component of the prostate and thereby providing presumably the outflow condition

---

Male Lower Urinary Tract Symptoms and Benign Prostatic Hyperplasia, First Edition.
Edited by Steven A. Kaplan and Kevin T. McVary.
© 2014 John Wiley & Sons, Ltd. Published 2014 by John Wiley & Sons, Ltd.

Table 11.1 α_1-Adrenoceptor antagonists and 5α-reductase inhibitor combination trial characteristics and subjective outcome measures

Trial	Years trial was performed	Patients, no.	Drug (dose)	Trial duration, mo	Primary end point	Age of patients and size of prostate at baseline, mean±SD	Inclusion criteria	Change of symptom score from baseline (IPSS or AUA-SS)			
								α1-Blocker	5-ARI	Placebo	Combination
VA-COOP [15]	1992–1995	1229	Terazosin (10mg) finasteride (5mg)	12	AUA-SS and Q_{max}	65±7yr and 37±1ml	Age 45-80yr AUA-SS >8 PSA ≤10ng/ml Q_{max} 4-15ml/s No limits on prostate size	**-6.1** Significant vs baseline VS 5-ARI vs placebo	**-3.2** Significant vs baseline	**-2.6** Significant vs baseline	**-6.2** Significant vs baseline vs 5-ARI vs placebo
ALFIN [17]	1994-1996	1051	Alfuzosin (2 × 5mg) finasteride (5mg)	6	IPSS and Q_{max}	63±6yr and 41±24ml	Age 50-75yr IPSS >7 PSA ≤10ng/ml Q_{max} 5–15ml/s No limits on prostate size	**-6.3** Significant vs baseline vs 5-ARI	**-5.2** Significant vs baseline	**n.a.**	**-6.1** Significant vs baseline vs 5-ARI
PREDICT [22]	2001-2007	1095	Doxazosin (4–8mg) finasteride (5mg)	12	IPSS and Q_{max}	63±7yr and 36±14ml (assessed by DRE)	Age 50-80yr IPSS >12 PSA ≤10ng/ml Qmax 5–15ml/s Prostatic enlargement assessed by DRE	**-83** Significant vs baseline vs 5-ARI vs placebo	**-6.6** Significant vs baseline	**-5.7** Significant vs baseline	**-8.5** Significant vs baseline vs 5-ARI vs placebo

Study	Years	N	Drug (dose)	Follow-up (mo)	Inclusion criteria	Primary endpoint				
MTOPS [19]	1995–2001	3047	Doxazosin (4–8 mg) finasteride (5 mg)	54–72	Age >50yr AUA-SS 8–30 PSA ≤10ng/ml Q_{max} 4–14ml/s No limits on prostate size	Clinical progression (as defined by, eg, an AUA score increase of 4 points)	−6.6 Significant vs baseline vs placebo vs 5-ARI	−5.6 Significant vs baseline vs placebo	−4.9 Significant vs baseline vs placebo	Significant vs baseline	−7.4 Significant vs baseline vs placebo vs 5-ARI vs α1-blocker
CombAT [28]	2003–2009	3195–3822	Tamsulosin (0.4mg) dutasteride (0.5mg)	24–48	Age >50yr IPSS >12 PSA 1.5–10ng/ml Q_{max} 5–15ml/s Prostate size >30ml	Time to first AUR or BPH-related surgery	−3.8 Significant vs baseline	−5.3 Significant vs baseline vs al-blocker	n.a. n.a.	−63 Significant vs baseline vs 5-ARI vs α1-blocker

α1-blocker = α1-adrenoceptor antagonist; 5-ARI = 5α-reductase inhibitor; ALFIN = Alfuzosin, Finasteride, and Combination in the Treatment of Benign Prostatic Hyperplasia; AUA-SS = American Urological Association symptom score; AUR = acute urinary retention; BPH = benign prostatic hyperplasia; CombAT = Combination of Avodart and Tamsulosin; DRE = digital rectal examination; IPSS = International Prostate Symptom Score; MTOPS = Medical Therapy of Prostatic Symptoms; Q_{max} = maximum flow rate of urine; PSA = prostate-specific antigen; n.a. = not assessed; PREDICT = Prospective European Doxazosin and Combination Therapy; SD = standard deviation; VA-COOP = Veteran Affairs Cooperative Study.

Table 11.2 α_1-Adrenoceptor antagonists and 5α-reductase inhibitor combination objective outcome measures*

	Change in Q_{max} from baseline (ml/s)				Change in prostate size from baseline			
	α1-Blocker	5-ARI	Placebo	Combination	α1-Blocker	5-ARI	Placebo	Combination
VA-COOP [15] (terazosin/ finasteride)	+2.7 Significant vs baseline vs 5-ARI vs placebo	+1.6 Significant vs baseline	+1.4 Significant vs baseline	+3.2 Significant vs baseline vs 5-ARI vs placebo	+0.5 ml Significant vs baseline	−6.1 ml Significant vs baseline vs 5-ARI vs placebo	+0.5 ml Significant vs baseline	−7 ml Significant vs baseline vs 5-ARI vs placebo
ALFIN [17] (alfuzosin/ finasteride)	+1.8 Significant vs baseline	+1.8 Significant vs baseline	n.a.	+2.3 Significant vs baseline	−0.2 ml n.s.	−4.3 ml Significant vs baseline vs α1-blocker	n.a.	−4.9 ml Significant vs baseline vs α1-blocker
PREDICT [22] (doxazosin/ finasteride)	+3.6 Significant vs baseline vs 5-ARI vs placebo	+1.8 Significant vs baseline	+1.4 Significant vs baseline	+3.8 Significant vs baseline vs 5-ARI vs placebo	n.a.	n.a.	n.a.	n.a.
MTOPS [19] (doxazosin/ finasteride)	+2.5 Significant vs baseline vs placebo	+2.2 Significant vs baseline vs placebo	+1.4 Significant vs baseline	+3.7 Significant vs baseline vs placebo vs 5-ARI vs α1-blocker	+24% n.r.	−19% n.r.	+24% n.r.	−19% n.r.
CombAT [28] (tamsulosin/ dutasteride)	+0.7 Significant vs baseline	+2.0 Significant vs baseline vs α1-blocker	n.a.	+2.4 Significant vs baseline vs 5-ARI vs α1-blocker	+4.6% Significant vs baseline	−28% Significant vs baseline vs α1-blocker	n.a.	−27.3% Significant vs baseline vs 5-ARI vs α1-blocker

Qmax=maximum flow rate of urine; 5-ARI=5α-reductase inhibitor; α_1-blocker=α1-adrenoceptor antagonist; ALFIN=Alfuzosin, Finasteride, and Combination in the Treatment of Benign Prostatic Hyperplasia; AUR=acute urinary retention; CombAT=Combination of Avodart and Tamsulosin; MTOPS=Medical Therapy of Prostatic Symptoms; n.a. = not assessed; n.r. = not reported; PREDICT=Prospective European Doxazosin and Combination Therapy; VA-COOP=Veteran Affairs Cooperative Study.

*Prostate size was given only as percentage value in some trials.

Table 11.3 α_1-Adrenoceptor antagonists and 5α-reductase inhibitor combination selected side effects

	al-Blocker, %								5ARI, %								Placebo, %								Combination, %							
	Headache	Dizziness and hypotension	Loss of libido	Impotence	Side effects, total	Severe side effects	Discontinuation rate due to side effects	AUR	Headache	Dizziness and hypotension	Loss of libido	Impotence	Side effects, total	Severe side effects	Discontinuation rate due to side effects	AUR	Headache	Dizziness and hypotension	Loss of libido	Impotence	Side effects, total	Severe side effects	Discontinuation rate due to side effects	AUR	Headache	Dizziness and hypotension	Loss of libido	Impotence	Side effects, total	Severe side effects	Discontinuation rate due to side effects	AUR
VA-COOP [15] (terazosin/finasteride)	6	26	3	6	n.r.	n.r.	7.0	n.r.	6	8	5	9	n.r.	n.r.	6.1	n.r.	3	7	1	5	n.r.	n.r.	1.9	n.r.	5	21	5	9	n.r.	n.r.	9.4	n.r.
ALFIN [17] (alfuzosin/finasteride)	2	1.7	0.6	2.2	27	1.7	7.8	0.6	1.2	1.2	1.7	6.7	26	2.9	5.9	0.3	n.a.	n.a.	n.a.	n.a.	n.a.	n.a.	n.a.	n.a.	1.4	2.3	2	7.4	26	2.3	8.1	0.3
PREDICT [22] (doxazosin/finasteride)	n.r.	15.6	3.6	5.8	n.r.	n.r.	11.6	0.4	n.r.	8	3.4	4.9	n.r.	n.r.	13.6	1.9	n.r.	7.4	1.9	10.5	n.r.	n.r.	11.9	2.6	n.r.	13.6	2.1	3.3	n.r.	n.r.	12.6	0
MTOPS [19] (doxazosin/finasteride)	n.r.	4.4*	1.5*	3.5*	27	n.r.	n.r.	1	n.r.	2.3*	2.3*	4.5*	24	n.r.	n.r.	<1	n.r.	2.2*	1.4*	3.3*	n.r.	n.r.	n.r.	2	n.r.	5.3*	2.5*	5.1*	18	n.r.	n.r.	<1
CombAT [28] (tamsulosin/dutasteride)	n.r.	2	2	5	19	<1	4	6.8	n.r.	<1	3	7	21	<1	4	2.7	n.r.	n.a.	n.a.	n.a.	n.a.	n.a.	n.a	2.7	n.r.	2	4	9	28	<1	6	2.2

α_1-Blocker=α1-adrenoceptor antagonist; 5-ARI=5α-reductase inhibitor; ALFIN=Alfuzosin, Finasteride, and Combination in the Treatment of Benign Prostatic Hyperplasia; AUR=acute urinary retention; CombAT=Combination of Avodart and Tamsulosin; MTOPS=Medical Therapy of Prostatic Symptoms; n.a. = not assessed; n.r. = not reported; PREDICT=Prospective European Doxazosin and Combination Therapy; VA-COOP=Veteran Affairs Cooperative Study.

*Rate per 100 person-years of follow-up.

and leading to symptom improvement [6–8]. No alternative mechanisms have been proposed, although effects on vascular endothelial growth factor have been reported but not linked to male LUTS per se [9,10]. Since AARBs begin to be effective within a week, whereas 5ARIs usually require at least 3 months to become effective, the combination of these two drug classes has generated considerable interest.

Small studies of short duration

Pushkar and colleagues published and/or presented data from a series of studies in which patients received combination therapy with finasteride and terazosin [11,12]. The investigators reported superior outcomes with combination therapy. The studies, however, lacked placebo control, and the outcome assessment was inconsistent.

Another study compared the efficacy of terazosin, finasteride, or a combination of both in 195 men with enlarged prostate glands [13]. All patients – those receiving terazosin ($n = 64$), finasteride ($n = 65$), or combination therapy ($n = 66$) – were well matched at baseline. Decreases in symptom scores of 4.9, 4.1, and 6.4 points from baseline were obtained at 12 months for the terazosin, finasteride, and combination therapy arms, respectively; the differences between the combination therapy group and both the finasteride and terazosin groups were significant, whereas the difference between the terazosin and finasteride groups was not. Improvements in flow rate of 1.2 mL/s, 4.0 mL/s, and 4.9 mL/s were obtained for the terazosin, finasteride, and combination therapy groups, respectively. The authors provided information on study patients with prostates of 40 mL or larger ($n = 33$). In the finasteride group, these patients had greater improvements in symptom score compared with those with prostates smaller than 40 mL ($n = 32$; −6.3 points vs −1.6 points; $P < 0.01$). However, prostate size did not influence the change in symptom score in the terazosin or combination therapy groups. Similarly, the improvement in peak urinary flow rate was greater for the patients in the finasteride group who had prostate volumes of 40 mL or more (5.4 mL/s vs 3.2 mL/s; $P < 0.05$). Although this study also lacked a placebo group, it differed from the previous studies in that it enrolled patients with particularly large prostates [on average 46.8 mL as measured by transrectal ultrasonography (TRUS)].

Placebo-controlled and direct comparator studies

In 1998, Debruyne and colleagues [14] reported results on behalf of the Alfuzosin vs. Finasteride vs. Comb Study Group. This randomized, double-blind, multicenter trial compared the effects of 6 months of therapy with a sustained-release formulation of the α_1-adrenergic receptor blocker alfuzosin, 5 mg twice daily ($n = 358$); finasteride, 5 mg once daily ($n = 344$); or both drugs in combination ($n = 349$) [14]. Patients in the alfuzosin, finasteride, and combination therapy groups had decreases from the baseline symptom score of 6.3, 5.2, and 6.1 points, respectively. The difference in score reduction was significant between the alfuzosin and finasteride groups ($P = 0.01$), as well as between the combination therapy and finasteride groups ($P = 0.03$). Improvements in peak flow rate (alfuzosin, 1.8 mL/s; finasteride, 1.8 mL/s; combination therapy, 2.3 mL/s) were not significantly different among treatment groups. Reductions in prostate volume of slightly more than 10% were obtained in the finasteride and combination therapy arms. Prostate-specific antigen (PSA) levels also decreased significantly in these two treatment arms, whereas no change was observed in the alfuzosin arm. This trial, as well as the previously mentioned studies, lacked a placebo group and, therefore, did not allow a systematic analysis of the effect of prostate volume on response to treatment.

The Veterans Affairs (VA) Cooperative Studies Benign Prostatic Hyperplasia Study Group conducted a 1-year, double-blind, placebo-controlled trial in men with BPH [15–20]. A total of 1229 men were randomized to receive placebo (n = 305); finasteride, 5 mg/day (n = 310); terazosin at a forced titration to 10 mg/day, with permission to reduce the dosage to 5 mg/day in the event of an adverse effect (n = 305); or a combination of finasteride and terazosin (n = 309).

At 52 weeks, symptom scores in the terazosin and combination groups were significantly lower than at baseline and lower than those in the placebo and finasteride groups. Changes in symptom score from baseline for the finasteride and placebo groups were also significant, but the difference between those groups was not. The same was true for the improvement in peak urinary flow rate. As expected, a prostate volume reduction and decrease in PSA level (by nearly 50%) were noted in the finasteride and combination arms only [18]. Several secondary analyses of the VA COOP study have been published. An analysis of bother and quality-of-life (QoL) measures found that group mean differences in symptom problem and BPH impact scores between the finasteride and placebo and between the terazosin and combination groups were not statistically or clinically significant. Group mean differences in all outcome measures were highly statistically significant between the terazosin and finasteride, and combination and finasteride groups. The percentages of subjects who rated improvement as marked or moderate with placebo, finasteride, terazosin, and

combination were 39, 44, 61, and 65%, respectively [19]. There were no differences in those patients enrolled with a baseline prostate volume of 50 mL or greater [19]. Filling and voiding subscores of the International Prostate Symptom Score (IPSS) were analyzed but found not to be clinically useful [16]. Johnson reported on nocturia episodes in the VA COOP study [15]. Of the 1078 men available for analysis 1040 (96.5%) had at least one episode of nocturia at baseline, and 38 (3.5%) had no more than one episode (baseline nocturia is an average of two measures). Of those 1040 men, 788 (75.8%) had two or more nocturia episodes. Overall, nocturia decreased from a baseline mean of 2.5 to 1.8, 2.1, 2.0, and 2.1 episodes in the terazosin, finasteride, combination, and placebo groups, respectively. Of men with two or more episodes of nocturia, a 50% reduction in nocturia was seen in 39%, 25%, 32%, and 22% in the terazosin, finasteride, combination, and placebo groups, respectively. Changes in nocturia were correlated with changes in reported bother from nocturia (Pearson correlation 0.48), BPH Impact Index (0.32), and overall satisfaction with urinary symptoms (0.33).

The Prospective European Doxazosin and Combination Therapy study group recently published data from a similar European multicenter, randomized, placebo-controlled trial, also lasting 52 weeks [21]. The study included 1095 patients with LUTS and BPH aged 50–80 years, each with an IPSS of 12 or higher, a maximum flow rate between 5 mL/s and 15 mL/s with a total voided volume of more than 150 mL, and an enlarged prostate as determined by digital rectal examination (DRE). Patients were randomized to receive placebo; finasteride, 5 mg; doxazosin titrated to response based on an IPSS improvement of 30% or more and an improvement of 3 mL or greater in maximum flow rate; or a combination of finasteride and doxazosin.

Similar to the results of the VA Cooperative Trial, both doxazosin and the combination of doxazosin and finasteride produced statistically significant improvements in all outcome parameters (IPSS, maximum flow rate, QoL score, and BPH Impact Index score) compared with placebo and finasteride alone ($P < 0.05$). Finasteride alone did not differ from placebo with respect to maximum flow rate and QoL score, and differed only marginally with respect to BPH Impact Index score and total IPSS ($0.05 \leq P < 0.10$).

There are two trials examining the combination of AARB and 5ARIs against monotherapy with an alpha blocker and in the case of the Medical Therapy of Prostatic Symptoms (MTOPS) study against placebo over a period of 4 years [Combination of Avodart and Tamsulosin (CombAT)] and 5.5 years (MTOPS) [22–24].

The MTOPS trial is not only the largest but also the longest study ever undertaken in the field of LUTS and clinical BPH [25]. Participants were men aged 50 years or older with an American Urological Association (AUA) symptom score of 8–30 and a maximum urinary flow rate of 4–15 mL/s with a voided volume of at least 125 mL. A total of 3047 patients were enrolled from 1993 through 1998 at 17 academic centers and were followed for 4–5 years (average: 4.5 years). Patients with a previous medical or surgical intervention for LUTS or BPH, supine blood pressure lower than 90/70 mm Hg, or a serum PSA level of greater than 10 ng/mL were excluded from the study.

Subjects were randomly assigned in a double-blind fashion to one of four treatment groups: placebo, doxazosin, finasteride, or combination therapy. Finasteride was administered as a 5 mg daily dose. The dosage of doxazosin was increased weekly from 1 mg daily to 2, 4, and 8 mg daily doses. Participants unable to tolerate the 8 mg dose of doxazosin were given a 4 mg dose; those unable to tolerate both the 8 mg and 4 mg doses were counted as having discontinued doxazosin therapy.

Quarterly assessments were conducted in the research centers; DREs, serum PSA measurements, and urinalyses were performed annually. Prostate volume was assessed at baseline and at the end of year 5 or end of the study, whichever came first.

In contrast with previous trials, the primary outcome in the MTOPS trial was overall clinical progression, defined as the occurrence of one of the following five events: an increase in the AUA symptom score of 4 or more points from baseline, acute urinary retention (AUR), renal insufficiency, recurrent urinary tract infection, or urinary incontinence. An increase in the AUA symptom score of 4 or more points was measured relative to score at the time of randomization and confirmed by readministration of the symptom index within 4 weeks. AUR was defined as the inability to urinate following a trial without catheter. Renal insufficiency had to be attributable to BPH and was defined as a serum creatinine level of at least 1.5 mg/dL and an increase relative to baseline of 50% or more. Recurrent urinary tract infection was defined as two or more infections within 1 year, separated by a negative urine culture, or urosepsis. Urinary incontinence was defined as self-reported socially or hygienically unacceptable involuntary loss of urine. All outcomes were reviewed by a clinical review committee unaware of treatment assignments. Secondary outcomes were the longitudinal change in AUA symptom score and maximum urinary flow rate. All analyses were conducted using the intention-to-treat principle, with life-table methods used to estimate the cumulative incidence of outcome events.

Of 4391 men screened for eligibility, 3747 were enrolled and randomly assigned to one of the four treatment groups. Among the treatment groups, the mean age at baseline ranged from 62.5 to 62.7 years, and the mean AUA symptom score ranged from 16.8 to 17.6 points. The maximum urinary flow rate ranged from 10.3 mL/s to 10.6 mL/s, and the TRUS-measured prostate volume ranged from 35.2 mL to 36.9 mL. Over a mean follow-up period of 4.5 years, 351 primary outcome events occurred, distributed as follows: approximately 78% due to a rise in the AUA symptom score of 4 or more points; 12% due to AUR; 9% due to urinary incontinence; and 1% due to recurrent urinary tract infection.

In this well-controlled study that included quarterly visits and yearly laboratory checks, renal insufficiency due to BPH did not develop in any patient. The rate of overall clinical progression in the subjects who received placebo was 4.5 per 100 person-years. Compared with placebo, doxazosin reduced the risk of progression by 39%; finasteride by 34%; and combination therapy by 66%. The risk reduction for both single and combination therapy compared with placebo was highly significant ($P < 0.01$), and the risk reduction for combination therapy was significant compared with either drug alone ($P < 0.001$).

The risk of AUR was significantly reduced in the finasteride and combination therapy groups compared with placebo. However, although doxazosin therapy delayed the time to AUR, it did not ultimately reduce the cumulative incidence compared with placebo. Similarly, finasteride and combination therapy significantly reduced the cumulative incidence of crossover to invasive therapy for BPH, whereas doxazosin slightly delayed but did not ultimately reduce crossover to invasive therapy [22]. Rates of urinary incontinence and urinary tract infection were too low in the treatment groups to perform meaningful analyses between treatments or with placebo.

Longitudinal change in AUA symptom score and maximum urinary flow rate were recorded following the intention-to-treat principle. Combination therapy produced the greatest improvements in symptom score (7.4 points) and peak urinary flow rate (5.1 mL/s). When interpreting the improvements in symptom score and flow rate for the placebo group (4.9 points and 2.8 mL/s, respectively), it is important to keep in mind that, in the intention-to-treat analysis, subjects who crossed over to active known therapy and/or had a surgical intervention for BPH were nonetheless counted as being in placebo group. Thus, taking into account the prolonged duration of this clinical trial, the estimation of changes in symptom score and flow rate may be overly optimistic, particularly in the placebo group, in which more patients than in any of the other treatment groups crossed over to active known therapy or had surgical intervention for their disease. A protocol analysis, eliminating patients who did not continue on placebo throughout the entirety of the study, would help elucidate the actual natural history of the disease in this group of patients.

A number-needed-to-treat (NNT) analysis was performed. The NNT to prevent a case of overall clinical progression was 8.4 with combination therapy, 13.7 with doxazosin, and 15.0 with finasteride. In men with serum PSA levels higher than 4.0 ng/mL (20% of the randomized patients) or baseline TRUS prostate volumes greater than 40 mL (30% of the randomized patients), the NNT was reduced in the combination therapy group (4.7 and 4.9, respectively) and the finasteride group (7.2 for both subgroups).

The initial results of the MTOPS trial have answered several important questions regarding the use of combination therapy for BPH. It has become clear that combination therapy is of significant value in the long-term management of patients with LUTS and clinical BPH, particularly those presenting at the onset with enlarged prostates or slightly elevated serum PSA levels, who are at risk for progression. Monotherapy with an alpha blocker (in this case, doxazosin) is effective in treating LUTS associated with clinical BPH and preventing symptomatic progression of the disease; however, it is less effective in preventing AUR and not at all effective in preventing crossover to surgical therapy.

The second large combination study of sufficient duration is the CombAT trial, a 4-year study randomizing over 4500 patients to treatments with tamsulosin, dutasteride, or a combination of both [24,26–29]. The absence of a placebo group is explained by ethical considerations, since the fate of prolonged placebo treatment had been demonstrated in the MTOPS trial.

Men aged ≥50 years with a BPH clinical diagnosis by medical history and physical examination, an IPSS of ≥12 points, prostate volume of ≥30 mL by TRUS, total serum PSA of ≥1.5 ng/mL, and Q_{max} of >5 mL/s and ≤15 mL/s with a minimum voided volume ≥125 mL were eligible for inclusion. Principal exclusion criteria were total serum PSA > 10.0 ng/mL, history or evidence of prostate cancer, previous prostatic surgery, history of AUR within 3 months prior to study entry, 5-ARI use within 6 months (or dutasteride within 12 months) prior to entry, or use of an alpha blocker or phytotherapy for BPH within 2 weeks prior to entry.

The importance of the inclusion criteria requiring a prostate volume of ≥30 mL by TRUS and a total serum PSA ≥1.5 ng/mL cannot be overstated, since they created baseline parameters quite different from MTOPS resulting in different and more severe outcomes as well. While age, IPSS, and maximum flow rate (MFR) were similar, the average prostate volume was 55.0 mL versus 36.3 mL (CombAT vs MTOPS), and the serum PSA 4.0 versus 2.4 ng/mL (CombAT vs MTOPS).

The improvements from baseline were −3.8 (tamsulosin), −5.3 (dutasteride), and −6.3 (combination). The difference from baseline was significant for all three treatment arms. Combination was superior compared with tamsulosin from 9 months and compared with dutasteride from 3 months on. Dutasteride (in the only study in which a 5ARI is superior to any AARB in this regard) was numerically superior to tamsulosin starting after 18 months [23].

The MFR followed a very similar pattern with an improvement of +0.7 for tamsulosin, +2.0 for dutasteride, and +2.4 for combination. Again, dutasteride proved numerically superior to tamsulosin starting after 6 months.

At month 48, the adjusted mean percentage change from baseline in total prostate volume was −27.3% for combination therapy, +4.6% ($P < 0.001$) for tamsulosin, and −28.0% ($P = 0.42$) for dutasteride. At month 48, the adjusted mean percentage change from baseline in transition zone volume in a subset of 656 men was −17.9% for combination therapy, +18.2% ($P < 0.001$) for tamsulosin, and −26.5% ($P = 0.053$) for dutasteride [23].

The time to first AUR or BPH-related surgery was significantly lower with combination therapy versus tamsulosin ($P < 0.001$); there were no significant differences between combination therapy and dutasteride ($P = 0.18$). Combination therapy reduced the relative risk of AUR or BPH-related surgery by 65.8% compared with tamsulosin and by 19.6% compared with dutasteride. The cumulative incidence of AUR or BPH-related surgery during the study is shown in the CombAT study. Starting at 8 months, a higher incidence of AUR or BPH-related surgery was seen in the tamsulosin arm compared with the combination and dutasteride arms; the margin of this difference increased with time to month 48 [23].

The time to first BPH clinical progression was significantly different in favor of combination therapy versus tamsulosin and dutasteride ($P < 0.001$ for both comparisons). Combination therapy reduced the relative risk of BPH clinical progression by 44.1% compared with tamsulosin and 31.2% compared with dutasteride. Symptom deterioration was the most common progression event

in each treatment group. The time to first symptom deterioration was significantly different in favor of combination therapy compared with tamsulosin and dutasteride ($P < 0.001$ for both comparisons). Combination therapy reduced the relative risk of symptom deterioration of IPSS ≥4 points by 41.3% versus tamsulosin and 35.2% versus dutasteride [23].

With the CombAT study, it is possible to examine outcomes stratified by baseline parameters such as prostate volume and serum PSA to determine at what level of prostate volume or serum PSA there is a measurable benefit of combination therapy or at what level dutasteride becomes superior to tamsulosin.

Figure 11.1 shows that with increasing prostate volume, there is an increase in the benefit of combination therapy over tamsulosin, as well as dutasteride over tamsulosin; however, the benefit of combination over

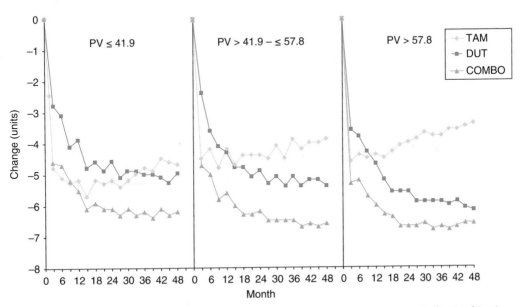

Figure 11.1 International Prostate Symptom Score over time for three treatment groups in the Combination of Avodart and Tamsulosin trial stratified by baseline prostate volume (PV) by tertiles (unpublished data on file at GSK). COMBO, combination; DUT, dutasteride; TAM, tamsulosin.

dutasteride diminishes. Very similar observations can be made for MFR stratified by prostate volume, and for both parameters IPSS and MFR stratified by tertiles of serum PSA. Similarly, when assessing the risk reduction for either AUR or BPH-related surgery, there is a statistically superior risk reduction comparing tamsulosin versus combination in the upper two tertiles of prostate volume, but not in the lowest tertile (Figure 11.2).

Crawford *et al.* [30] studied the placebo group in MTOPS and found that the risk of various definitions of progression was related to baseline median prostate volume (<> 31 mL) and baseline median serum PSA (<>1.6 ng/mL; Figure 11.3). With these data, it is possible to draft recommendations regarding the appropriateness of combination medical therapy to prevent symptomatic progression and/or progression to AUR and surgery in men with larger glands and/or higher serum PSA values.

Adverse events of α_1-blocker/5α-reductase inhibitor combination therapy (Table 11.3)

α_1-Adrenoceptor-specific adverse events, such as dizziness, hypotension, or rhinitis occurred significantly more frequently in α_1-blocker and combination therapy than in 5ARI therapy. Antiandrogenic adverse events, such as impotence, decreased libido, or reduction in semen volume, occurred significantly more often in 5ARI and combination treatments than in α_1-blocker therapy groups [20–22]. Consequently, adverse events were more prevalent in patients with combination therapy than in any monotherapy group. Adverse events seem to be additive and not synergistic. Severe adverse events were not observed in either group [20–22]. Discontinuation rates were similar between treatment groups (11.6–13.6%) [21].

Within 2 years of treatment, drug-related adverse events occurred more often in the combination therapy group (24%) than in

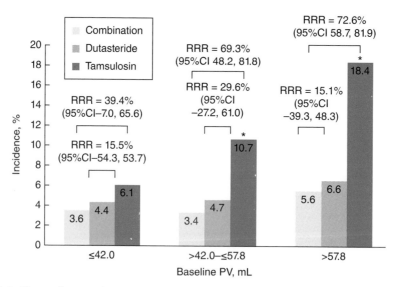

Figure 11.2 Incidence of acute urinary retention or benign prostatic hyperplasia-related surgery for three treatment groups in the Combination of Avodart and Tamsulosin study stratified by baseline prostate volume (PV) by tertiles. *$P < 0.001$ versus combination therapy (unpublished data on file at GSK).

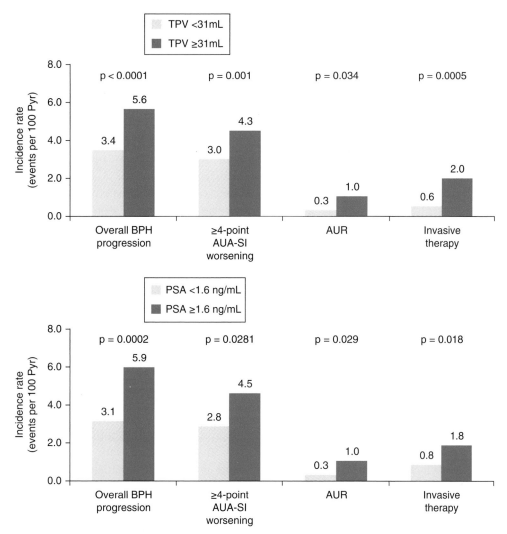

Figure 11.3 Incidence rates of overall, symptomatic progression, acute urinary retention and invasive therapy in the Medical Therapy of Prostatic Symptoms study by baseline median prostate volume and serum prostate-specific antigen (PSA). AUA-SI, American Urological Association Symptom Index; AUR, acute urinary retention; BPH, benign prostatic hyperplasia; TPV, total prostate volume. Crawford [30]. Reproduced with permission of Elsevier.

either the tamsulosin (16%) or dutasteride (18%) groups. However, the occurrence of a serious drug-related adverse event (<1% in each treatment arm) or withdrawal from the trial (<5% in each treatment arm) was similar between the groups [24]. After 4 years of treatment, 6% of patients with combination therapy, 4% with tamsulosin, and 4% with dutasteride discontinued the study due to drug-related adverse events [23].

However, it should not be forgotten that 60–80% of BPH/LUTS patients are sexually active [31]. Both drugs, 5ARI as well as α_1-blocker, might have sexual-related side effects [e.g. loss of libido (5ARI) and retrograde ejaculation (α_1-blockers)]. When α_1-blockers and 5ARI are combined, these potential side effects might add up and affect the sex life of the patient. This should not be overlooked in discussing potential side effects with individual patients.

Alpha adrenergic receptor blocker + antimuscarinics

A recent systematic review and associated tables (Tables 11.4,11. 5) serve as the basis for this section [1]. The first clinical study on α_1-blocker/antimuscarinic combination therapy was published by Saito and Yamada in 1999 [32]. They administered tamsulosin and propiverine to patients with enlarged prostates and increased the frequency of any cause (including neurogenic bladders). Following this landmark study, clinical studies with more homogeneous study populations were performed on α_1-blocker/antimuscarinic combination [33–45] (Table 11.2). The majority are add-on studies, where an antimuscarinic is added to α_1-blocker therapy. Only one study included from the beginning on, next to the α_1-blocker and α_1-blocker/antimuscarinic groups, an antimuscarinic only group [34]. All studies defined an upper limit of postvoid residual volume (PVR) and a lower limit of Q_{max} as study inclusion criteria. As such, statements concerning the safety of the combination are valid only for patients with a PVR of <200 mL and a Q_{max} above 5 mL/s.

All studies on α_1-blocker/antimuscarinic combination therapy have only a short follow-up time, usually 12 weeks, and no study assessed this combination for more than 4 months. Therefore, it is currently unknown as to whether long-term α_1-blocker/antimuscarinic combination is useful, safe, and/or effective.

Subjective outcomes of α_1-blocker/ antimuscarinic combination therapy

Add-on studies reported significant IPSS reductions when patients were treated with α_1-blocker or α_1-blocker/antimuscarinic combination, especially reductions of the IPSS subscore, which determines storage symptoms (questions 2, 4, and 7) [41,42,45]. A mean reduction of 3 IPSS points was observed in 74.4% of patients when oxybutinin was given as an add-on but only in 65% of patients receiving placebo add-ons [37]. Reports on antimuscarinics as add-on therapy regarding the patients' QoL are controversial, but most studies state that add-on therapy does not significantly improve QoL compared with placebo [41,42,45]. However, different inclusion criteria in the studies and different time periods regarding duration of previous α_1-blocker use make outcome parameters difficult to compare (Table 11.2).

The effects of add-on tolterodine were, regardless of initial PSA values, dependent on prostate size [43]. Another study reported that IPSS reduction with propiverine was more pronounced in patients with a Q_{max} of <15 mL/s at baseline [44]. However, data on specific patient groups that might profit from add-on treatment are scarce. Particularly, low case numbers and a high patient heterogeneity in existing trials make it difficult to determine which LUTS patient benefits most from an add-on antimuscarinic therapy.

The Tolterodine and Tamsulosin in Men with LUTS Including OAB: Evaluation of Efficacy and Safety Study was the only trial in which an antimuscarinic monotherapy treatment arm was included. TIMES reported that only patients treated with combination therapy showed a significant treatment benefit as defined by patient perception but not patients treated with either tamsulosin,

Table 11.4 α₁-Adrenoceptor antagonist and antimuscarinic combination: International Prostate Symptom Score outcome and trial characteristics

Trial	Level of evidence no	Patients, no	Drug (dose)	Duration, mo	Inclusion criteria	Time during which an α₁-blocker was given prior to add-on antimuscarinic, wk	Total IPSS reduction from baseline (IPSS *storage* symptom reduction, where assessed separately)			
							α₁-Blocker	Antimuscarinic	Placebo	Combination
Studies in which α1-blocker, antimuscarinic, or a combination of both was tested from the start										
TIMES	Ib	879	Tamsulosin (0.4 mg) tolterodine	3	Age >40 yr Qma. >5 ml/s **PVR <200 ml** IPSS >12 >8 voids/24 h PSA ≤10 ng/ml		7.8 (3.4) Significant vs baseline vs placebo	6.8 (3.4) Significant vs baseline	6.2 (2.8) Significant vs baseline	8.0 (4.2) Significant vs baseline vs placebo
Studies in which al-blocker/antimuscarinic or al-blocker/placebo was tested from the start										
Lee et al.	Ib	228	Doxazosin (4 mg) propiverine (20 mg)	2	Age 50–80 yr >8 voids/24 h urodynamically obstructed (Abrams-Griffith >20) **PVR <30% bladder capacity**			7.4 (3.8) Significant vs baseline	73 (2.9) Significant vs baseline	
Studies in which antimuscarinic or placebo was tested as add-on to an al-blocker										
MacDiarmid et al.	Ib	409	Tamsulosin (0.4 mg) oxybutinin (10 mg)	3	Age >45 yr Qma. >8 ml/s **PVR <150 ml** IPSS >13 IPSS storage subset >8 PSA ≤4 ng/ml	≥4		6.9 (3.7) Significant vs baseline vs placebo	5.2 (2.4) Significant vs baseline	
VICTOR	Ib	397	Tamsulosin (0.4 mg) solifenacin (5 mg)	4	Age >45 yr Qma. >5 ml/s **PVR <100 ml** IPSS >13 >8 voids/24 h PSA ≤10 ng/ml	≥4		5.4 (2.8) Significant vs baseline	4.9 (2.3) Significant vs baseline	

(Continued)

Table 11.4 Continued

Trial	Level of evidence	Patients, no	Drug (dose)	Duration, mo	Inclusion criteria	Time during which an α1-blocker was given prior to add-on antimuscarinic, wk	Total IPSS reduction from baseline (IPSS *storage* symptom reduction, where assessed separately)			
							α1-Blocker	Antimuscarinic	Placebo	Combination
ADAM	Ib	652	Any a1-blocker tolterodine (4 mg)	3	Age >45 yr no limit on Qma. **PVR <200 ml** >8 voids/24 h >1 urgency episode/24 h PSA <10 ng/ml	≥4		4.8 (2.7) Significant vs baseline vs placebo	43 (2.2) Significant vs baseline	Significant vs baseline
ASSIST	Ib	638	Tamsulosin (0.2 mg) solifenacin (2.5–5 mg)	3	Age >50 yr Qma. >5 ml/s **PVR <50 ml** >8 voids/24 h >2 urgency episodes/24 h	≥6		3.5 (2.4) Significant vs baseline vs placebo	3.1 (1.8) Significant vs baseline	Significant vs baseline
TAABO	Ib	214	Tamsulosin (0.2 mg) propiverine (10–20 mg)	3	Age >50 yr Qma. 5–15 ml/s **PVR <100 ml** IPSS >8 >8 voids/24 h >1 urgency episodes/24 h	8		(2.2) Significant vs baseline	(1.1) Significant vs baseline	Significant vs baseline
Oelke et al.	Ib	1849	Propiverine (30 mg) with or without al-blocker (any)	3	Age >40 yr Qma. >10 ml/s **PVR <100 ml** IPSS <20 >8 voids/24 h prostate size <40 ml	Unknown	≥15 ml/s	5.1 Significant vs baseline	4.6 Significant vs baseline	Significant vs baseline
						Unknown	<15 ml/s	53 Significant vs baseline	3.7 Significant vs baselin	Significant vs baselin

α1-Blocker=α1-adrenoceptor antagonist; ADAM=Add-on study of Detrol LA to Alpha-blockers in men; ASSIST=Add-on therapy of Solifenacin Succinate in men for BPH with OAB symptoms treated by Tamsulosin; BPH=benign prostatic hyperplasia; IPSS=International Prostate Symptom Score; LUTS=lower urinary tract symptoms; OAB=overactive bladder; PVR=postvoid residual; PSA=prostate-specific antigen; Q_{max}=maximum flow rate of urine; TAABO=Trial of combination treatment of an Alpha-blocker plus an Anticholinergic for BPH with OAB; TIMES=Tolterodine and Tamsulosin in men with LUTS; VICTOR=Vesicare in combination with Tamsulosin in OAB residual symptoms.

Table 11.5 α_1-Adrenoceptor antagonist and antimuscarinic combination side effects, postvoid residual volume increase, and acute urinary retention

Trial	α1-Blocker alone, %				Antimuscarinic alone, %				Placebo alone, %				α1-Blocker/antimuscarinic, %				α1-Blocker/placebo, %				PVR and Q_{max} limitations of study patients
	Side effects (dry mouth)	Clinically significant* increase in PVR (mean increase, ml)	Acute urinary retention	Study discontinuation due to side effects	Side effects (dry mouth)	Clinically significant* increase in PVR (mean increase, ml)	Acute urinary retention	Study discontinuation due to side effects	Side effects (dry mouth)	Clinically significant* increase in PVR (mean increase, ml)	Acute urinary retention	Study discontinuation due to side effects	Side effects (dry mouth)	Clinically significant* increase of PVR (mean increase, ml)	Acute urinary retention	Study discontinuation due to side effects	Side effects (dry mouth)	Clinically significant* increase in PVR (mean increase, ml)	Acute urinary retention	Study discontinuation due to side effects	
TIMES [42]	27.9 (6.9)	0 (0.1)	0	3.2	19.9 (7.4)	0 (5.2)	1.8	2.3	16.8 (2.2)	0 (−3.6)	1.8	3.1	47.1 (20.8)	0 (6.4)	0.8	8.8					<200 ml and >5 ml/s
Lee et al. [45]													42.7 (18.3)	1.4 (20.7)	0	4.9	18.9 (5.8)	0 (n.r.)	0	1.4	<30% bladder capacity
MacDiarmid et al. [45]													42.6 (15.3)	2.9 (18)	0	10.3	42.6 (4.8)	0.5 (7)	0	9.7	<150 ml and >8 ml/s
VICTOR [48]													45 (7)	n.r. (−13.5)	3	7	39 (3)	n.r. (0)	0	4	<100 ml and >5 ml/s
ADAM [49]													34.7 (9.7)	0 (13.6)	0.9	4	27.6 (5.6)	0 (1)	0.6	2.5	<200 ml and no Q_{max} limit
ASSIST [50]													55.9 (11.3)	6.1 (22.6)	1.9	4.7	42.1 (2.8)	0.9 (5.9)	0	2.8	<50 ml and >5 ml/s
TAABO [53]													13.1 (3.2)	2.4 (n.r.)	0.8	7.4	0 (0)	0 (n.r.)	0	0	<100 ml and 5–15 ml/s

α1-Blocker = α1-adrenoceptor antagonist; ADAM = Add-on study of Detrol LA to Alpha-blockers in men; ASSIST = Add-on therapy of Solifenacin Succinate in men for BPH with OAB symptoms treated by Tamsulosin; BPH = benign prostatic hyperplasia; IPSS = International Prostate Symptom Score; LUTS = lower urinary tract symptoms; n.r. = not reported; OAB = overactive bladder; PVR = postvoid residual; PSA = prostate-specific antigen; Q_{max} = maximum flow rate of urine; TAABO = Trial of combination treatment of an Alpha-blocker plus an Anticholinergic for BPH with OAB; TIMES = Tolterodine and Tamsulosin in men with LUTS; VICTOR = Vesicare in combination with Tamsulosin in OAB residual symptoms.

*Clinically significant increase in PVR depending on the study, defined as increase requiring catheterization or increase >300 ml or increase >50% of initial PVR or over the initially defined PVR threshold for exclusion.

tolterodine, or placebo alone (80% vs 71% and 65%, and 62%, respectively) [34]. Similarly, following the 12 weeks of treatment, only combination therapy significantly improved total IPSS and QoL, whereas tolterodine alone did not differ from the placebo. Interestingly, after the same treatment period, tamsulosin alone did improve total IPSS but without any significant effects on the IPSS QoL item [34]. IPSS storage subscore was only significantly reduced in the combination group [38]. However, in men with a PSA of <1.3 ng/mL or a prostate size of <29 mL, tolterodine alone was also able to significantly reduce storage symptoms [36,39]. As such, TIMES indicates that in the short term, men with enlarged prostates in particular benefit from α_1-blocker/antimuscarinic combination therapy. In men with small prostates, antimuscarinics alone are also sufficient [34].

Objective outcomes of α_1-blocker/antimuscarinic combination therapy

Studies in which antimuscarinics were assessed as add-ons to α_1-blockers showed no significant differences in Q_{max} increase between treatment groups [33,41,42,45]. Add-on combination therapy, when compared with α_1-blockers alone, showed a significantly higher reduction in 24 h voiding frequency [33,41,42,44,45] (e.g. 23.5% vs −14.3% [33]) and urgency episodes per day [40–42,44] (e.g. 2.9 vs 1.8 [41]).

TIMES reported that in patients with a prostate size of >29 mL, only combination therapy significantly reduced the 24 h voiding frequency (2.8 vs 1.7 with tamsulosin alone, 1.4 with tolterodine alone, or 1.6 with placebo). In patients with a prostate size of <29 mL, tolterodine alone also reduced the 24 h voiding frequency (tamsulosin/tolterodine

2.2, tolterodine 1.9, vs placebo 1.1, and tamsulosin 1.6) [39]. The significant frequency reduction began 1 week after the start of treatment [34].

The α_1-blocker/antimuscarinic combination does not seem to influence Q_{max} but improves other objective outcome parameters such as 24 h frequency and urgency episodes. Similar to other subjective outcome parameters, combination therapy appears to be as efficacious as with antimuscarinics alone in men with small prostates (<30 mL).

Adverse events of α_1-blocker/ antimuscarinic combination therapy

Although several studies have found a significant increase in PVR with antimuscarinics (alone or in combination), most studies in fact have not found a significant increase in AUR with antimuscarinics [33,34,37,41, 42,44,45] (Table 11.2). For example, when oxybutinin was given to patients who had already received tamsulosin, the mean PVR increased by 18.2 mL, whereas the placebo increased PVR by 7.8 mL. No AURs occurred either in the oxybutinin/tamsulosin or in the placebo/tamsulosin group [37]. Only a few studies reported a higher frequency of AUR in patients treated with antimuscarinic add-on compared with placebo add-on, ranging from 1.9 to 3% [40,42]. However, studies including a placebo group only (patients who did not receive any active compounds) also reported an occurrence of AUR around 1.8% (Table 11.2). Considering the natural occurrence rate of AUR in patients with LUTS, the AUR rate with antimuscarinics seems even more irrelevant. But it should not be forgotten that all studies used an upper PVR limit of 200 mL and a Q_{max} above 5 mL/s at the time of inclusion (Table 11.2). Men with an increased risk for

AUR were excluded from the trials. As such, the results from these trials and subsequent recommendations can only be applied and given to/for patients with a similar low-risk profile. In general, caution (regular evaluation of PVR) is recommended when prescribing antimuscarinics to patients with an increased risk of developing AUR. Interestingly, prostate size and serum PSA concentration at study initiation had no influence on AUR development during antimuscarinic treatment [39,43].

Study discontinuation occurred more frequently in patients with add-on combination therapy than in patients with placebo add-on (4.7–7% and 1.5–4% respectively [33,40,42]). Other studies found no differences in discontinuation rates due to drug-related adverse events [34,37] (Table 11.2). Antimuscarinic adverse events such as dry mouth or constipation occurred in the combination therapy group more often than with α_1-blocker monotherapy [33,34,40–42]. For example, "dry mouth" occurred in 15.3% of patients taking oxybutinin and tamsulosin, but in only 4.8% of patients taking tamsulosin and placebo [37]. However, in most studies, side effects were mild and improved on drug discontinuation [33,40].

Similar to α_1-blocker/5ARI combination therapy, adverse events do not seem to be a decisive criterion, since the types of adverse events are identical with either monotherapy and do not potentiate.

Astellas has sponsored a 12-week randomized trial using different dosages of solifenacin with 0.4 mg tamsulosin against placebo (SATURN trial, Astellas NCT00510406, men 45 years or older, Inclusion Criteria: male patients with LUTS associated with BPH diagnosed >3 months, IPSS score >13, voiding and storage symptoms, maximum flow rate of >4 mL/s and <15 mL/s Exclusion

Criteria: postvoid residual volume >200 mL, symptomatic urinary tract infection), followed by an optional open label extension of 52 weeks [NEPTUNE, Astellas NCT01021332, men 45 years or older, participated in SATURN inclusion criteria: completion of 12-week double-blind treatment in Study 905-CL-055 exclusion criteria: any significant PVR volume (>150 mL)]. If these trials are positive, this may mark the introduction of a combination tablet of tamsulosin plus flexible dosing of solifenacin to the market and, thus, the second combination tablet in the area of male LUTS and BPH.

Alpha adrenergic receptor blocker + phosphodiesterase type 5 inhibitor

Clinical studies

There are five studies employing a combination of a PDE5 inhibitor (sildenafil, tadalafil, or vardenafil) with an AARB (tamsulosin and alfuzosin [46–50]). These studies do not feature a placebo control arm, are of short duration, and have a limited number of patients enrolled. The sample size and power calculation are often missing (Table 11.6).

In the Kaplan study, IPSS improved significantly in all groups (alfuzosin: 17.3 ± 4.3 vs 14.6 ± 3.7 points; $P = 0.01$; sildenafil: 16.9 ± 4.1 vs 14.9 ± 4.2 points; $P = 0.03$; combination: 17.8 ± 4.7 vs 13.5 ± 4.2; $P = 0.002$). The mean IPSS remained in the moderate LUTS category for all groups. Alfuzosin significantly ($P < 0.05$) improved Q_{max} (11.7%), whereas sildenafil alone did not. Combination therapy produced near-additive improvements in IPSS (24.1%), Q_{max} (21.1%), and erectile-dysfunction measures [46].

Bechara *et al.* noted significant improvements in IPSS and IPSS-QoL with both

Table 11.6 Studies of alpha adrenergic receptor blockers and phosphodiesterase type 5 inhibitors in the treatment of male lower urinary tract symptoms

Study	Baseline characteristics			Treatment		
	Age (years)	Body mass index	International Prostate Symptom Score	Drug	Dosage (mg)	Pills/week
Kaplan et al. [46]	63.4	25.4	17.3	n = 67; 12 weeks Sildenafil versus alfuzosin versus combination	25	7
Bechara et al. [47]	63.7	–	19.4	n = 30; 45 days + 45 days Tadalafil versus tamsulosin Cross-over design	20	7
Liguori et al. [50]	61.3	–	15	n = 66; 12 weeks Tadalafil versus alfuzosin versus combination	20	7
Tuncel et al. [48]	58.8	–	15.4	n = 60; 8 weeks Sildenafil versus tamsulosin versus combination	25	4
Gacci et al. [49]	68	25.7	19.6	n = 60; 12 weeks Vardenafil versus tamsulosin	10	7

treatments but greater improvements with the drug combination. Both regimens similarly improved Q_{max} and decreased the PVR volume from baseline with no significant differences between treatment with tamsulosin alone and treatment with tamsulosin and tadalafil. The International Index of Erectile Function (IIEF) domain score improved with tamsulosin and tadalafil but not with tamsulosin alone [47].

In the Liguori study, IIEF-EF scores were improved in all groups (increases of 15%, 36%, and 37% from baseline for the alfuzosin, tadalafil, and combination groups, respectively). All groups had an increase in peak urine flow (increases of 22%, 10%, and 29.6% from baseline for the alfuzosin, tadalafil, and combination groups, respectively), as well as a significant decrease in IPSS score (decreases of 27%, 8%, and 42% from baseline, respectively). All changes were

statistically significant compared with baseline values ($P < 0.05$), with the exception of the change in IPSS score in the tadalafil-only group [50].

In the small study by Tuncel et al., IPSS, Q_{max}, PVR volume, Sexual Health Inventory for Male (SHIM) scores, and questions number 3 and 4 of the IIEF significantly improved in each group. The improvement in symptom score was more evident in both the combination (40.1%) and tamsulosin-only (36.2%) groups as compared with the sildenafil-only group (28.2%; $P < 0.001$). Improvements in Q_{max} and PVR volume were greater in both the tamsulosin-only and combination group compared with the sildenafil-only group. SHIM scores showed a significantly greater improvement in both the sildenafil-only (65%) and combination (67.4%) group than in patients who received tamsulosin only (12.4%; $P < 0.001$), and increases in the IIEF scores were greater in the sildenafil-only and combination group than tamsulosin only. This study showed that treatment with the combination of tamsulosin and sildenafil was not superior to monotherapy with tamsulosin [48].

Gacci *et al.* found a between-group significant difference from baseline to 12 weeks in the following: (1) Q_{max} (placebo: +0.07, vardenafil: +2.56, $P = 0.034$); (2) Qave (placebo: −0.15, vardenafil: +1.02, $P = 0.031$); (3) irritative-IPSS subscores (placebo: −1.67, vardenafil: −3.11, $P = 0.039$); and (4) IIEF (placebo: +0.06, vardenafil: +2.61, $P = 0.030$). No patient reported any serious (grade ≥2) adverse event (AE). There were no differences in the incidence of common, treatment-related AEs between men undergoing combined therapy or those using tamsulosin alone [49].

Meta-analysis

In the meta-analysis performed by Gacci *et al.* the combination of the two medications significantly improved IPSS [−1.8 (−3.7 to 0.0); $P = 0.05$] and IIEF score [+3.6 (+3.1 to +4.1); $P < 0.0001$] as well as Q_{max} [+1.5 mL/s (+0.9 to +2.2); $P < 0.0001$] when compared with the use of alpha blockers alone (Figure 11.4) [51]. In studies comparing the effect of combination therapy of PDE5-Is plus alpha blocker versus alpha blocker alone, seven of 103 AEs (6.8%) were reported in men treated with combined therapy and five of 99 AEs (5.1%) in men treated with alpha blocker alone [49].

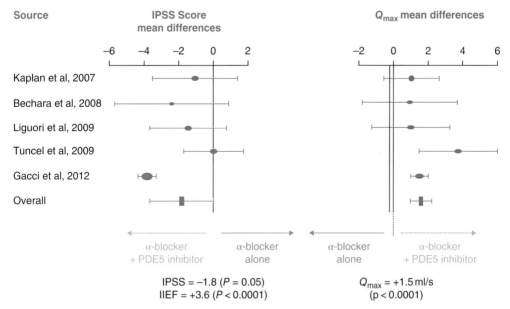

Figure 11.4 International Prostate Symptom Score (IPSS) and maximum flow rate changes in studies combining alpha adrenergic receptor blockers and phosphodiesterase type 5 (PDE5) inhibitors [51]. IIEF, International Index of Erectile Function. Gacci M, *et al.* A systematic review and meta-analysis on the use of phosphodiesterase 5 inhibitors alone or in combination with alpha-blockers for lower urinary tract symptoms due to benign prostatic hyperplasia. *Eur Urol.* 2012;61(5):994–1003. Epub 2012/03/13. Reproduced with permission of Elsevier.

Dos and don'ts

- Combination therapy with an alpha blocker and 5-alpha reductase inhibitor should be reserved for larger prostates. The best results appear to be in those with a prostate volume of >40 mL.
- Antimuscarinics, albeit safe in men, are usually prescribed in combination with an alpha blocker.
- The role of combination therapy with a PDE5-I and an alpha blocker remains to be fully elucidated.

Bibliography

1 Fullhase C, Chapple C, Cornu JN, De Nunzio C, Gratzke C, Kaplan SA, et al. Systematic review of combination drug therapy for non-neurogenic male lower urinary tract symptoms. Eur Urol. 2013;64(2):228–43. Epub 2013/02/05.

2 Schwinn DA, Roehrborn CG. Alpha1-adrenoceptor subtypes and lower urinary tract symptoms. Int J Urol. 2008;15(3):193–9. Epub 2008/02/29.

3 Roehrborn CG, Schwinn DA. Alpha1-adrenergic receptors and their inhibitors in lower urinary tract symptoms and benign prostatic hyperplasia. J Urol. 2004;171(3):1029–35. Epub 2004/02/10.

4 Schwinn DA. The role of alpha1-adrenergic receptor subtypes in lower urinary tract symptoms. BJU Int. 2001;88 Suppl 2:27–34; discussion 49–50.

5 Smith MS, Schambra UB, Wilson KH, Page SO, Schwinn DA. Alpha1-adrenergic receptors in human spinal cord: specific localized expression of mRNA encoding alpha1-adrenergic receptor subtypes at four distinct levels. Brain Res Mol Brain Res. 1999;63(2):254–61.

6 Marks LS, Hess DL, Dorey FJ, Luz Macairan M, Cruz Santos PB, Tyler VE. Tissue effects of saw palmetto and finasteride: use of biopsy cores for in situ quantification of prostatic androgens. Urology. 2001;57(5):999–1005.

7 Marks LS, Partin AW, Dorey FJ, Gormley GJ, Epstein JI, Garris JB, et al. Long-term effects of finasteride on prostate tissue composition. Urology. 1999;53(3):574–80. Epub 1999/03/30.

8 Marks LS, Partin AW, Gormley GJ, Dorey FJ, Shery ED, Garris JB, et al. Prostate tissue composition and response to finasteride in men with symptomatic benign prostatic hyperplasia. J Urol. 1997;157(6): 2171–8. Epub 1997/06/01.

9 Memis A, Ozden C, Ozdal OL, Guzel O, Han O, Seckin S. Effect of finasteride treatment on suburethral prostatic microvessel density in patients with hematuria related to benign prostate hyperplasia. Urol Int. 2008;80(2):177–80. Epub 2008/03/26.

10 Pareek G, Shevchuk M, Armenakas NA, Vasjovic L, Hochberg DA, Basillote JB, et al. The effect of finasteride on the expression of vascular endothelial growth factor and microvessel density: a possible mechanism for decreased prostatic bleeding in treated patients. J Urol. 2003; 169(1):20–3.

11 Pushkar D, Kosko J, Loran O. Peak flow and IPSS changes in patients treated with a combination of finasteride and terazosin after withdrawing terazosin. Br J Urol. 1997;80(Suppl 2):208.

12 Pushkar D, Kosko D, Loran O, Kan A, Sapozhnikov I, Tevlin K. A trial of the use of finasteride and terazosin in patients with benign prostatic hyperplasia. Urol Nefrol. 1995;4:32–5.

13 Savage SJ, Spungen AM, Galea G, Britanico J, Vapnek JM. Combination medical therapy for symptomatic benign prostatic hyperplasia. Can J Urol. 1998;5(3):578–84. Epub 2001/04/18.

14 Debruyne FM, Jardin A, Colloi D, Resel L, Witjes WP, Delauche-Cavallier MC, et al. Sustained-release alfuzosin, finasteride and the combination of both in the treatment of benign prostatic hyperplasia. European ALFIN Study Group. Eur Urol. 1998;34(3):169–75.

15 Johnson TM, 2nd, Jones K, Williford WO, Kutner MH, Issa MM, Lepor H. Changes in nocturia from medical treatment of benign prostatic hyperplasia: secondary analysis of the Department of Veterans Affairs Cooperative Study Trial. J Urol. 2003;170(1):145–8. Epub 2003/06/11.

16 Barry MJ, Williford WO, Fowler FJJ, Jones KM, Lepor H. Filling and voiding symptoms in the American Urological Association Symptom Index: the value of their distinction in a veterans affairs randomized trial of medical therapy in men with a clinical diagnosis of benign prostatic hyperplasia. J Urol. 2000;164(5):1559–64.

17 Lepor H, Jones K, Williford W. The mechanism of adverse events associated with terazosin: an analysis of the Veterans Affairs cooperative study. J Urol. 2000;163(4):1134–7. Epub 2000/03/29.

18 Brawer MK, Lin DW, Williford WO, Jones K, Lepor H. Effect of finasteride and/or terazosin on serum PSA: results of VA Cooperative Study #359. *Prostate.* 1999;39(4):234–9. Epub 1999/05/27.

19 Lepor H, Williford WO, Barry MJ, Haakenson C, Jones K. The impact of medical therapy on bother due to symptoms, quality of life and global outcome, and factors predicting response. Veterans Affairs Cooperative Studies Benign Prostatic Hyperplasia Study Group. *J Urol.* 1998;160(4): 1358–67. Epub 1998/09/29.

20 Lepor H, Williford WO, Barry MJ, Brawer MK, Dixon CM, Gormley G, *et al.* The efficacy of terazosin, finasteride, or both in benign prostatic hyperplasia. Veterans Affairs Cooperative Studies Benign Prostatic Hyperplasia Study Group. *N Engl J Med.* 1996;335(8):533–9. Epub 1996/08/22.

21 Kirby RS, Roehrborn C, Boyle P, Bartsch G, Jardin A, Cary MM, *et al.* Efficacy and tolerability of doxazosin and finasteride, alone or in combination, in treatment of symptomatic benign prostatic hyperplasia: the Prospective European Doxazosin and Combination Therapy (PREDICT) trial. *Urology.* 2003;61(1):119–26. Epub 2003/02/01.

22 McConnell JD, Roehrborn CG, Bautista OM, Andriole GL, Jr., Dixon CM, Kusek JW, *et al.* The long-term effect of doxazosin, finasteride, and combination therapy on the clinical progression of benign prostatic hyperplasia. *N Engl J Med.* 2003;349(25):2387–98. Epub 2003/12/19.

23 Roehrborn CG, Siami P, Barkin J, Damiao R, Major-Walker K, Nandy I, *et al.* The effects of combination therapy with dutasteride and tamsulosin on clinical outcomes in men with symptomatic benign prostatic hyperplasia: 4-year results from the CombAT study. *Eur Urol.* 2010;57(1): 123–31. Epub 2009/10/15.

24 Roehrborn CG, Siami P, Barkin J, Damiao R, Major-Walker K, Morrill B, *et al.* The effects of dutasteride, tamsulosin and combination therapy on lower urinary tract symptoms in men with benign prostatic hyperplasia and prostatic enlargement: 2-year results from the CombAT study. *J Urol.* 2008;179(2): 616–21; discussion 21. Epub 2007/12/18.

25 Bautista OM, Kusek JW, Nyberg LM, McConnell JD, Bain RP, Miller G, *et al.* Study design of the Medical Therapy of Prostatic Symptoms (MTOPS) trial. *Control Clin Trials.* 2003;24(2):224–43. Epub 2003/04/12.

26 Becher E, Roehrborn CG, Siami P, Gagnier RP, Wilson TH, Montorsi F. The effects of dutasteride, tamsulosin, and the combination on storage and voiding in men with benign prostatic hyperplasia and prostatic enlargement: 2-year results from the Combination of Avodart and Tamsulosin study. *Prostate Cancer Prostatic Dis.* 2009;12(4):369–74. Epub 2009/11/11.

27 Barkin J, Roehrborn CG, Siami P, Haillot O, Morrill B, Black L, *et al.* Effect of dutasteride, tamsulosin and the combination on patient-reported quality of life and treatment satisfaction in men with moderate-to-severe benign prostatic hyperplasia: 2-year data from the CombAT trial. *BJU Int.* 2009;103(7):919–26. Epub 2009/02/26.

28 Roehrborn CG, Siami P, Barkin J, Damião R, Becher E, Miñana B, *et al.* The influence of baseline parameters on changes in international prostate symptom score with dutasteride, tamsulosin, and combination therapy among men with symptomatic benign prostatic hyperplasia and an enlarged prostate: 2-year data from the CombAT study. *Eur Urol.* 2009;55(2):461–71. Epub 2008/11/18.

29 Chung BH, Roehrborn CG, Siami P, Major-Walker K, Morrill BB, Wilson TH, *et al.* Efficacy and safety of dutasteride, tamsulosin and their combination in a subpopulation of the CombAT study: 2-year results in Asian men with moderate-to-severe BPH. *Prostate Cancer Prostatic Dis.* 2009;12(2):152–9. Epub 2008/09/25.

30 Crawford ED, Wilson SS, McConnell JD, Slawin KM, Lieber MC, Smith JA, *et al.* Baseline factors as predictors of clinical progression of benign prostatic hyperplasia in men treated with placebo. *J Urol.* 2006;175(4):1422–6; discussion 6–7. Epub 2006/03/07.

31 Rosen RC, Wei JT, Althof SE, Seftel AD, Miner M, Perelman MA. Association of sexual dysfunction with lower urinary tract symptoms of BPH and BPH medical therapies: results from the BPH Registry. *Urology.* 2009;73(3):562–6. Epub 2009/01/27.

32 Saito H, Yamada, T. A comparative study of the efficacy and safety of tamsulosin hydrochloride (Harnal capsules) alone and in combination with propiverine hydrochloride (BUP-4 tablets) in patients with prostatic hypertrophy associated with pollakiuria and/or urinary incontinence. *Jpn J Urol Surg.* 1999;12(4):525–36.

33 Lee KS, Choo MS, Kim DY, Kim JC, Kim HJ, Min KS, *et al.* Combination treatment with propiverine hydrochloride plus doxazosin controlled release gastrointestinal therapeutic system formulation

for overactive bladder and coexisting benign prostatic obstruction: a prospective, randomized, controlled multicenter study. *J Urol.* 2005;174(4 Pt 1):1334–8. Epub 2005/09/08.

34 Kaplan SA, Roehrborn CG, Rovner ES, Carlsson M, Bavendam T, Guan Z. Tolterodine and tamsulosin for treatment of men with lower urinary tract symptoms and overactive bladder: a randomized controlled trial. *JAMA.* 2006;296(19): 2319–28. Epub 2006/11/16.

35 Rovner ES, Kreder K, Sussman DO, Kaplan SA, Carlsson M, Bavendam T, *et al.* Effect of tolterodine extended release with or without tamsulosin on measures of urgency and patient reported outcomes in men with lower urinary tract symptoms. *J Urol.* 2008;180(3):1034–41. Epub 2008/07/22.

36 Roehrborn CG, Kaplan SA, Kraus SR, Wang JT, Bavendam T, Guan Z. Effects of serum PSA on efficacy of tolterodine extended release with or without tamsulosin in men with LUTS, including OAB. *Urology.* 2008;72(5):1061–7; discussion 7. Epub 2008/09/27.

37 MacDiarmid SA, Peters KM, Chen A, Armstrong RB, Orman C, Aquilina JW, *et al.* Efficacy and safety of extended-release oxybutynin in combination with tamsulosin for treatment of lower urinary tract symptoms in men: randomized, double-blind, placebo-controlled study. *Mayo Clin Proc.* 2008;83(9):1002–10. Epub 2008/09/09.

38 Kaplan SA, Roehrborn CG, Chancellor M, Carlsson M, Bavendam T, Guan Z. Extended-release tolterodine with or without tamsulosin in men with lower urinary tract symptoms and overactive bladder: effects on urinary symptoms assessed by the International Prostate Symptom Score. *BJU Int.* 2008;102(9):1133–9. Epub 2008/05/31.

39 Roehrborn CG, Kaplan SA, Jones JS, Wang JT, Bavendam T, Guan Z. Tolterodine extended release with or without tamsulosin in men with lower urinary tract symptoms including overactive bladder symptoms: effects of prostate size. *Eur Urol.* 2009;55(2):472–9. Epub 2008/06/28.

40 Kaplan SA, McCammon K, Fincher R, Fakhoury A, He W. Safety and tolerability of solifenacin add-on therapy to alpha-blocker treated men with residual urgency and frequency. *J Urol.* 2009;182(6):2825–30. Epub 2009/10/20.

41 Chapple C, Herschorn S, Abrams P, Sun F, Brodsky M, Guan Z. Tolterodine treatment improves storage symptoms suggestive of overactive bladder in men treated with alpha-blockers. *Eur Urol.* 2009; 56(3):534–41. Epub 2008/12/17.

42 Yamaguchi O, Kakizaki H, Homma Y, Takeda M, Nishizawa O, Gotoh M, *et al.* Solifenacin as add-on therapy for overactive bladder symptoms in men treated for lower urinary tract symptoms – ASSIST, randomized controlled study. *Urology.* 2011;78(1):126–33. Epub 2011/05/24.

43 Chapple CR, Herschorn S, Abrams P, Wang JT, Brodsky M, Guan Z. Efficacy and safety of tolterodine extended-release in men with overactive bladder symptoms treated with an alpha-blocker: effect of baseline prostate-specific antigen concentration. *BJU Int.* 106(9):1332–8. Epub 2010/05/26.

44 Oelke M, Murgas S, Baumann I, Schnabel F, Michel MC. Efficacy of propiverine ER with or without alpha-blockers related to maximum urinary flow rate in adult men with OAB: results of a 12-week, multicenter, non-interventional study. *World J Urol.* 29(2):217–23. Epub 2011/02/18.

45 Nishizawa O, Yamaguchi O, Takeda M, Yokoyama O. Randomized controlled trial to treat benign prostatic hyperplasia with overactive bladder using an alpha-blocker combined with anticholinergics. *LUTS.* 2011;3:29–35.

46 Kaplan SA, Gonzalez RR, Te AE. Combination of alfuzosin and sildenafil is superior to monotherapy in treating lower urinary tract symptoms and erectile dysfunction. *Eur Urol.* 2007;51(6):1717–23. Epub 2007/01/30.

47 Bechara A, Romano S, Casabe A, Haime S, Dedola P, Hernandez C, *et al.* Comparative efficacy assessment of tamsulosin vs tamsulosin plus tadalafil in the treatment of LUTS/BPH. Pilot study. *J Sex Med.* 2008;5(9):2170–8. Epub 2008/07/22.

48 Tuncel A, Nalcacioglu V, Ener K, Aslan Y, Aydin O, Atan A. Sildenafil citrate and tamsulosin combination is not superior to monotherapy in treating lower urinary tract symptoms and erectile dysfunction. *World J Urol.* 2010;28(1):17–22. Epub 2009/10/27.

49 Gacci M, Vittori G, Tosi N, Siena G, Rossetti MA, Lapini A, *et al.* A randomized, placebo-controlled study to assess safety and efficacy of vardenafil 10 mg and tamsulosin 0.4 mg vs tamsulosin 0.4 mg alone in the treatment of lower urinary tract symptoms secondary to benign prostatic hyperplasia. *J Sex Med.* 2012;9(6):1624–33. Epub 2012/04/19.

50 Liguori G, Trombetta C, De Giorgi G, Pomara G, Maio G, Vecchio D, *et al*. Efficacy and safety of combined oral therapy with tadalafil and alfuzosin: an integrated approach to the management of patients with lower urinary tract symptoms and erectile dysfunction. Preliminary report. *J Sex Med.* 2009;6(2):544–52. Epub 2009/01/14.

51 Gacci M, Corona G, Salvi M, Vignozzi L, McVary KT, Kaplan SA, *et al*. A systematic review and meta-analysis on the use of phosphodiesterase 5 inhibitors alone or in combination with alpha-blockers for lower urinary tract symptoms due to benign prostatic hyperplasia. *Eur Urol.* 2012;61(5): 994–1003. Epub 2012/03/13.

CHAPTER 12

Complementary Therapy

Aaron E. Katz & Anne Darves-Bornoz

Garden City, New York, NY, USA

Key points

- The use of phytotherapy for benign prostatic hyperplasia (BPH) is extremely popular, especially in Europe.
- The active ingredients in most phytochemicals are thought to be isoflavones, β-sitosterol, and fatty acids.
- *Serona repens* and pygeum are among the most commonly used complementary therapies for BPH.
- Nutrients such as zinc, amino acids, and essential fatty acids are beneficial for lower urinary tract symptoms (LUTS).

The popularity of herbal and nutritional medicine is increasing, and the science behind it is advancing. One study showed that as many as 34% of people use unconventional therapies (medical interventions not taught widely at US medical schools or generally available at US hospitals), mainly for chronic conditions such as BPH [1]. A study analyzing self-reported questionnaires on the health and supplement use of 61,587 participants showed a strong association between saw palmetto use and the diagnosis of an enlarged prostate (odds ratio: 3.33; 95% confidence interval: 3.00–3.72) [2]. Many patients are not satisfied with available pharmacological or surgical therapies for BPH due to potential adverse effects and have turned to natural therapies, as they are readily available over the counter without prescription. Many of these agents are commonly prescribed in Europe for LUTS and are gaining popularity in the US. Advantages of natural therapies may include better patient compliance, less anxiety among patients, improved safety, and lower cost.

The National Institute of Health has recognized the importance and practicality of natural therapies and has allocated funds to alternative medicine research. It is important that physicians be aware of a therapy's safety, dosage, efficacy, and mechanism of action. When researching natural therapies, the following criteria should be considered:

- enough health-conferring ingredient to have an effect;
- a known mechanism of action;
- evidence that it relieves symptoms;
- demonstrated safety;
- quality of product (provides what it says it will);
- low cost;
- once-daily administration, if possible.

Many peer-reviewed publications now exist that assess these parameters, and these will be discussed below.

Male Lower Urinary Tract Symptoms and Benign Prostatic Hyperplasia, First Edition.
Edited by Steven A. Kaplan and Kevin T. McVary.
© 2014 John Wiley & Sons, Ltd. Published 2014 by John Wiley & Sons, Ltd.

Phytotherapy

Phytochemicals are plant-derived substances and are among the most commonly used alternative treatments for BPH. Some of the more commonly used plants are listed in Table 12.1. Extracts are derived from the roots, seeds, fruit, or bark of these plants and are available for purchase in supermarkets, health stores, and online. Most companies manufacture extracts that contain numerous mixtures of the plants listed in Table 12.1 and are marketed as prostate health supplements. These extracts contain many compounds such as, but not limited to, those listed in Table 12.2. The active ingredients have been

suggested to be β-sitosterol, isoflavones, and fatty acids. Some of the mechanisms of action of these phytotherapeutics include 5α-reductase inhibition, antiproliferative, and anti-inflammatory effects. It is important to note that not all extracts of the same plant contain the same amount of differing compounds due to the variability in the extracting process. This makes clinical trials of monotherapy difficult, as all extracts from the same plant are not alike and could lead to differing results. This should also be taken into consideration when choosing a product.

Common compounds in phytochemicals

β-Sitosterol

β-Sitosterol is one of the most abundant dietary phytosterols found in many vegetables and legumes. It is also thought to be one of the key active ingredients in many of the prostate phytotherapeutics including pygeum, saw palmetto, and South African star grass, and as such it is also found in many of the combination products marketed for prostate health. The proposed mechanism of action for β-sitosterol is inhibition of 5α-reductase [3] in addition to being a potent antiproliferative agent. It has been found to inhibit several growth factors including TGF-β in human prostate stromal cells *in vitro* [4].

Azuprostat is a product that contains β-sitosterol from South African star grass (*Hypoxis rooperi*), pine (*Pinus*), and spruce (*Picea*). In a randomized, double-blind, placebo-controlled clinical trial, the safety and efficacy of this product were assessed. A total of 177 men diagnosed with BPH were supplemented with 130 mg over 7 months. A significant improvement in International Prostate Symptom Score (IPSS) was found

Table 12.1 Common phytochemicals used for benign prostatic hyperplasia

Species name	Common name	Common trademark
Serona repens/Sabal serrulata	American dwarf palm/saw palmetto berry	Permixon
Pygeum africanum	Pygeum	Tadenan
Urtica dioica et urens	Stinging nettle	
Hypoxis rooperi	South African star grass	Harzol
Secale cerale	Rye pollen	Cernilton
Curcubita pepo L.	Pumpkin seeds	

Table 12.2 Common compounds within phytochemical extracts

Phytosterols	Phytoestrogens
B-sitosterol	Fatty acids
Campesterol	Isoflavones:
Stimasterol	• formononetin
	• genistein
	• biochanin A
	• daidzein

between the supplemented and control group ($P < 0.01$). A significant improvement was also found in PFRs and PVRs between the two groups [5]. Another double-blind placebo-controlled clinical trial examined β-sitosterol supplementation in men with 6 months of treatment and 18 months of follow-up. Significant change in the IPSS was again found between the β-sitosterol and placebo group ($P < 0.01$) [6]. A systematic review of the use of β-sitosterol for BPH was carried out by Wilt and associates in 1999, in which they found a significant improvement in LUTS when treated with β-sitosterol [7].

Isoflavones

Isoflavones are phytochemicals also termed phytoestrogens secondary to their estrogenic activity. They are a principal dietary source of phytoestrogens and are primarily found in legumes such as soybeans, chickpeas, red clover, lentils, beans, and groundnuts. Epidemiologic studies have linked a low incidence of BPH and prostate cancer with diets rich in isoflavones. Increased risk of BPH and prostate cancer among Western men has been postulated to be a result of decreased consumption of isoflavone-containing foods. A case-control study assessed the risk between different diets and surgically treated BPH. In this study, a significant and inverse relationship was found between BPH and intake of total vegetables, dark yellow vegetables, and tofu [8].

The four main active isoflavones are formononetin and its demethylated product, daidzein, and biochanin A and its demethylated product, genistein. There are several proposed mechanisms of action of isoflavones (Table 12.3), acting on both glandular epithelium and stroma. Using isoflavone doses higher than those found *in vivo*, it was demonstrated that formononetin, daidzein,

biochanin A, and genistein inhibit 5α-reductase in genital skin fibroblasts [9]. This suggests that isoflavones may work similarily to finasteride. Uridine 5′-diphospho-glucuronosyl-transferase is an enzyme responsible for conjugating and inactivating steroid hormone in tissues. All four isoflavones were found to stimulate this enzyme activity in prostate cancer cells *in vitro*, thus increasing the amount of inactivated testosterone [10]. Growth of prostate stromal cells is stimulated by estrogen [11], and aromatase is an enzyme responsible for estrogen synthesis. A study carried out by Campbell and Kurzer demonstrated that biochanin A inhibits aromatase activity [12]. Biochanin A has also been shown to inhibit the dimerization of the estrogen receptor, thus inhibiting the biological activity of estradiol [13]. Similarly, genistein competes with estradiol for binding to the estrogen receptors at expected circulating concentrations on a human breast-cancer cell line. Prolonged exposure to genistein on this cell line resulted in downregulation of estrogen-receptor mRNA [14].

Selected phytotherapeutic agents

Saw palmetto (*Serona repens*)

The extract of African dwarf palm, *Serona repens*, is certainly the most widely used alternative treatment for BPH worldwide. There are more than 100 varieties of saw palmetto extract, with over 70 available in the US [15]. The saw palmetto plant grows in swampy areas in Southeastern US. It has dark berries from which the extract is derived. Native Americans used the berries for genitourinary symptoms. It was later used for ovarian dysfunction, dysmenorrhea, cystitis, and relief of LUTS. It was an official

Table 12.3 Mechanisms of action of isoflavones

Herb/nutrient	Proposed mechanism	Dosage	Side effects
Saw palmetto	Antiandrogenic, anti-inflammatory, and a proapoptotic effect	160 mg twice a day	Possible gastrointestinal discomfort, rarely dizziness and headache, possible decreased libido, and gynecomastia
Pygeum	Anti-inflammatory, antiestrogenic, antiproliferative	50 mg twice daily or 100 mg once daily	Possible gastrointestinal discomfort
Stinging nettle	Antiproliferative, anti-inflammatory	120 mg twice a day; often used in combination with saw palmetto	Possible gastrointestinal discomfort, allergic skin reaction
South African star grass	5α-Reductase inhibition, antiproliferative	Marketed as Harzol, containing 20 mg of beta-sitosterol three times daily	Mild gastrointestinal discomfort
Cernilton	Urethral smooth muscle relaxation, antiproliferative	126 mg three times a day	Mild to moderate heartburn and nausea
Pumpkin seeds	Antiandrogenic (blocks dihydrotestosterone at prostate)	160 mg of pumpkin seed oil three times daily; or recommend eating pumpkin seeds	None reported
Flaxseed	Anti-inflammatory	Tbsp. of flaxseed oil daily, or 2–4 tbsp. of ground flaxseed daily	Diarrhea at high doses, possible increased risk of bleeding (stop before surgery)
β-Sitosterol	5α-Reductase inhibition, antiproliferative	20 mg three times daily	Mild gastrointestinal discomfort
Zinc	5α-Reductase inhibition	30–60 mg daily (with 2–3 mg of copper)	Immune system suppression with long-term doses over 100 mg

drug in the United States Pharmacopoeia and National Formulary but was later removed in the 1950s due to a lack of evidence for saw palmetto's active ingredient [15].

Several different mechanisms of action have been proposed for saw palmetto. It is difficult to study, as the different extracts have different components and may not mimic each other pharmacologically; however, many *in vitro* and *in vivo* studies have been carried out to propose mechanisms of saw palmetto. The main three mechanisms proposed are an antiandrogenic, anti-inflammatory, and proapoptotic effect. It was first found in 1984 to have a dose-dependent

inhibition of 5α-reductase in human foreskin fibroblast [16], suggesting that saw palmetto works similarly to the commonly prescribed 5α-reductase inhibitors. Weisser *et al.* again found a dose-dependent inhibition of 5α-reductase enzyme activity in the epithelium and stroma of human BPH cell lines. In this study, they found the fatty acids in the extract to have the strongest pharmacologic effect [17]. It has been indicated that an inflammatory process is present in BPH with the migration of monocytes, T-lymphocytes, and B-lymphocytes. It is suggested that saw palmetto inhibits the migration of these inflammatory cells, as *in vitro* inhibition of the synthesis of cyclo-oxygenase and 5-lipoxygenase by saw palmetto has been documented [18]. Lastly, proapoptotic properties have been proposed as the mechanism of action for saw palmetto. Saw palmetto increases the bax-to-bcl2 expression ratio and caspase-3 activity in patients [19], thus inducing apoptosis. Apoptosis is a natural defense of overproliferation, but the prostate does not undergo apoptosis normally to a high degree [20], and thus the induction by saw palmetto may be of benefit.

There have been several randomized controlled trials showing the efficacy of saw palmetto. In 1998, a meta-analysis of 18 of these trials was carried out involving 2939 men. Compared with placebo, men treated with saw palmetto had decreased urinary-tract symptom scores, decreased nocturia, increased peak flow rate, and improved self-rating of urinary tract symptoms. Compared with finasteride, saw palmetto had similar effects of IPSS and peak flow rates. Adverse effects with *serona repens* were rare and infrequent, and erectile dysfunction occurred less than with finasteride [21]. It was again shown that saw palmetto causes less sexual dysfunction than finasteride in a review carried out by the same group in 2002 [22].

More recently, a National Institute of Health-funded prospective trial, the Complementary and Alternative Medicines for Urological Symptoms trial, was carried out to compare escalating doses of saw palmetto extract with placebo in 369 subjects. No significant difference was found in symptom scores between the saw palmetto and placebo groups [23]. However, one of the authors still recommends the use of saw palmetto in men with LUTS, as it has been beneficial to many patients in his practice. Further clinical trials with saw palmetto are needed, as only one extract was investigated; and as mentioned earlier, different extracts vary in their components.

Pygeum (*Pygeum africanum*)

Pygeum africanum is derived from the bark of the African plum tree. It is commonly used in France under the trade name Tadenan and is now widely available over the counter in the United States. The African plum tree has been overharvested due to the demand of its extract and in 1995 was listed as an endangered species by the Convention on International Trade of Endangered Species. Compositional analysis shows pygeum is made of antioxidant, ferrulic esters, and β-sitoserol [24]. It has several proposed mechanisms of action, including anti-inflammatory and antiproliferative effects. Pygeum, as well as saw palmetto, was shown to inhibit neutrophil production of leukotriene and lipoxygenase metabolites in two different studies [25,26]. Additional *in vitro* studies have shown that pygeum inhibits human and rat prostate proliferation by inhibiting basic fibroblastic growth factor and epidermal growth factor [27]. Pygeum has also been found to have antiestrogenic effects. Pretreatment with Tadenan in rats significantly reduced the obstructive effects of DHT on micturition and reduced the DHT-induced enlargement of prostate [28]. A meta-analysis of 18 randomized controlled trials involving 1582 men was analyzed to assess the efficacy of pygeum. Men using pygeum were more than twice as likely to report an improvement in LUTS (relative risk 2.1; 95% confidence interval 1.4–3.1). Nocturia was decreased by 19%, and peak urine flow increased by 23%. Adverse effects in men supplementing with pygeum were mild and comparable with those taking placebo [29]. This study, as well as several others, suggests positive results for the use of pygeum in BPH; however, further placebo-controlled trials are needed with standardized urologic symptom scale scores. The Tadenan-IPSS trial intended to do this and began in 1996, but the results of this study were never released or published.

Stinging nettle (*Urtica dioica et urens*)

Nettle root extract is commonly used in Germany where at least 16 different preparations exist. These preparations contain a mixture of lectins, phenols, sterols (including β-sitosterol), and lignans [30]. The mechanism of action of stinging nettle is unknown but is thought to involve anti-inflammatory and antiproliferative effects [31].

In a randomized, placebo-controlled, double-blind, multicenter trial, the use of stinging nettle was found to reduce IPSS scores by 53%. The study included 257 subjects assigned to either placebo or PRO (160/120), which is a combination of extract from sabal fruit (160 mg) and nettle root (120 mg). Peak and average urinary flow significantly increased by 19%, and residual urine volume decreased by 44% [32].

South African star grass (*Hypoxis rooperi*)

The extracts of South African star grass are marketed as Harzol. Its main active ingredient is thought to be β-sitosterol (contains 20 mg), among other phytosterols. Therefore, its mechanism of action is believed to be through 5α-reductase inhibition and antiproliferative [3,4].

In 1995, Berges *et al.* completed a multicenter, randomized, double-blinded, placebo-controlled trial of 200 patients. The subjects took Harzol three times a day for 6 months. Significant improvements in IPSS, quality of life, PVRs, and PFRs were reported. The IPSS score improved by 7.4 units compared with 2.3 units in the placebo group [33]. The same

group followed up with the subjects after 18 months, at which point the beneficial effects of Harzol were still reported in the group that was treated for only 6 months. This suggests that intermittent treatment with Harzol may be sufficient [6].

Rye pollen (*Secale cerale*)

The pollen from *Secale cerale* is a registered pharmaceutical in Japan, Argentina, Korea, and Western Europe. It is commonly used for treatment of BPH and prostatitis. Cernilton is the most popular trademarked preparation of this flower pollen and has been on the market for nearly 40 years. It is produced by the Swedish company AB Cernelle and is a mix of rye pollen from several different plants grown in the southern part of the country. Rye pollen is thought to work by relaxing the urethral smooth muscle. It was shown to do this in mouse and pig tissue by acting on α adrenergic receptors [34]. It has also been shown to inhibit prostatic cell growth in human tissues *in vitro* [35].

In a Japanese study, 79 patients with BPH were treated with 126 mg of Cernilton three times a day. After 12 weeks, symptom scores decreased significantly. The maximum flow rate increased significantly from 9.3 mL/s to 11.0 mL/s, and average flow rate from 5.1 mL/s to 6.0 mL/s. Twenty-eight of the subjects were treated for more than 1 year and showed a significant decreased in prostatic volume from 33.2 mL to 26.5 mL [36]. Due to this study, the recommended dose of Cernilton is 126 mg three times a day.

A systematic review of four rye pollen trials was carried out [37]. In total, 444 men were enrolled in two placebo-controlled and two comparative trials. A self-reported decrease in LUTS was found compared with placebo (IPSS was not used). Furthermore, an improvement in nocturia was found with Cernilton use.

Pumpkin seeds (*Curcubita pepo* L.)

Pumpkin seed oil has been shown to act by inhibiting 5α-reductase [38,39]. Pumpkin seeds, or pepitas, are popular in Gemany. A randomized, placebo-controlled 12-month trial examined the effect of pumpkin seeds on LUTS and BPH. A total of 476 men participated. IPSS improved by 6.8 points with pumpkin seeds, 1.2 points higher than that of the placebo group [40].

Flaxseed lignans

Secoisolaricieresinol diglucoside (SDG) is a phytoestrogen found in flax thought to improve LUTS. A randomized, double-blind, placebo-controlled trial was conducted in 2008 with 87 subjects and assessed the efficacy of flaxseed lignan extract containing 33% SDG on the treatment of BPH. IPSS decreased and quality-of-life score improved in subjects taking SDG extract compared with the placebo group. The observed decreases in IPSS correlated with plasma concentrations of total lignans. The doses studied in this trial were 300 and 600 mg/day of SDG [41].

Nutrients

Zinc

Men with BPH and prostate cancer have been found to have lower levels of zinc in their blood and prostatic secretions [42]. Prostatic fluid contains high amounts of zinc, suggesting an important role for the gland, and is thought to work by inhibiting 5α-reductase. In a randomized trial of 4770 participants, the presence and symptoms were assessed over 7 years and were followed for medical or surgical treatment of BPH. Zinc was shown to have a possible protective role for BPH [43].

In an unpublished study of 19 men with BPH, the subjects took 150 mg of zinc daily for 2 months and then lowered their dose to 50–100 mg daily; 74% of the men in this preliminary study experienced a decrease in prostate size [44].

Amino acids

One group found that prostatic fluid is rich in amino acids glycine, glutamic acid, and alanine. Patients with BPH were given this combination 760 mg three times daily for 2 weeks, and then given 380 mg three times daily for an additional 10 weeks. After 3 months, 50% of the men reported reduced urgency and frequency, compared with only 15% in the placebo group [45].

Fatty acids

Essential fatty acids are known to reduce inflammation, and it is likely through this mechanism that they benefit men with BPH. In an Italian case-control study, the diets of 1369 patient with BPH and 1451 controls were assessed. An inverse relation between essential fatty acid liolenic acid and linoleic acid consumption and risk of BPH was found (odds ratio 0.71% and 0.73%, respectively) [46]. Flaxseed and fish oil are good sources of essential fatty acids.

Exercise

A high level of physical activity appears to protect men against BPH. A study found that men who did more physical activity had decreased BPH symptoms, decreased diagnosis of BPH, and decreased amount of surgery. Subjects who walked for 2–3 h per week decreased their risk of BPH by 25% compared with men who did not exercise [47].

Table 12.4 Summary of alternative treatment options for benign prostatic hyperplasia

Glandular activity	Stromal activity
5-α-Reductase inhibition	17-β-Hydroxysteroid dehydrogenase inhibition
Increased uridine	Aromatase inhibition
5′-diphosphoglucuronosyltransferase activity	Estrogen-receptor antagonism

Dos and don'ts

- Consider phytotherapy for patients with mild IPSS scores (Table 12.4).
- Phytotherapy is not recommended for patients in retention to replace alpha blockade.
- Recommend a saw palmetto extract that has been standardized to contain 85–95% fatty acids and sterols.
- Consider combining phytotherapy with alpha blockade. Combinations may have clinical benefit over either one alone.

Bibliography

1 Eisenberg DM, Kessler RC, Foster C, Norlock FE, Calkins DR, Delbanco TL. Unconventional medicine in the United States. Prevalence, costs, and patterns of use. *N Engl J Med*. 1993;328(4):246–52. PubMed PMID: 8418405.

2 Gunther S, Patterson RE, Kristal AR, Stratton KL, White E. Demographic and health-related correlates of herbal and specialty supplement use. *J Am Diet Assoc*. 2004;104(1):27–34. PubMed PMID: 14702580.

3 Cabeza M, Bratoeff E, Heuze I, Ramirez E, Sanchez M, Flores E. Effect of beta-sitosterol as inhibitor of 5 alpha-reductase in hamster prostate. *Proc West Pharmacol Soc*. 2003;46:153–5. PubMed PMID: 14699915. Epub 2004/01/01.eng.

4 Kassen A, Berges R, Senge T. Effect of beta-sitosterol on transforming growth factor-beta-1 expression and translocation protein kinase C alpha in human prostate stromal cells *in vitro*. *Eur Urol*. 2000;37(6):735–41. PubMed PMID: 10828677. Epub 2000/06/01.eng.

5 Klippel KF, Hiltl DM, Schipp B. A multicentric, placebo-controlled, double-blind clinical trial of beta-sitosterol (phytosterol) for the treatment of benign prostatic hyperplasia. German BPH-Phyto Study group. *Br J Urol*. 1997;80(3):427–32. PubMed PMID: 9313662. Epub 1997/10/06.eng.

6 Berges RR, Kassen A, Senge T. Treatment of symptomatic benign prostatic hyperplasia with beta-sitosterol: an 18-month follow-up. *BJU Int*. 2000;85(7):842–6. PubMed PMID: 10792163. Epub 2000/05/03.eng.

7 Wilt TJ, MacDonald R, Ishani A. Beta-sitosterol for the treatment of benign prostatic hyperplasia: a systematic review. *BJU Int*. 1999;83(9):976–83. PubMed PMID: 10368239. Epub 1999/06/15.eng.

8 Ambrosini GL, de Klerk NH, Mackerras D, Leavy J, Fritschi L. Dietary patterns and surgically treated benign prostatic hyperplasia: a case control study in Western Australia. *BJU Int*. 2008;101(7):853–60. PubMed PMID: 18070188.

9 Evans BA, Griffiths K, Morton MS. Inhibition of 5 alpha-reductase in genital skin fibroblasts and prostate tissue by dietary lignans and isoflavonoids. *J Endocrinol*. 1995;147(2):295–302. PubMed PMID: 7490559.

10 Sun XY, Plouzek CA, Henry JP, Wang TT, Phang JM. Increased UDP-glucuronosyltransferase activity and decreased prostate specific antigen production by biochanin A in prostate cancer cells. *Cancer Res*. 1998;58(11):2379–84. PubMed PMID: 9622078.

11 Matzkin H, Soloway MS. Immunohistochemical evidence of the existence and localization of aromatase in human prostatic tissues. *The Prostate*. 1992;21(4):309–14. PubMed PMID: 1281323.

12 Campbell DR, Kurzer MS. Flavonoid inhibition of aromatase enzyme activity in human preadipocytes. *J Steroid Biochem Mol Biol*. 1993;46(3):381–8. PubMed PMID: 9831487.

13 Collins BM, McLachlan JA, Arnold SF. The estrogenic and antiestrogenic activities of phytochemicals with the human estrogen receptor expressed in yeast. *Steroids*. 1997;62(4):365–72. PubMed PMID: 9090797.

14 Wang TT, Sathyamoorthy N, Phang JM. Molecular effects of genistein on estrogen receptor mediated pathways. *Carcinogenesis*. 1996;17(2):271–5. PubMed PMID: 8625449.

15 Buck AC. Is there a scientific basis for the therapeutic effects of *Serenoa repens* in benign prostatic hyperplasia? Mechanisms of action. *J Urol*. 2004;172 (5 Pt 1):1792–9. PubMed PMID: 15540722.

16 Sultan C, Terraza A, Devillier C, Carilla E, Briley M, Loire C, et al. Inhibition of androgen metabolism and binding by a liposterolic extract of "*Serenoa repens* B" in human foreskin fibroblasts. *J Steroid Biochem*. 1984;20(1):515–9. PubMed PMID: 6708534.

17 Weisser H, Tunn S, Behnke B, Krieg M. Effects of the sabal serrulata extract IDS 89 and its subfractions on 5 alpha-reductase activity in human benign prostatic hyperplasia. *The Prostate*. 1996;28(5):300–6. PubMed PMID: 8610056.

18 Vela Navarrete R, Garcia Cardoso J, Lopez Farre A, Barat A, Manzarbeitia F, Ramirez M, et al. [Benign prostatic hyperplasia: biological significance of lymphohistiocytic infiltration of the adenoma.] *Actas Urol Esp*. 2002;26(3):163–73. PubMed PMID: 12053516.

19 Vela-Navarrete R, Escribano-Burgos M, Farre AL, Garcia-Cardoso J, Manzarbeitia F, Carrasco C. *Serenoa repens* treatment modifies bax/bcl-2 index expression and caspase-3 activity in prostatic tissue from patients with benign prostatic hyperplasia. *J Urol*. 2005;173(2):507–10. PubMed PMID: 15643230.

20 Colombel M, Vacherot F, Diez SG, Fontaine E, Buttyan R, Chopin D. Zonal variation of apoptosis and proliferation in the normal prostate and in benign prostatic hyperplasia. *Br J Urol*. 1998;82(3):380–5. PubMed PMID: 9772874.

21 Wilt TJ, Ishani A, Stark G, MacDonald R, Lau J, Mulrow C. Saw palmetto extracts for treatment of benign prostatic hyperplasia: a systematic review. *J Am Med Assoc*. 199811;280(18):1604–9. PubMed PMID: 9820264. Epub 1998/11/20.eng.

22 Wilt T, Ishani A, Mac Donald R. *Serenoa repens* for benign prostatic hyperplasia. *Cochrane Database Syst Rev*. 2002(3):CD001423. PubMed PMID: 12137626. Epub 2002/07/26.eng.

23 Barry MJ, Meleth S, Lee JY, Kreder KJ, Avins AL, Nickel JC, et al. Effect of increasing doses of saw palmetto extract on lower urinary tract symptoms: a randomized trial. *J Am Med Assoc*. 2011;306(12):1344–51. PubMed PMID: 21954478. Pubmed Central PMCID: PMC3326341. Epub 2011/09/29.eng.

24 Gruenwald J. *Physician's desk reference (PDR) for herbal medicines*. 1st ed. Jaenicke C, editor. Montvale, NJ: Physicians Desk Reference Inc; 1998.

25 Paubert-Braquet M, Cave A, Hocquemiller R, Delacroix D, Dupont C, Hedef N, et al. Effect of Pygeum africanum extract on A23187-stimulated production of lipoxygenase metabolites from human polymorphonuclear cells. *J Lipid Mediat Cell Signal*. 1994;9(3):285–90. PubMed PMID: 7921787.

26 Paubert-Braquet M, Mencia Huerta JM, Cousse H, Braquet P. Effect of the lipidic lipidosterolic extract of *Serenoa repens* (Permixon) on the ionophore A23187-stimulated production of leukotriene B4 (LTB4) from human polymorphonuclear neutrophils. *Prostaglandins Leukot Essent Fatty Acids*. 1997;57(3):299–304. PubMed PMID: 9384520.

27 Yablonsky F, Nicolas V, Riffaud JP, Bellamy F. Antiproliferative effect of *Pygeum africanum* extract on rat prostatic fibroblasts. *J Urol*. 1997;157(6):2381–7. PubMed PMID: 9146675. Epub 1997/06/01.eng.

28 Choo MS, Bellamy F, Constantinou CE. Functional evaluation of Tadenan on micturition and experimental prostate growth induced with exogenous dihydrotestosterone. *Urology*. 2000;55(2):292–8. PubMed PMID: 10688098.

29 Wilt T, Ishani A, Mac Donald R, Rutks I, Stark G. Pygeum africanum for benign prostatic hyperplasia. *Cochrane Database Syst Rev*. 2002 (1):CD001044. PubMed PMID: 11869585.

30 Fagelman E, Lowe FC. Herbal medications in the treatment of benign prostatic hyperplasia (BPH). *Urol Clin N Am*. 2002;29(1):23–9, vii. PubMed PMID: 12109350. Epub 2002/07/12.eng.

31 Durak I, Biri H, Devrim E, Sozen S, Avci A. Aqueous extract of *Urtica dioica* makes significant inhibition on adenosine deaminase activity in prostate tissue from patients with prostate cancer. *Cancer Biol Ther*. 2004;3(9):855–7. PubMed PMID: 15254411. Epub 2004/07/16.eng.

32 Lopatkin N, Sivkov A, Walther C, Schlafke S, Medvedev A, Avdeichuk J, et al. Long-term

efficacy and safety of a combination of sabal and urtica extract for lower urinary tract symptoms—a placebo-controlled, double-blind, multicenter trial. *World J Urol.* 2005;23(2):139–46. PubMed PMID: 15928959. Epub 2005/06/02.eng.

33 Berges RR, Windeler J, Trampisch HJ, Senge T. Randomised, placebo-controlled, double-blind clinical trial of beta-sitosterol in patients with benign prostatic hyperplasia. Beta-sitosterol Study Group. *Lancet.* 1995;345(8964):1529–32. PubMed PMID: 7540705. Epub 1995/06/17.eng.

34 Kimura M, Kimura I, Nakase K, Sonobe T, Mori N. Micturition activity of pollen extract: contractile effects on bladder and inhibitory effects on urethral smooth muscle of mouse and pig. *Planta Med.* 1986;April:148–51. PubMed PMID: 3725935.

35 Habib FK, Ross M, Buck AC, Ebeling L, Lewenstein A. *In vitro* evaluation of the pollen extract, cernitin T-60, in the regulation of prostate cell growth. *Br J Urol.* 1990;66(4):393–7. PubMed PMID: 1699627.

36 Yasumoto R, Kawanishi H, Tsujino T, Tsujita M, Nishisaka N, Horii A, *et al.* Clinical evaluation of long-term treatment using cernitin pollen extract in patients with benign prostatic hyperplasia. *Clin Ther.* 1995;17(1):82–7. PubMed PMID: 7538904. Epub 1995/01/01.eng.

37 MacDonald R, Ishani A, Rutks I, Wilt TJ. A systematic review of Cernilton for the treatment of benign prostatic hyperplasia. *BJU Int.* 2000; 85(7):836–41. PubMed PMID: 10792162. Epub 2000/05/03.eng.

38 Tsai YS, Tong YC, Cheng JT, Lee CH, Yang FS, Lee HY. Pumpkin seed oil and phytosterol-F can block testosterone/prazosin-induced prostate growth in rats. *Urol Int.* 2006;77(3):269–74. PubMed PMID: 17033217. Epub 2006/10/13.eng.

39 Gossell-Williams M, Davis A, O'Connor N. Inhibition of testosterone-induced hyperplasia of the prostate of Sprague-Dawley rats by pumpkin seed oil. *J Med Food.* 2006;9(2):284–6. PubMed PMID: 16822218. Epub 2006/07/11.eng.

40 DB. nd der interdisziplinä rer Arbeitskreis Prostata. Placebokontrollierte Langzeittherapiestudie mit Kü rbissamenextrakt bei BPH-bedingten Miktionsbeschwerden. *J Clin Endocrinol Metab.* 2000;56:139–46.

41 Zhang W, Wang X, Liu Y, Tian H, Flickinger B, Empie MW, *et al.* Effects of dietary flaxseed lignan extract on symptoms of benign prostatic hyperplasia. *J Med Food.* 2008;11(2):207–14. PubMed PMID: 18358071.

42 Gomez Y, Arocha F, Espinoza F, Fernandez D, Vasquez A, Granadillo V. [Zinc levels in prostatic fluid of patients with prostate pathologies.] *Invest Clin.* 2007;48(3):287–94. PubMed PMID: 17853788. Epub 2007/09/15.

43 Kristal AR, Arnold KB, Schenk JM, Neuhouser ML, Goodman P, Penson DF, *et al.* Dietary patterns, supplement use, and the risk of symptomatic benign prostatic hyperplasia: results from the prostate cancer prevention trial. *Am J Epidemiol.* 2008;167(8):925–34. PubMed PMID: 18263602. Epub 2008/02/12.eng.

44 Bush IM BE, Nourkayhan S. *Zinc and the prostate.* Presented at the Annual Meeting of the American Medical Association; 1974.

45 Damrau F. Benign prostatic hypertrophy: amino acid therapy for symptomatic relief. *J Am Geriatr Soc.* 1962;10:426–30. PubMed PMID: 13883328. Epub 1962/05/01.eng.

46 Bravi F, Bosetti C, Dal Maso L, Talamini R, Montella M, Negri E, *et al.* Macronutrients, fatty acids, cholesterol, and risk of benign prostatic hyperplasia. *Urology.* 2006;67(6):1205–11. PubMed PMID: 16765180. Epub 2006/06/13.eng.

47 Platz EA, Kawachi I, Rimm EB, Colditz GA, Stampfer MJ, Willett WC, *et al.* Physical activity and benign prostatic hyperplasia. *Arch Intern Med.* 1998;158(21):2349–56. PubMed PMID: 9827786. Epub 1998/11/25.eng.

CHAPTER 13

Open Simple Prostatectomy

Annika Herlemann[1], Matthias Oelke[2] & Christian Gratzke[1]

[1]Department of Urology, LMU Munich, Munich, Germany
[2]Department of Urology, Hannover Medical School, Hannover, Germany

---

Key points

- Open prostatectomy is indicated in patients with large prostate adenomas exceeding 80–100 cm³ or those with indication for prostatic surgery and concomitant bladder diverticula or bladder stones [1].
- Complications of open prostatectomy include bleeding/blood transfusion, urinary incontinence, erectile dysfunction, retrograde ejaculation, urinary tract infection, urethral stricture, and deep venous thrombosis/embolism [1].
- Advantages of open prostatectomy over transurethral resection of the prostate (TURP) are a lower retreatment rate, complete removal of the prostatic adenoma under direct vision, and no risk of transurethral resection syndrome [1].
- the Disadvantages compared with TURP are midline incision, longer hospitalization time, and increased potential for perioperative hemorrhage [1].
- Before performing an open prostatectomy, the presence of prostate cancer should be excluded [1].

Introduction

Traditionally, open simple prostatectomy (OSP; i.e. transvesical or retropubic enucleation of the prostate adenoma) has been considered as the standard treatment option for patients with lower urinary tract symptoms (LUTS) due to benign prostatic enlargement (BPE) and benign prostatic obstruction (BPO) [2]. Today, transurethral approaches using mainly resection and vaporization techniques have replaced open surgery in the Western world; for large adenomas, transurethral enucleation of the prostate using various energy sources such as the holmium (holmium enucleation of the prostate) or thulium laser (thulium enucleation of the prostate) is considered to be superior to open surgery due to its minimally invasive nature and low adverse-event profile [3]. However, in most countries with fewer health-care resources, limited access to endoscopic equipment, or lack of endourological experience, simple open prostatectomy remains the standard of care for patients with prostates exceeding 80–100 cm³ [4], as opposed to many developed countries where it is performed in 13–40% of all cases [5,6].

Two main approaches for OSP emerged at the end of the 19th until the middle of the 20th century, the suprapubic transvesical (Freyer) and retropubic transcapsular (Millin)

---

procedures [7,8]. While open prostatectomy is invasive and, compared with the transurethral enucleation procedures, requires a lower vertical midline incision as well as longer hospitalization and reconvalescence time, it results in excellent functional outcome and low reoperation rates [4,9–11]. Indications for open prostatectomy include the treatment of adenomas greater than 80–100 cm³, and coexistent pathological conditions such as bladder diverticula, bladder stones, or inguinal hernias; however, the latter pathologies of the lower urinary tract are not limited to large prostates [2].

- adenomas greater than 80–100 cm³;
- coexistent pathological conditions such as:
  - bladder diverticulum;
  - bladder stones;
  - inguinal hernia;
- prior urethral stricture reconstruction surgery;
- need for concomitant bladder surgery:
  - reconstruction of bladder neck;
  - ureteral reimplantation.

Open surgery may also be indicated in patients who are unfit for transurethral surgery, for example, if those patients who cannot be positioned in lithotomy position for TURP, in cases of orthopedic pathologies in the hip, in those with complex urethral conditions, or in cases of hypospadia repair or urethral strictures. Progress in laparoscopic urological expertise has led to the development of laparoscopic as well as robotic simple prostatectomy [12–17]. There is growing evidence that these less invasive techniques are equally effective and safe options compared with open prostatectomy. All surgical techniques have to be compared with the gold standard in the treatment of LUTS, which is TURP.

Open simple prostatectomy

Open prostatectomy involves the surgical enucleation of the prostate via a suprapubic or retropubic incision in the lower abdomen, or via a perineal route. The first technique described was the perineal approach more than 2000 years ago, which was performed until suprapubic transvesical prostatectomy was first undertaken by Eugene Fuller in New York in 1894 and popularized by Peter Freyer in London at the beginning of the 20th century [18]. In 1945, Terrence Millin introduced the retropubic transcapsular prostatectomy and published the results of his first 20 patients operated on with this procedure (Table 13.1) [8].

Table 13.1 Advantages of the various open approaches of prostatectomies

Suprapubic OSP	Retropubic OSP	Perineal OSP
Good exposure of the bladder neck and ureteral orifices in patients with median prostatic lobe, bladder stones or diverticulum	Good visualization of the prostate during enucleation as well as direct view of the proximal urethra	Treatment of concomitant prostatic abscess and cysts
	Minimal trauma to the bladder	Ability to avoid the lower abdomen or retropubic space
	Direct access to the prostatic fossa for postenucleation haemostasis	Less postoperative pain

OSP, open simple prostatectomy.

Surgical techniques

Suprapubic transvesical prostatectomy (Freyer)

This technique is characterized by an extra-peritoneal transverse or vertical incision of the anterior abdominal and bladder wall [1,2,19]. The use of temporary sutures lateral to the bladder incision, usually at 3 and 9 o'clock positions, is recommended to expose the bladder lumen. After identification of the ureteral orifices and placement of temporary ureteral catheters in patients with prostate lobes close to the ureteral orifices, the bladder neck mucosa is incised from the 5- to 7-o'clock position (Figure 13.1A) [19]. The index finger is then placed in the urethra and pressed ventrally against the pubic bone in the midline, the finger sweeps firmly to fracture the anterior commissure of the prostate, and the plane between the surgical capsule and the adenoma/transition zone can be defined (Figure 13.1B) [19]. The adenoma is then circumferentially separated from the capsule by digital dissection. Both lobes of the adenoma are separated in this fashion up to the area of the bladder neck (Figure 13.1C) [19]. Special attention is necessary when the transition zone is separated from the prostatic apex in order to prevent injury to the external urethral sphincter [2]. To provide good haemostasis, the enucleated and now empty prostatic fossa should be tightly packed with gauze and compressed with a swab for 5–10 min [19]. After removal of the swab and gauze, sutures of the main prostatic arteries should be placed at the 5 and 7 o'clock positions, even if no active bleeding is evident. During suturing, the surgeon should pay attention to the ureteral orifices. The bladder neck may be closed with a running suture of fast-resorbing material (e.g. Catgut or Vicryl-rapid) in cases of severe bleeding.

Before closing the bladder, a transurethral and suprapubic catheter should be inserted under vision [1,19]. Traction of the urethral catheter balloon should be removed after a couple of hours to avoid ischemic necrosis of the glans penis [1].

The main advantage of the transvesical removal of the transition zone is the good exposure of the bladder neck and ureteral orifices in patients with large prostatic median lobes, bladder stones, or bladder diverticula [2].

Retropubic transcapsular prostatectomy (Millin)

After horizontal or vertical incision of the anterior abdominal wall and exposure of the ventral circumference of the prostate, the anterior prostatic capsule is incised with a steel or electric knife approximately 1 cm distal to the bladder neck deep enough to expose the plane between the fibrous external capsule and prostate adenoma (transition zone). Once the surgeon has identified the right plane between the transition zone and capusule, they should proceed, separating the tissues with Metzenbaum scissors [1,19]. Afterwards, the adenoma can be liberated bluntly with scissors or the index finger. By cutting the urethra distally, the adenoma can be removed without injury to the external urethral sphincter. To avoid late complications such as bladder neck stricture, a resection of the trigone may be considered in some cases. In analogy with the suprapubic technique, the empty prostatic fossa may be packed with gauze and compressed with a swab for 5–10 min to ensure haemostasis [1,19]. After removal of the gauze, the prostatic capsule is finally closed after the insertion of a transurethral catheter and visual placement of the catheter ballon in the bladder. Urine should be drained for 3–4 days.

(A)

SPP bladder mucosal incision

Bladder neck

Prostatic intravesical adenoma

Bladder mucosal incision 5 to 7 o'clock

(B)

Suprapubic prostatectomy finger adenoma enucleation

Rectum

Prostate apex

(C)

Suprapubic prostatectomy finger enucleation of prostate adenoma

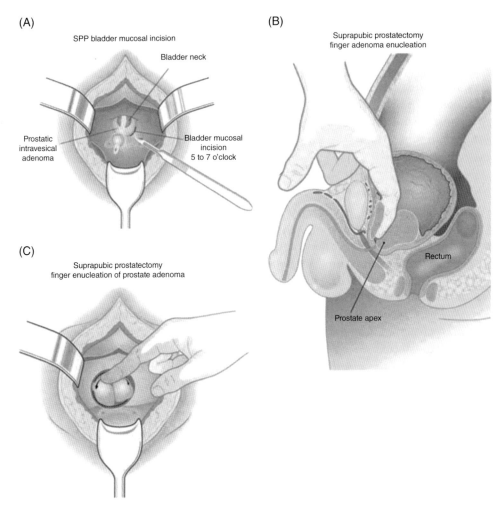

Figure 13.1 (A) Incision of the bladder neck mucosa only from the 5- to 7-o'clock position. (B) At the apex, the index finger sweeps ventrally to fracture the anterior prostatic commissure. (C) Both lobes of the adenoma are separated in this fashion up the area of the bladder neck. Modlin C. Open Benign Prostatectomy in Novick AC et al. (eds). Operative Urology at the Cleveland Clinic. 2006 Humana Press. Reproduced with permission of Humana Press Inc.

The advantages of the retropubic transcapsular approach compared with the suprapubic technique include minimal trauma of the bladder, better visualization of the prostate during enucleation, direct view of the proximal urethra, and direct access to the prostatic fossa for postenucleation haemostasis [2].

Simple perineal prostatectomy

This rare approach might be indicated in selected patients in whom transurethral surgery is contraindicated, who have had extensive abdominal, pelvic, or retroperitoneal surgery, or who do not qualify for the above-mentioned techniques [19]. The perineal approach is similar to radical perineal prostatectomy for prostate cancer with the exception that the prostatic capsule is only incised and the transition zone enucleated [19]. Treatment of concomitant prostatic abscess and cysts, the ability to avoid the lower abdomen or retropubic space, and less postoperative pain are the advantages of the perineal approach [2,19].

Perioperative antibiotic prophylaxis

Controversies still exist about the necessity for prophylactic antibiotics during urologic procedures [20]. However, in cases of opening the urinary tract, a single perioperative parenteral dose of antibiotics (e.g. second- or third-generation cephalosporine) is recommended [2]. In open prostatectomy, the risk of postoperative infection is particularly increased. Thus, a known urinary tract infection should be treated prior to surgery.

Postoperative management

In case of significant bleeding postoperatively, traction may be applied to the indwelling transurethral catheter in order to compress the bladder neck and prostatic fossa. In addition, continuous bladder irrigation through the suprapubic (inflow) and transurethral catheters (outflow) [1] is recommended to avoid clot formation. In case of excessive bleeding, re-exploration is advised. Bladder irrigation may be discontinued if haematuria is resolved, and the bladder catheter may be removed on the second day after surgery if the urine is clear [1]. In case the bladder neck is closed with a running suture during the operation, the catheter balloon can be retracted into the prostatic fossa under X-ray control after approximately 1 week and finally removed when the urine is clear.

Functional outcomes

Open prostatectomy results in excellent functional results with low morbidity and mortality. In a large prospective study including more than 900 patients, the mean operative time was 80.8 ± 34.2 min, while the mean enucleated tissue weight was 84.8 ± 44 g. Incidental carcinoma of the prostate was found on histological examination in 3.1% of this PSA-screened population. Postvoid residual volume and urinary flow rate improved significantly at discharge [10]; postvoid residual urine decreased from 145.1 ± 152.8 mL to 17.5 ± 34.8 mL, and maximum urinary flow rate increased from 10.6 ± 6.4 mL/s to 23.1 ± 10.5 mL/s. Similar outcomes for functional results at the time of patients' discharge were reported by Adam and colleagues in a retrospective study [21]. In a small prospective study, Tubaro *et al.* showed a decrease in symptoms, as measured with the International Prostate Symptom Score (IPSS) from 19.9 ± 4.4 to 1.5 ± 2.7, and an increase in quality of life 1 year after surgery (QoL score decreased from 4.9 ± 1 to 0.2 ± 0.4) [9]. In this study, the maximum flow rate improved from 9.1 ± 5.3 to 29.0 ± 8.9 mL/s, while postvoid residual urine decreased from 128 ± 113 to 8 ± 18 mL. These excellent functional results were documented up to 5 years, as shown in prospective and retrospective analyses [4,11,22]. At 5 years, the IPSS dropped from 21.0 ± 3.6 to 3.0 ± 1.7, while maximum urinary flow rates increased from 3.6 ± 3.8 to 24.4 ± 7.4 mL/s [22]. Postvoid residual volume decreased from 292 ± 191 mL to 5.3 ± 11.2 mL.

Postoperative urodynamic changes were also assessed over time [4]. The authors showed relief of BPO starting at a 3-month follow-up and reaching a plateau at 24 months (Schäfer grade = linPURR 3.1 at baseline versus 0.8 at month 12 post surgery). Based on these data, it is obvious that open prostatectomy

Table 13.2 Surgical outcome after open simple prostatectomy [2]

Studies	Duration (weeks)	Patients (n)	Change in symptoms (International Prostate Symptom Score)		Change in Q_{max}		Change in postvoid residual		Change in prostate volume		Level of evidence
			Absolute	%	mL/s	%	mL/s	%	mL/s	%	
Kuntz et al. [9]	260	32	−18.2	86	21.4	677	−287	98			1b
Skolarikos et al. [8]	78	60	−12.5	63	7	86	−77	86	−86	88	1b
Naspro et al. [7]	104	39	−13.2	62	15.9	291					1b
Varkarakis et al. [12]	151	232	−23.3	84	16.5	329	−104	90			3
Gratzke et al. [13]		868			13	218	−128	88	−85	88	2b

Oelke 2013 [2]. Reproduced with permission of Elsevier.

Table 13.3 Morbidity and mortality rates of open simple prostatectomy [2]

	Perioperative mortality (%)	Postoperative stress incontinence (%)	Reoperation for benign prostatic obstruction (%)
Kuntz et al. [9]	0	0	0
Skolarikos et al. [8]	0		0
Naspro et al. [7]	0	2.5	0
Varkarakis et al. [12]	0	0	
Gratzke et al. [13]	0.2		

Oelke 2013 [2]. Reproduced with permission of Elsevier.

provides long-lasting functional improvements and increased quality of life (Table 13.2).

Morbidity and mortality

Over the years, open prostatectomy has seen a steady decrease in morbidity and mortality. The most important perioperative complications are surgical revisions due to severe bleeding (0–3.7%), blood transfusions (0–24%) and urinary tract infections (UTI; 2.6–12.9%) [4,10,22]. Mortality rates were described as low as 0–0.2%. Late complications included bladder neck or urethral strictures requiring surgical treatment (up to 6.7%) and dysuria (up to 3.3%). Erectile function as measured with the erectile function domain of the International

Index of Erectile Function questionnaire, showed no significant reduction in the follow-up period (Table 13.3) [4].

Minimally invasive alternatives of simple prostatectomy

Laparoscopic simple prostatectomy

Feasibility of laparoscopic simple prostatectomy (LSP) was first described in 2002 by Mariano and coworkers [15]. Four years later, the same group reported the results of 60 patients who had undergone laparoscopic prostatectomy [16]. The average prostate weight was 144.50±41.74g, with a mean operation time of 138.48±23.38 min and estimated blood loss of 330.98±149.52 mL. No patients required blood transfusions or conversion to open surgery, and the postoperative complication rate was low. Erectile function was preserved in all those patients who were potent before surgery, and no patient reported de novo urinary incontinence. As with most laparoscopic approaches, a short hospital stay and early return to normal activity were considered to be the main advantages. To date, reports from several centers have confirmed the technical feasibility and safety of LSP [13,23–27].

In a nonrandomized, comparative study, 280 consecutive patients underwent prostatectomy either by the laparoscopic extraperitoneal transcapsular (Millin) or by the open transvesical (Freyer) approach. There was no significant difference in uroflow rate, mean IPSS, operative blood loss, total time of continuous bladder irrigation, or complication rate between the groups. The mean operation time was significantly longer in the laparoscopy group, while the hospital stay and length of catheterization were significantly shorter [14].

Robot-assisted simple prostatectomy

The first reports on robot-assisted simple prostatectomy (RASP) were published by Sotelo and coworkers in 2008 based on their experience of seven patients [12, 17]. The mean operative time was 205 min, hospital stay 1.4 days, Foley catheter duration 7 days, and drain removal after 3.75 days. No serious complications were documented. Still, a blood transfusion was necessary in one patient secondary due to injury to the epigastric artery. On pathological examination, the average prostate weight was 50.48g. Considerable

improvements from baseline were noted in IPSS (22 vs 7.25) and maximum urinary flow (17.75 vs 55.5 mL/s).

In 2012, a technical modification during the reconstructive part of the RASP was described by Coelho and coworkers and analyzed in six consecutive patients [28]. Following the resection of the adenoma and instead of performing the classical "trigonization" of the bladder neck and closure of the prostatic capsule, three modified steps were proposed: plication of the posterior prostatic capsule, a modified van Velthoven continuous vesicourethral anastomosis, and, finally, suture of the anterior prostatic capsule to the anterior bladder wall (Figure 13.2). The mean patient age was 69 years, mean estimated blood loss 208 mL, mean operative time 90 min, and mean weight of the surgical specimen 145 g. The potential advantages of this modified technique include reduced blood loss, lower blood transfusion rates, and shorter hospitalization length without the need for postoperative continuous bladder irrigation.

In comparison with OSP, several principal concerns remain when applying RASP: the learning curve of this technique remains considerably high, and the costs of RASP significantly exceed those of OSP. Furthermore, very large prostates could pose a problem for the ability to perform this technique safely due to increased blood loss. The need for large incisions for prostate extraction to remove these adenomas may limit the usefulness of the approach as well [29]. Very recently, it was advocated that in high-volume centers with surgeons experienced in robotic surgery, the indication for robot-assisted simple prostatectomy should be extended, considering that bipolar TURP costs in patients with large-volume prostates have similar costs to RASP [30].

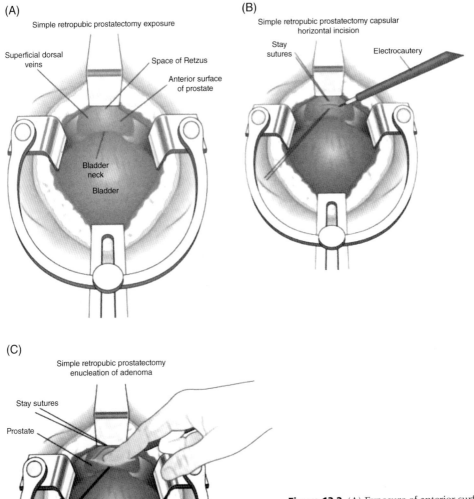

Figure 13.2 (A) Exposure of anterior surface of the prostate and bladder neck. (B) Horizontal incision through the prostatic capsule with a steel or electric knife. (C) Index finger is inserted through this incision and the adenoma enucleated with a sweeping motion. Modlin C. Open Benign Prostatectomy in Novick AC et al. (eds). Operative Urology at the Cleveland Clinic. 2006 Humana Press. Reproduced with permission of Humana Press Inc.

Still, advocates of the robotic approach postulate several advantages such as three-dimensional vision, six degrees of freedom in the instrument movements, and downscaling of movements, which are thought to allow the surgeon greater precision and vision. While a number of feasibility studies have been reported [31,32], it will be interesting to see whether this technique will gain broader acceptance in the

Dos and don'ts

- Before OSP, a known urinary tract infection should be treated. In addition, a single perioperative parenteral dose of antibiotics (e.g. second- or third-generation cephalosporine) is recommended.

- In suprapubic and retropubic prostatectomy, to achieve good hemostasis it is useful to pack the prostatic fossa with (warm) gauze after removal of the prostatic tissue.

- After removal of prostatic tissue during suprapubic transvesical prostatectomy, sutures of the main prostatic arteries should be placed at the 5 and 7 o'clock positions, even if no active bleeding is evident, while avoiding harming the ureteral orifices.

- During retropubic transcapsular prostatectomy, resection of the trigone may be considered to avoid late complications such as bladder neck strictures.

future. Therefore, a larger, multicenter, randomized trial of RASP is required before recommending this technique as standard practice [17].

Single-port transvesical enucleation of the prostate

Initially published by Sotelo and coworkers, today various reports have described the feasibility of single-port transvesical enucleation of the prostate (STEP) techniques (laparoscopic or robot-assisted), whereas no randomized trials comparing STEP with the open approach have been published so far [33]. Exclusively performed in specialized centers, STEP has shown good functional results but longer operation times and higher morbidity rates. In a recent series of 34 patients, the mean operative time was 116 min; the authors reported one death, a patient with bowel injury, and one with severe bleeding [34–37].

Bibliography

1 Han M, Alfert H, Partin A. Retropubic and suprapubic open prostatectomy. In: Walsh PCR, Vaughan ED, Wein AJ, editors. *Campbell's urology. 8.* Philadelphia, PA: Saunders; 2002. pp. 1423–33.

2 Oelke M, Bachmann A, Descazeaud A, Emberton M, Gravas S, Michel MC, et al. EAU guidelines on the treatment and follow-up of non-neurogenic male lower urinary tract symptoms including benign prostatic obstruction. *Eur Urol.* 2013;64(1):118–40.

3 Herrmann TR, Liatsikos EN, Nagele U, Traxer O, Merseburger AS. EAU guidelines on laser technologies. *Eur Urol.* 2012;61(4):783–95.

4 Naspro R, Suardi N, Salonia A, Scattoni V, Guazzoni G, Colombo R, et al. Holmium laser enucleation of the prostate versus open prostatectomy for prostates >70 g: 24-month follow-up. *Eur Urol.* 2006;50(3):563–8.

5 Bruskewitz R. Management of symptomatic BPH in the US: who is treated and how? *Eur Urol.* 1999;36(Suppl 3):7–13.

6 Serretta V, Morgia G, Fondacaro L, Curto G, Lo bianco A, Pirritano D, et al. Open prostatectomy for benign prostatic enlargement in southern Europe in the late 1990s: a contemporary series of 1800 interventions. *Urology.* 2002;60(4):623–7.

7 Freyer PJ. One thousand cases of total enucleation of the prostate for radical cure of enlargement of that organ. *Br Med J.* 1912;868.

8 Millin T. Retropubic prostatectomy; a new extravesical technique; report of 20 cases. *Lancet.* 1945;2(6380):693–6.

9 Tubaro A, Carter S, Hind A, Vicentini C, Miano L. A prospective study of the safety and efficacy of suprapubic transvesical prostatectomy in patients with benign prostatic hyperplasia. *J Urol.* 2001;166(1):172–6.

10 Gratzke C, Schlenker B, Seitz M, Karl A, Hermanek P, Lack N, et al. Complications and early postoperative outcome after open prostatectomy in patients with benign prostatic enlargement: results of a prospective multicenter study. *J Urol.* 2007;177(4):1419–22.

11 Varkarakis I, Kyriakakis Z, Delis A, Protogerou V, Deliveliotis C. Long-term results of open trans-vesical prostatectomy from a contemporary series of patients. *Urology*. 2004;64(2):306–10.

12 Sotelo R, Clavijo R, Carmona O, Garcia A, Banda E, Miranda M, *et al.* Robotic simple prostatectomy. *J Urol*. 2008;179(2):513–5.

13 Baumert H, Ballaro A, Dugardin F, Kaisary AV. Laparoscopic versus open simple prostatectomy: a comparative study. *J Urol*. 2006;175(5): 1691–4.

14 McCullough TC, Heldwein FL, Soon SJ, Galiano M, Barret E, Cathelineau X, *et al.* Laparoscopic versus open simple prostatectomy: an evalua-tion of morbidity. *J Endourol/Endourol Soc*. 2009; 23(1):129–33.

15 Mariano MB, Graziottin TM, Tefilli MV. Laparoscopic prostatectomy with vascular con-trol for benign prostatic hyperplasia. *J Urol*. 2002;167(6):2528–9.

16 Mariano MB, Tefilli MV, Graziottin TM, Morales CM, Goldraich IH. Laparoscopic prostatectomy for benign prostatic hyperplasia—a six-year experience. *Eur Urol*. 2006;49(1):127–31; discus-sion 31–2.

17 Merseburger AS, Herrmann TR, Shariat SF, Kyriazis I, Nagele U, Traxer O, *et al.* EAU guide-lines on robotic and single-site surgery in urology. *Eur Urol*. 2013;64(2):277–91.

18 Freyer P. One thousand cases of total enucleation of the prostate for radical cure of enlargement of that organ. *Br Med J*. 1912;868.

19 Modlin C. Open benign prostatectomy. In: Novick A, editor. *Operative urology at the Cleveland Clinic*. Totowa, NJ: Humana Press; 2006. pp. 315–22.

20 Grabe M, Bjerklund-Johanse TE, Botto H, Cek M, Naber KG, Pickard RS, *et al. Guidelines on urological infections*; 2013. Available from: http://www. uroweborg

21 Adam C, Hofstetter A, Deubner J, Zaak D, Weitkunat R, Seitz M, *et al.* Retropubic trans-vesical prostatectomy for significant prostatic enlargement must remain a standard part of urology training. *Scand J Urol Nephrol*. 2004;38(6):472–6.

22 Kuntz RM, Lehrich K, Ahyai SA. Holmium laser enucleation of the prostate versus open prostatec-tomy for prostates greater than 100 grams: 5-year follow-up results of a randomised clinical trial. *Eur Urol*. 2008;53(1):160–6.

23 Nadler RB, Blunt LW, Jr., User HM, Vallancien G. Preperitoneal laparoscopic simple prostatectomy. *Urology*. 2004;63(4):778–9.

24 van Velthoven R, Peltier A, Laguna MP, Piechaud T. Laparoscopic extraperitoneal adenomectomy (Millin): pilot study on feasibility. *Eur Urol*. 2004;45(1):103–9; discussion 9.

25 Yun HK, Kwon JB, Cho SR, Kim JS. Early experi-ence with laparoscopic retropubic simple prosta-tectomy in patients with voluminous benign prostatic hyperplasia (BPH). *Korean J Urol*. 2010;51(5):323–9.

26 Castillo OA, Bolufer E, Lopez-Fontana G, Sanchez-Salas R, Foneron A, Vidal-Mora I, *et al.* [Laparoscopic simple prostatectomy (adenomectomy): experi-ence in 59 consecutive patients.] *Actas Urol Esp*. 2011;35(7):434–7.

27 Thaidumrong T, Akarasakul D. Laparoscopic retropubic simple prostatectomy for large benign prostatic hyperplasia: first case report in Thailand. *J Med Assoc Thai*. 2013;96(Suppl 3):S104–8.

28 Coelho RF, Chauhan S, Sivaraman A, Palmer KJ, Orvieto MA, Rocco B, *et al.* Modified technique of robotic-assisted simple prostatectomy: advantages of a vesico-urethral anastomosis. *BJU Int*. 2012; 109(3):426–33.

29 Sutherland DE, Perez DS, Weeks DC. Robot-assisted simple prostatectomy for severe benign prostatic hyperplasia. *J Endourol/Endourol Soc*. 2011;25(4):641–4.

30 Matei DV, Brescia A, Mazzoleni F, Spinelli M, Musi G, Melegari S, *et al.* Robot-assisted simple prostatectomy (RASP): does it make sense? *BJU Int*. 2012;110(11 Pt C):E972–9.

31 Yuh B, Laungani R, Perlmutter A, Eun D, Peabody JO, Mohler JL, *et al.* Robot-assisted Millin's retro-pubic prostatectomy: case series. *Can J Urol*. 2008; 15(3):4101–5.

32 John H, Bucher C, Engel N, Fischer B, Fehr JL. Preperitoneal robotic prostate adenomectomy. *Urology*. 2009;73(4):811–5.

33 Sotelo RJ, Astigueta JC, Desai MM, Canes D, Carmona O, De Andrade RJ, *et al.* Laparoendoscopic single-site surgery simple prostatectomy: initial report. *Urology*. 2009;74(3):626–30.

34 Desai MM, Fareed K, Berger AK, Astigueta JC, Irwin BH, Aron M, *et al.* Single-port transvesical enucleation of the prostate: a clinical report of 34 cases. *BJU Int*. 2010;105(9):1296–300.

35 Oktay B, Vuruskan H, Koc G, Danisoglu ME, Kordan Y. Single-port extraperitoneal transvesical

adenomectomy: initial operative experience. *Urol Int*. 2010;85(2):131–4.

36 Fareed K, Zaytoun OM, Autorino R, White WM, Crouzet S, Yakoubi R, *et al*. Robotic single port suprapubic transvesical enucleation of the prostate (R-STEP): initial experience. *BJU Int*. 2012;110(5):732–7.

37 Lee JY, Han JH, Moon HS, Yoo TK, Choi HY, Lee SW. Single-port transvesical enucleation of the prostate for benign prostatic hyperplasia with severe intravesical prostatic protrusion. *World J Urol*. 2012;30(4):511–7.

CHAPTER 14

Minimally Invasive Therapies

Mauro Gacci, Matteo Salvi & Arcangelo Sebastianelli

Department of Urology, University of Florence, Careggi Hospital, Florence, Italy

Key points

- The surgical treatment of lower urinary tract symptoms (LUTS)/benign prostatic hyperplasia (BPH) continues to evolve, in particular due to the emerging role of mini-invasive techniques.
- Most of the techniques are based on the induction of a coagulative necrosis with consequent reduction in prostate size.
- The minimal need for anesthetics, short hospitalization time required, and minimal incidence of adverse events, in particular with regard to sexual activity, are some of the advantages of these procedures.
- Prolonged catheterization, need for patient selection, minimal effects on urinary flow rate at uroflowmetry, and high risk of retreatment are the limitations.
- Several biases, including study designs, patients features, intervention characteristics, outcome measures, and follow-up, strongly affect the overall quality of the evidence currently available in literature.

Overview

LUTS due to BPH are a common condition in elderly males [1]. LUTS are characterized by storage symptoms, including urgency, frequency, and nocturia, and voiding symptoms including a weak stream and incomplete voiding [2]. Sexual dysfunction, characterized by decreased libido, erectile dysfunction, difficulties reaching orgasm, and ejaculatory disorders, is frequently comorbid in men affected by LUTS/BPH [3].

The progressive worsening of both urinary and sexual function in men with BPH can have a remarkable impact on quality of life [4]. The main objectives of every treatment for BPH are the relief of symptoms and related bother, the prevention of disease progression, and the concomitant decline in the risk of treatment-related adverse events.

All medical and surgical treatments for BPH, even if they can completely restore urinary function, carry the potential risk of affecting sexual function, although the occurrence and severity of sexual dysfunction vary among treatments [5]. Patients slightly bothered by initial urinary symptoms can benefit from conventional medical treatment, while men affected by moderate to severe LUTS, refractory to any drugs, with an impairment of overall quality of life, are usually treated by surgical procedure [6,7].

Conventional surgery of the prostate, in addition to requiring hospitalization and

Male Lower Urinary Tract Symptoms and Benign Prostatic Hyperplasia, First Edition.
Edited by Steven A. Kaplan and Kevin T. McVary.

several days of catheterization, can expose patients to the risk of intraoperative complications, including blood loss, urinary tract infection, or transurethral resection syndrome. Moreover, long-term adverse events, affecting urinary function (persistent urgency, reduced continence, urethral stricture) or sexual activity (permanent ejaculatory dysfunction, worsening of erectile dysfunction), can also occur after surgery for LUTS/BPH [8].

Therefore, several minimally invasive procedures have been recently developed with the aim to reduce the length of stay and number of days of catheterization, and minimize early and late complications, as well as achieving symptom relief. In fact, there is an ongoing evolution of all technologies available for the treatment of LUTS/BPH, and newer devices are being introduced for clinical practice. Long-term safety and efficacy, in addition to the overall cost analysis, must be taken into account, to define the durability and utility of these procedures [9,10].

Transurethral needle ablation of the prostate

Transurethral needle ablation (TUNA) of the prostate was used for the first time in 1993 by Shulmann *et al.* and subsequently introduced in the United States in 1996 for the treatment of men affected by LUTS secondary to BPH, with prostate sizes of 20–50 cm³ [11]. In recent years, TUNA has been increasingly used in clinical practice and has been considered a potential alternative to conventional surgery for symptomatic BPH [12]. Over the years, new TUNA catheters have been developed (TUNA II and TUNA III).

The TUNA system includes the delivery of radio-frequency waves from a generator through two adjustable needles located at the end of disposable monopolar catheters, inserted into the prostate under endoscopic control. The low-level radio-frequency energy (460 kHz) creates a localized heating effect of up to 115 °C, resulting in areas of coagulative necrosis. The preservation of the urethra and other contiguous structures is guaranteed by Teflon sheaths advanced over the needles. The technique is repeated, placing the needles in different areas of the prostate once the coagulative effect has been achieved, usually every 5 min. The procedure is performed under local or regional anesthesia and generally lasts between 30 and 60 min, depending on the prostate size. An indwelling catheter is used up to a maximum of 3 days [13].

In 2003, Zlotta *et al.* [14,15] conducted a multicenter study for the long-term evaluation of TUNA clinical outcomes in BPH men: 188 consecutive patients were followed for 5 years in three different centers. At a mean follow-up of 63 months, the International Prostate Symptom Score (IPSS), a validated questionnaire to assess the urinary symptoms, decreased from 20.9 to 8.7 ($P<0.001$), demonstrating a remarkable clinical effectiveness. Moreover, the maximum flow rate at uroflowmetry increased from 8.6 mL/s to 12.1 mL/s ($P<0.001$). Overall, 78% and 24% of patients showed improved (at least 50%) urinary symptoms (IPSS) and maximum flow rate, respectively. Conversely, 23.3% of patients required additional treatment.

In 2006, a systematic review and meta-analysis based on data from 35 studies (26 noncomparative and nine comparative) assessing TUNA in symptomatic BPH was conducted by Bouza *et al.* [12]: Median lobe hypertrophy was considered the exclusion criterion for TUNA in most of the studies included in the review [16–23].

Among the 26 noncomparative studies, 13 (868 patients) provided data 1 year after surgery, reporting an average reduction in urinary symptoms (Symptom Index −12.6, $P = 0.000$), with a 59% improvement over pretreatment values. Moreover, 14 studies (959 patients) provided data on quality-of-life score reduction (−2.6, $P = 0.000$) and on maximum flow rate improvement (4.4 mL/s, $P = 0.000$).

Five comparative randomized studies including 336 patients [167 treated with TUNA vs 169 with transurethral resection of prostate (TURP)], in addition to four nonrandomized comparative studies, demonstrated a 3-month clinical efficacy of TUNA comparable with that reported after TURP in terms of relief of urinary symptoms and improvement in quality of life, but not in maximum flow rate at uroflowmetry. In particular, the mean change in Symptom Index was −12.1 for TUNA and −15.5 for TURP (55% vs 71% of improvement, respectively), with comparable outcomes in terms of quality of life score, at 12 months' follow-up: −4.0 for TUNA and −4.3 for TURP (49% vs 56%, respectively). However, the improvement in maximum flow rate at uroflowmetry achieved at 12 months was most remarkable after TURP compared with TUNA: 12.2 vs 6.5 and (160% vs 76% respectively).

Safety was assessed in 1204 patients enrolled in 26 studies [12]. The most frequent adverse event was hematuria (337 patients, 28%), but only 16 patients had severe hematuria, with just one requiring blood transfusion. Transitory urinary retention was described in 279 patients (23%). Other common adverse events such as dysuria, irritative symptoms, and urinary tract infections were described in 167 (14%), 117 (10%), and 43 (4%) of cases, respectively. Adverse events on sexual function were occasionally reported: four patients complained of erectile dysfunction (0.3%), three

of retrograde ejaculation (0.2%), and only one loss of ejaculation (0.08%). The low impact of TUNA on sexual function was confirmed by Frieben in a review of 2010 [23]. Overall 237 patients out of 1036 patients enrolled in 17 trials required further treatments with a retreatment rate of 19.1% (95% CI: 18.7–39.7).

Transurethral microwave thermotherapy

In 1980, Magin *et al.*, and 5 years later Harada *et al.*, showed in their experimental study that microwaves could create high temperatures in prostatic tissue without damaging surrounding tissue [24]. Currently available devices in the field of microwave thermotherapy include the Prostatron™ device (Urologix, Minneapolis, MN, USA), Targis™ (Urologix, Minneapolis, MN, USA), CoreTherm™ (ProstaLund, Lund, Sweden), and TMx-2000™ (TherMatrx Inc, Northbrook, ILL, USA) [25]. The main differences between the various devices are the structure of the urethral applicators and the cooling systems.

Transurethral microwave thermotherapy (TUMT) technology is based on the use of microwave energy to induce oscillation of water molecules and ions; in the microwave field, the electrical dipoles oscillate, and electrical charges move back and forth, thereby producing heat. Depending on the power setting and type of device, temperatures of 45–80 °C can be achieved in the prostate gland, inducing coagulative necrosis of tissues and denervation of alpha-receptors, and reducing smooth muscle tone.

An antenna mounted within a transurethral catheter, through which cooling fluid circulates, is used to perform the procedure, while urethral and rectal thermometers are needed to control the temperature to prevent any excessive heat causing damage to surrounding structures. The procedure lasts 30–60 min and can be performed under local anesthesia and oral analgesia together with sedation for high-energy protocols. Postoperative catheterization ranges from 1 to 12 weeks [26,27].

In a multicenter study of 541 patients, Trock *et al.* [28] reported a remarkable effect on LUTS [−11.5 American Urological Association (AUA) symptoms score, +55%] and an improvement in maximum flow rate (+4 mL/s, +51%) at 3 months. This effect was maintained for at least 4 years (−8.9, +42% and +2.7, +35%, respectively). In a systematic review comparing TUMT with TURP, based on data from 540 men in six randomized trials, Hoffman *et al.* [29] observed a restoration of urinary function (decrease in IPSS score of 65% vs 77%) with a concomitant increase in maximum flow rate of 70% vs 119%, after 6 months or more.

TUMT was performed as an outpatient procedure not requiring hospitalization, although with a longer catheterization time compared with TURP (7–15 days, vs 2–4 days). TUMT had a considerably lower morbidity rate compared with TURP, and retrograde ejaculation was significantly more common after TURP vs TUMT (57.6% vs 22.2%), as well as blood transfusions (5.7% vs 0%). However, the occurrence of retreatment for persistent LUTS due to BPH was significantly more common after TUMT. Several studies reported retreatment rates of 19.8–29.3% after high-energy TUMT at 5 years [30–32].

In conclusion, TUMT can help to achieve symptom relief, comparable with TURP, with a lower improvement at urodynamic evaluation. This procedure is associated with a lower morbidity risk but a higher retreatment rate, compared with TURP [1,25]. TUMT may be considered as a treatment option in men with moderate to severe symptoms, without complications, refractory to medical treatment [33].

Transurethral ethanol ablation of the prostate

The use of dehydrated ethanol for prostatic ablation originates from previous clinical evidence of its efficacy on the treatment of various lesions such as thyroid adenoma and hepatic tumors, or the ablation of renal cysts for over 10 years [34,35].

Transurethral ethanol ablation of the prostate (TEAP) is a procedure based on the use of liquid or gel ethanol (95–98%) to carry out chemical ablation of prostatic tissue. Ethanol, through dehydration of cells, protein denaturation, and thrombotic closure of arterioles and venules, induces coagulative necrosis of prostatic tissues. Ethanol can be injected transurethrally, transperineally, or transrectally, but the transurethral approach is most commonly performed; 20–22 Ga is used in the specific delivery system (InecTx™ in the USA and Prostaject™ in Europe), and there is no consensus about the number, site, and volume of injection: Depending on the prostate volume, two or three series of 2–4–8–10 o'clock injections are usually carried out; the distal limit is the verumontanum. The total amount of injected ethanol varies from 2 to 20 mL, and the volume of injected ethanol is slightly correlated with the size of tissue necrosis [36]. Continuous irrigation flow through a cystoscope and bladder emptying after each injection can help to avoid bladder and urethra mucosa injuries. The procedure is performed under general or regional anesthesia, or sometimes under local anesthesia supplemented by sedation. The whole procedure lasts 10–30 min, and the mean indwelling catheterization time is 7 days [37].

In a prospective multicenter trial on 115 patients, Grise *et al.* [38] found a significant reduction in urinary symptoms (IPSS: –50%) and prostate volume (–16%) with an improvement in maximum flow rate at uroflowmetry (+35%) at 12 months' follow-up. The most commonly reported adverse events were irritative voiding symptoms (26%), urinary retention/recatheterization (17%), and hematuria (16%). Two patients reported serious adverse events after treatment at two different centers, both involving a report of bladder necrosis. During the 1-year follow-up, 7% of patients required a transurethral resection of the prostate (TURP).

In 2008, Magno *et al.* found a significant improvement in urinary symptoms (IPSS: –13.3), maximum flow rate at uroflowmetry (+6.23), and postvoid residual volume 12 months after this procedure. The following year, in a noncontrolled study, Sakr *et al.* reported an equivalent improvement in urinary symptoms and uroflowmetry parameters, with a reduction in prostatic volume [39]. El-Husseiny *et al.*, in a long-term follow-up study at 54 months [40], found that (23%) patients showed an insufficient response and needed alternative treatment: Surgical treatment in the form of either TURP or prostatic stent insertion was carried out in 19% patients. Goya *et al.* followed 17 patients for more than 3 years (median follow-up for 4.3 years) and reported a retreatment rate of 41% [41].

Randomized-controlled trials with long-term follow-up comparing ethanol injections with TURP do not exist in the literature, and so data on TEAP are incomplete. It seems promising in terms of the reduction in LUTS scores, PVR, and prostatic volume, and improvement of uroflowmetry parameters, but its safety and long-term efficacy are still unknown.

Botulinum toxin A

Botulinum toxin A (BTX-A), an exotoxin produced by the *Clostridium botulinum* bacterium, has recently evolved from a deadly poison to a pharmaceutical agent with great potential. It was clinically used for the first time in 1987 in patients with cranial–cervical dystonia, including blepharospasm [42]. Since then, it has been used to treat various skeletal muscle spasticity and bladder disorders such as overactive bladder. Its mechanism of action involves an inhibition of neurotransmitters (e.g. acetylcholine or norepinephrine) released at the neuromuscular junction, leading to muscular paralysis.

Recently, intraprostatic injection of botulinum toxin A has been investigated as a minimally invasive alternative to oral medications in men with BPH-related LUTS. The rationale for this investigation was that the function of the prostate is rooted in its neural regulation. Even if the precise mechanism of action is not fully understood, it has been hypothesized that BTX-A can reduce LUTS directly or indirectly by inducing chemical denervation and apoptosis of epithelial cells, leading to tissue atrophy and prostate size reduction. Moreover, inhibition of sensory neurons, reduction in afferent signals to the central nervous system, and/or relaxation of smooth muscle cells by the downregulation of 1A adrenergic receptors [43] have been claimed as further mechanisms of action.

BTX-A can be injected into the prostatic parenchyma transperineally, transurethrally, or transrectally, using a 21–23 gauge needle

Table 14.1 Characteristics, efficacy, safety, and costs of minimally invasive procedures analysed

		Transurethral needle ablation	Transurethral microwave thermotherapy	Transurethral ethanol ablation of the prostate	Botulinum toxin A
Method		Radio-frequency coagulative necrosis	Microwave coagulative necrosis	Intraprostatic injection	Intraprostatic injection
Hospital stay		Day case	Day case	Day case	Day case
Duration of catheterization		3 days	1–2 weeks	7 days	–
Efficacy	IPSS	−12.0 to −12.6	−8.2 to −11.5[a]	−10.8 to −13.3	−5.6 to −6.6
	Q_{max}	4.1–6.5	2.7–4	4.8–6.2	2.0–2.4
	QoL	−2.6 to −4.0	−2.1 to −3.5	−1.9 to −2.7	−1.1 to −1.4
Safety	Urinary retention	19–23%	18–22%	14–17%	3–5%
	Dysuria	11–14%	22–35%	23–26%	2–5%
	Infection	3–5%	4–8%	4–7%	1–6%
	Blood transfusion	0–0.3%	0–0.3%	0–0.2%	0%
	Erectile dysfunction	0–0.3%	0–1.5%	0%	0%
	Retrograde ejaculation	0–0.2%	0–22.2%	0%	0%
	Retreatment within 5 years	17–20%	19–29%	15–22%	100%
Costs [48]	Average cost per procedure ($)	3765	3948	–	125–400[b]
	Expected cost for 24 months ($)	6179	5461–5699	–	1590–3390

Q_{max}, maximum flow rate; QoL, International Prostate Symptoms Score (IPSS) quality of life.
[a]American Urological Association Symptom Score.
[b]Per injection.

under ultrasound visualization. Different therapeutic doses (100–300 units Botox™ or 300–600 units Dysport™) and dilutions (25–50 units Botox™/mL or 75 units Dysport™/mL) have been used in various studies. Doses of 100 units Botox™ have been suggested for prostate sizes of <30 mL, 200 units for sizes between 30 mL and 60 mL, and 300 units for sizes of >60 mL. The majority of patients are treated without anesthesia, under local anesthesia, or under sedation. Each treatment lasts 20 min [44].

In 1998, Doggweiler conducted the first preclinical studies on murine prostates, and in 2003, the first injection of BTX-A in human prostate was reported [45,46]. In their study, Maria and colleagues injected 200 U of BTX-A into the prostate using a perineal approach with ultrasound guidance. Although only a small cohort of patients was followed up for 2 months after injection, the initial results were impressive, with significant improvements in AUA symptom scores compared with placebo. In patients who received BTX-A, the symptom score was reduced by 65% compared with baseline values, while no significant differences were observed in patients who received saline solution.

Dos and don'ts

- Mini-invasive procedures, including TUNA, TUMT, TEAP, and BTX-A, are possible treatment options for uncomplicated LUTS/BPH. Other emerging devices are under investigation.
- TUNA appears to be a relatively safe technique with low and generally mild side effects above all with regard to sexual function, minimal anesthetic requirements, short duration, and short hospital stay required.
- TUMT is a suitable treatment option for the patient who has moderate to severe symptoms and a desire to avoid more invasive therapy such as conventional TURP.
- Both TUNA and TUMT have been investigated for a long time, providing data for systematic review.
- TEAP is effective in partially relieving LUTS secondary to BPH. No randomized controlled trials with long-term follow-up exist, and so TEAP remains investigational.
- Intraprostatic injection of BTX-A appears to be a promising therapeutic option capable of improving both objective and subjective outcomes in symptomatic BPH patients without interfering with sexual function. The long-term safety and efficacy of BTX-A remain unknown.

In 2012, Marberger *et al.* [47] conducted the largest placebo-controlled randomized multicenter phase 2 dose-ranging study to investigate the utility of onabotulinumtoxinA (BoNT-ONA) for the treatment of LUTS/BPH. A total of 380 patients were evaluated, but only 265 patients completed the 72-week follow-up. Three different doses of BoNT-ONA were compared with placebo. A significant improvement in urinary symptoms from baseline to 12 weeks was observed: IPSS −5.5, −6.6, −6.3, and −5.6 for placebo, BoNT-ONA 100 U, BoNT-ONA 200 U and BoNT-ONA 300 U respectively, with no significant differences between placebo and BoNT-ONA in contrast with Maria *et al.*'s study. Only in a subgroup of patients previously treated with α-blocker was any remarkable difference reported between placebo and BoNT-ONA 200 U (IPSS: −3.5±6.1 vs −6.6±5.9 respectively; $P=0.023$).

The maximum flow rate during the uroflowmetry was also significantly improved from baseline through week 72 ($P=0.029$) but no significant differences between groups were found (2.3, 2.0, 2.4, and 2.0 mL/s in the placebo, BoNT-ONA 100-U, BoNT-ONA 200-U, and BoNT-ONA 300-U groups, respectively).

The same results were reported for the urinary-related quality-of-life improvement (IPSS quality-of-life question scores, mean change from baseline: −1.3, −1.2, −1.4, and −1.1 points).

The occurrence of adverse events was similar across the treatment groups, most of them local and related to the procedure. Hematuria, hematospermia, and micturition urgency were most commonly reported. No significant changes in sexual function, as measured by International Index of Erectile Function score, were observed at any time.

Bibliography

1 AUA Practice Guidelines Committee. AUA guideline on the management of benign prostatic hyperplasia. Diagnosis and treatment recommendations. *J Urol.* 2003;170:530–47.

2 Rosenberg MT, Staskin DR, Kaplan SA, MacDiarmid SA, Newman DK, Ohl DA. A practical guide to the evaluation and treatment of male lower urinary tract symptoms in the primary care setting. *Int J Clin Pract.* 2007;61(9):1535–46. Epub 2007 Jul 11.

3 Gacci M, Eardley I, Giuliano F, Hatzichristou D, Kaplan SA, Maggi M, *et al.* Critical analysis of the relationship between sexual dysfunctions

and lower urinary tract symptoms due to benign prostatic hyperplasia. *Eur Urol.* 2011;60(4):809–25.

4 Hoesl CE, Woll EM, Burkart M, Altwein JE. Erectile dysfunction (ED) is prevalent, bothersome and underdiagnosed in patients consulting urologists for benign prostatic syndrome (BPS). *Eur Urol.* 2005;47(4):511–7. Epub 2005 Jan 15.

5 Lowe FC. Treatment of lower urinary tract symptoms suggestive of benign prostatic hyperplasia: sexual function. *BJU Int.* 2005;95(Suppl 4):12–8.

6 Giuliano F. Impact of medical treatments for benign prostatic hyperplasia on sexual function. *BJU Int.* 2006;97(Suppl 2):34–8; discussion 44–5.

7 Gacci M, Bartoletti R, Figlioli S, Sarti E, Eisner B, Boddi V, *et al.* Urinary symptoms, quality of life and sexual function in patients with benign prostatic hypertrophy before and after prostatectomy: a prospective study. *BJU Int.* 2003;91(3):196–200.

8 Rosen RC, Wei JT, Althof SE, Seftel AD, Miner M, Perelman MA, *et al.* Association of sexual dysfunction with lower urinary tract symptoms of BPH and BPH medical therapies: results from the BPH Registry. *Urology.* 2009;73(3):562–6.

9 Gonzalez RR, Kaplan SA. First-line treatment for symptomatic benign prostatic hyperplasia: is there a particular patient profile for a particular treatment? *World J Urol.* 2006;24(4):360–6.

10 McVary KT, Roehrborn CG, Avins AL, Barry MJ, Bruskewitz RC, Donnell RF, *et al.* Update on AUA guideline on the management of benign prostatic hyperplasia. *J Urol.* 2011;185:1793–803.

11 Schulman CC, Zlotta AR, Rasor JS, Hourriez L, Noel JC, Edwards SD. Transurethral needle ablation (TUNA): safety, feasibility and tolerance of a new office procedure for treatment of benign prostatic hyperplasia. *Eur Urol.* 1993;24:415–23.

12 Bouza C, López T, Magro A, Navalpotro L, Amate JM. Systematic review and meta-analysis of transurethral needle ablation in symptomatic benign prostatic hyperplasia. *BMC Urol.* 2006;6:14. doi:10.1186/1471-2490-6-14.

13 Heaton JP. Radiofrequency thermal ablation of the prostate: the TUNA technique. *Tech Urol.* 1995;1:3–10.

14 Schulman CC, Zlotta AR. Transurethral needle ablation of the prostate for treatment of benign prostatic hyperplasia: early clinical experience. *Urology.* 1995;45(1):28–33.

15 Zlotta AR, Giannakopoulos X, Maehlum O, Ostrem T, Schulman CC. Long-term evaluation of transurethral needle ablation of the prostate

(TUNA) for treatment of symptomatic benign prostatic hyperplasia: clinical outcome up to five years from three centers. *Eur Urol.* 2003;44(1):89–93.

16 Elterman L, Ekbal S. An open prospective study of safety and efficacy of transurethral needle ablation in patients with trilobar benign prostatic hyperplasia [abstract]. *J Urol.* 1999;161:s304.

17 Naslund MJ, Benson RC, Cohen ES, Gutierrez-Aceves J, Issa MM. Transurethral needle ablation for BPH in patients with median lobe enlargement-report of a prospective multicenter study [abstract]. *J Urol.* 2000;163:s270.

18 Issa MM. Transurethral needle ablation of the prostate: report of initial United States clinical trial. *J Urol.* 1996, 156:413–19.

19 Daehlin L, Gustavsen A, Nilsen AH, Mohn J. Transurethral needle ablation for treatment of lower urinary tract symptoms associated with benign prostatic hyperplasia: outcome after 1 year. *J Endourol.* 2002;16:111–5.

20 Schulman CC, Zlotta AR, Rasor JS, Hourriez L, Noel JC, Edwards SD. Transurethral needle ablation (TUNA): safety, feasibility and tolerance of a new office procedure for treatment of benign prostatic hyperplasia. *Eur Urol.* 1993;24:415–23.

21 Holmes MA, Stewart J, Boulton JB, Chambers RM. Transurethral needle ablation of the prostate: outcome at 1 year. *J Endourol.* 1999;13:745–50.

22 Namasivayam S, Eardley I, Bryan NP, Hastie KJ, Chapple CR. 3 year prospective follow-up of 91 men treated with transurethral needle ablation of prostate(TUNA) [abstract]. *J Urol.* 1999;161:s390.

23 Frieben RW, Lin HC, Hinh PP, Berardinelli F, Canfield SE, Wang R. The impact of minimally invasive surgeries for the treatment of symptomatic benign prostatic hyperplasia on male sexual function: a systematic review. *Asian J Androl.* 2010;12:500–8.

24 Magin RL, Fridd CW, Bonfiglio TA, Linke CA. Thermal destruction of the canine prostate by high intensity microwaves. *J Surg Res.* 1980;29(3): 265–75.

25 Oelke M, Bachmann A, Descazeaud A, Emberton M, Gravas S, Michel MC, *et al.* EAU guidelines on the treatment and follow-up of non-neurogenic male lower urinary tract symptoms including benign prostatic obstruction. *Eur Urol.* 2013;64(1):118–40.

26 Naspro R, Salonia A, Colombo R, Cestari A, Guazzoni G, Rigatti P, *et al.* Update of the minimally invasive therapies for benign prostatic hyperplasia. *Curr Opin Urol.* 2005;51:49–53.

27 Rubenstein J, McVary KT. Transurethral microwave thermotherapy of the prostate (TUMT). *Emedicine*; 2005 [updated 2006; cited 2011]. Available from: http://www.emedicine.com/med/topic3070.htm

28 Trock BJ, Brotzman M, Utz WJ, Ugarte RR, Kaplan SA, Larson TR, *et al.* Long-term pooled analysis of multicenter studies of cooled thermotherapy for benign prostatic hyperplasia results at three months through four years. *Urology*. 2004;63(4):716–21.

29 Hoffman RM, MacDonald R, Monga M, Wilt TJ. Transurethral microwave thermotherapy versus transurethral resection for treating benign prostatic hyperplasia: a systematic review. *BJU Int.* 2004;94:1031–6.

30 Floratos DL, Kiemeney LA, Rossi C, Kortmann BB, Debruyne FM, de La Rosette JJ. Long-term followup of randomised transurethral microwave thermotherapy versus transurethral prostatic resection study. *J Urol* 2001;165(5):1533–8.

31 Thalmann GN, Mattei A, Treuthardt C, Burkhard FC, Studer UE. Transurethral microwave therapy in 200 patients with a minimum followup of 2 years: urodynamic and clinical results. *J Urol* 2002;167(6):2496–501.

32 Miller PD, Kastner C, Ramsey EW, Parsons K. Cooled thermotherapy for the treatment of benign prostatic hyperplasia: durability of results obtained with the Targis System. *Urology* 2003;61(6):1160–4.

33 McVary KT, Roehrborn CG, Avins AL, Barry MJ, Bruskewitz RC, Donnell RF, *et al.* Update on AUA guideline on the management of benign prostatic hyperplasia. *J Urol.* 2011;185(5):1793–803.

34 Livraghi T, Festi D, Monti F, Salmi A, Vettori C. US-guided percutaneous alcohol injection of small hepatic and abdominal tumors. *Radiology.* 1986;161:309–12.

35 Banner M. Percutaneous renal cyst ablation. In: Banner M, editor. *Radiologic interventions uroradiology.* Baltimore, MD: Williams & Wilkins; 1998. pp. 73–7.

36 Plante MK, Gross AL, Kliment J, *et al.* Intraprostatic ethanol chemoablation via transurethral and transperineal injection. *BJU Int.* 2003;91(1):94–8.

37 Magno C, Mucciardi G, Galì A, Anastasi G, Inferrera A, Morgia G. Transurethral ethanol ablation of the prostate (TEAP): an effective minimally invasive treatment alternative to traditional surgery for symptomatic benign prostatic hyperplasia (BPH) in high-risk comorbidity patients. *Int Urol Nephrol.* 2008;40:941–6.

38 Grise P, Plante M, Palmer J, Martinez-Sagarra J, Hernandez C, Schettini M, *et al.* Evaluation of the transurethral ethanol ablation of the prostate (TEAP) for symptomatic benign prostatic hyperplasia (BPH): A European multi-center evaluation. *Eur Urol.* 2004;46:496–502.

39 Sakr M, Eid A, Shoukry M, Fayed A. Transurethral ethanol injection therapy of benign prostatic hyperplasia: four-year follow-up. *Int J Urol.* 2009;16(2):196–201.

40 El-Husseiny T, Buchholz N. Transurethral ethanol ablation of the prostate for symptomatic benign prostatic hyperplasia: long-term follow-up. *J Endourol.* 2011;25(3):477–80.

41 Goya N, Ishikawa N, Ito F, Kobayashi C, Tomizawa Y, Toma H. Transurethral ethanol injection therapy for prostatic hyperplasia: 3-year results. *J Urol.* 2004;172(3):1017–20.

42 Jankovic J, Orman J. Botulinum A toxin for cranial-cervical dystonia: a double-blind, placebo controlled study. *Neurology.* 1987;37:616–23.

43 Smith CP, Franks ME, McNeil BK, Ghosh R, de Groat WC, Chancellor MB, *et al.* Effect of botulinum toxin A on the autonomic nervous system of the rat lower urinary tract. *J Urol* 2003;169:1896–900.

44 Cruz F, Dinis P. Resiniferatoxin and botulinum toxin type A for treatment of lower urinary tract symptoms. *Neurourol Urodyn.* 2007;26(Suppl 6):920–7.

45 Doggweiler R, Zermann DH, Ishigooka M, Schmidt RA. Botox-induced prostatic involution. *Prostate.* 1998;37(1):44–50.

46 Maria G, Brisinda G, Civello IM, Bentivoglio AR, Sganga G, Albanese A. Relief by botulinum toxin of voiding dysfunction due to benign prostatic hyperplasia: results of a randomized, placebo-controlled study. *Urology.* 2003;62:259–65.

47 Marberger M, Chartier-Kastler E, Egerdie B, Lee KS, Grosse J, Bugarin D, *et al.* A randomized double-blind placebo-controlled phase 2 dose-ranging study of onabotulinumtoxina in men with benign prostatic hyperplasia. *Eur Urol.* 2013;63(3): 496–503.

48 Stovsky MD, Griffiths RI, Duff SB. A clinical outcomes and cost analysis comparing photoselective vaporization of the prostate to alternative minimally invasive therapies and transurethral prostate resection for the treatment of benign prostatic hyperplasia. *J Urol.* 2006;176(4 Pt 1):1500–6.

CHAPTER 15

Holmium Laser Prostatectomy

Simon van Rij[1] & Peter J. Gilling[2]
[1]Tauranga Hospital, Tauranga, New Zealand
[2]University of Auckland, Urology BOP Limited, Tauranga, New Zealand

Key points

- Traditional transurethral resection of the prostate (TURP) surgery is being performed far less frequently for benign prostatic hyperplasia (BPH) and is being replaced by alternative energy sources and techniques such as HoLEP.
- The holmium laser's wavelength makes it an ideal laser for endoscopic BPH and stone surgery.
- The holmium laser enucleation of the prostate (HoLEP) technique has developed incrementally and is an endoscopic version of open prostatectomy, utilizing much of the same equipment as traditional endoscopic surgery.
- HoLEP can be used to treat any size of prostate gland and is particularly useful in large prostates due to its relatively bloodless nature and the use of saline as irrigation fluid.
- The published rates of morbidity from HoLEP are low, with most patients being discharged on the first postoperative day and with no catheter *in situ*.
- HoLEP has been rigorously compared with traditional BPH surgery in both randomized controlled trials and meta-analyses, and has been shown to have similar outcomes and with less morbidity. Durability has been confirmed with low rates of reintervention.
- HoLEP can be safely performed on patients taking anticoagulant medication.
- Proficiency in the HoLEP technique entails a learning curve, which can be minimized with the appropriate training and mentorship.

Introduction

There has been a marked change in the treatment of BPH with the advent of new technologies. Focusing on the surgical management of this condition, the current guidelines from both the American Urological Association (AUA) and European Association of Urology endorse a number of different options for both patient and clinician [1,2]. Traditionally TURP was used for patients with prostate glands smaller than 80 g, and for larger prostate glands, open prostatectomy. However, there has been a marked shift to other forms of treatment, with laser treatment of BPH making up 44% of all procedures for BPH in 2011 compared with 11% in 2004 [3]. The key reason for this change has been the introduction of new laser techniques, with similar outcomes but less morbidity compared with traditional surgery. The use of the holmium laser, and in particular the HoLEP procedure, is at the forefront of this technology.

Male Lower Urinary Tract Symptoms and Benign Prostatic Hyperplasia, First Edition.
Edited by Steven A. Kaplan and Kevin T. McVary.
© 2014 John Wiley & Sons, Ltd. Published 2014 by John Wiley & Sons, Ltd.

Laser physics

The holmium:yttrium aluminium garnet (YAG) laser (Lumenis Tel Aviv, Israel) has a wavelength of 2140 nm. This and its pulsed wave form make it an ideal laser for prostate surgery. At this wavelength, tissue down to a depth of 0.4 mm can be vaporized, with coagulation of the tissue 3–4 mm below the vaporization area. The wavelength is strongly absorbed by tissue water, and because of these properties, precise incision of the prostate with minimal bleeding is possible. Normal saline can be used as the irrigation fluid, which can mitigate the risk of TURP syndrome. Unlike other lasers used for the treatment of BPH, the holmium laser is versatile and can also be used for other urological procedures, in particular the management of stones and strictures anywhere in the urinary system. These properties enabled the first use of the holmium laser for BPH surgery in 1994 [4].

History

The initial procedure used a combination of the holmium laser to vaporize a channel in the prostate and the Nd:YAG laser to coagulate the remainder. However, by utilizing the coagulation ability of the "defocused" holmium laser, the procedure could be performed solely with the holmium laser. This procedure, termed holmium laser ablation of the prostate (HoLAP), utilized either a side-firing or end-firing fiber and a 60 W laser. This procedure was found to be effective and durable compared with TURP [5]. Like all ablative techniques, however, there were several limitations to this procedure. No tissue could be collected for histologic analysis, the procedure was time-consuming, the

ablation produced a variable channel, and it was less well suited to larger prostate glands. The next advance in the technology was the procedure called holmium laser resection of the prostate tissue (HoLRP). This utilized the bloodless incisional properties of the holmium laser to "resect" prostate tissue into pieces for retrieval rather than ablation. More tissue was removed, the procedure was quicker, tissue was available for analysis, and larger glands could be treated [6]. Trials comparing HoLRP with TURP were performed and showed similar outcomes between the two, with decreased morbidity in the HoLRP arm [7]. However, the relatively inefficient process of removing small pieces of tissue led researchers to develop the current technique, holmium laser enucleation of the prostate (HoLEP), which will be described in more detail.

Holmium laser enucleation of the prostate technique

The HoLEP technique is aimed at removing the entire transition zone of the prostate endoscopically. This is, in principle, similar to an open prostatectomy but without the major morbidity of open prostatectomy. Rather than removing the tissue in small pieces, the laser is used to enucleate each prostate lobe in its entirety. The lobes are then morcellated inside the bladder for endoscopic removal and histological analysis. A key advantage of this is that it can be applied to any sized prostate gland, including extremely large glands (>200 g). Whereas other techniques have size limits due to the degree of bleeding or the amount of irrigation fluid used, this is not the case with HoLEP in experienced hands [8]. The technique has been developed over time into a reproducible procedure that is now performed all over the world.

Equipment

The high-powered VersaPulse™ holmium laser (Lumenis, Tel Aviv, Israel) is used with a power setting of 2.0 J at 50 Hz (100 W). A modified 27Ch continuous flow resectoscope with an inner laser fiber channel is used with a 30° telescope. A 550 μm end firing fiber is employed through a 6F ureteric catheter placed down the fiber channel of the resectoscope. Normal saline (0.9%) is used for irrigation, and the patient is placed in lithotomy, similar to the positioning employed during TURP. For the morcellation process, there are a number of different products now available. A long nephroscope is placed down the outer working sheath (with an adaptor), and the morcellator hand piece is placed through this. The morcellator uses a hand piece with reciprocating blades attached to a suction pump to morcellate and hence remove the prostate tissue.

Procedure

A detailed understanding of the anatomy of the enlarged prostate and its landmarks is important before commencing HoLEP. Care is taken to ensure that no tissue beyond the veru is removed to avoid the risk of sphincter damage; the uretric orifices are also visualized throughout the procedure to ensure they are not damaged. The HoLEP procedure lends itself to modular training that has been shown to improve the time to reach competency [9]. By breaking down the procedure into a number of steps of varying difficulty, each step can be mastered individually under supervision and then combined for complete learning.

Bladder neck incision

The urethra is well lubricated and calibrated. First, one or two incisions are made at the 7 and 5 o'clock positions from the bladder neck to the verumontanum. It is important to attain the correct depth down to the surgical capsule to facilitate removal of the lobes in the next step. If these are too superficial, the adenoma will not peel away easily; if they are too deep they will cause perforation of the capsule.

Median lobe enucleation

A transverse incision is made proximal to the verumontanum to connect the two bladder neck incisions. In a retrograde fashion, the median lobe is then dissected off the capsule by extending the transverse incision at the level of the surgical capsule up to the bladder neck. The lobe is then detached at the bladder neck and remains in the bladder until later on.

Lateral lobe enucleation

The same principle is employed for the lateral lobes. The initial bladder neck incisions are extended at the apex laterally up to the 2–3 o'clock (9–10) position, often described as "hockey stick incisions" for the curved path they take at the apex. A further incision is made at 12 o'clock from the bladder neck to just proximal to the veromontanum; this splits the anterior commisure. Similar to the inferior incision, the incision is brought around laterally at the apex to connect the inferior and superior incisions. The connecting of the two incisions is one of the most demanding steps of the procedure. This is more difficult in a large gland, since the distance between incisions is greater. If not done properly, a large amount of tissue can potentially be left behind, or multiple incisions will be made that will not allow the lobe to be removed as one. Once the incisions are connected, the lobe is peeled away at the level of the surgical capsule in a retrograde manner. Both lobes are placed in the bladder along with the median lobe

Haemostasis

Before commencing morcellation, it is important to have excellent haemostasis. Due to the properties of the laser, this is mostly done during the enucleation process because of the coagulation that occurs in association with the incision. However, for persistent sites of bleeding, "defocusing" the laser fiber by moving it slightly away from the tissue coagulates all vessels encountered eventually. Decompressing the bladder once or twice helps uncover bleeding.

Morcellation

The equipment is slightly altered to allow the morcellator to be inserted into the bladder (see above). Inadvertent bladder injury is very rare when key principles are followed. The bladder must always remain full while morcellating, and to avoid its collapse due to the suction, a steady flow is required. The use of a double inflow of irrigation will facilitate this. Second, visualization of the mobile prostate lobe tissue is important. Good haemostasis and visually monitoring both the morcellator and the tissue at all times is necessary. Finally, keeping the morcellator at the level of the bladder neck and trigone angled up slightly towards the dome of the bladder minimizes any inadvertent injury to the bladder. Once the morcellator has removed the bulk of the prostate tissue, any small residual fragments can be removed by a manual evacuator such as a Toomey syringe or a modified loop using a resectoscope. Depending on the degree of bleeding, either a two-way 20F or three-way 22F catheter is positioned, and slow irrigation is applied if desired, though many patients will leave the theatre on free drainage. A diuretic can be helpful.

Modifications

Modifications to the technique have been developed to cater for different scenarios. In those with smaller prostate glands (<30 g) a bladder neck incision or median lobe enucleation alone has been shown to be highly successful. Those men who present at the time of surgery with bladder stones can have these fragmented and evacuated during the same procedure.

Patient selection

Choosing the appropriate patient for surgery is just as important as performing the surgery appropriately. Patient workup and diagnosis for HoLEP should follow the standard pathway for any patient being considered for surgical treatment of BPH. In those deemed fit for BPH surgery, there are no specific contraindications to the HoLEP procedure such as the size of the gland. Knowing the size of the prostate gland is important, as this influences the consent process with the patient, the probable length of surgery, technical difficulty, and potential complications. Many men who require surgical treatment for BPH take some form of antiplatelet or anticoagulation medicine. There is now increased awareness of the potential significant risk of stopping these medications even for a short period. In particular, stopping aspirin can lead to cardiovascular complications often unseen by the urologist who does not deal with these complications if they arise. Review panels have advised that men undergoing TURP may stop aspirin due to the risk of heavy bleeding from the procedure [10].

However, HoLEP patients can remain on aspirin due to the low bleeding risk and the decreased risk of cardiovascular complications [11]. As the population continues to age, and more men are on anticoagulation medications, patients should be counselled about the cardiovascular risk of stopping these medications when deciding on what BPH treatment to have.

Outcomes

To assess the outcomes of HoLEP or any other new surgical technique, they must be compared with the current standard procedures. This must be done rigorously using the highest possible level of evidence to justify the introduction and ongoing usage of this technique. A meta-analysis of randomized trials, properly performed, provides this high level of evidence to answer treatment questions. In assessing outcomes for BPH surgery, the important factors include the effectiveness of the surgery both subjectively and objectively, the morbidity associated with the procedure including complications, and finally the durability of the procedure. These are also meaningful to the patient rather than just surrogate end-points for clinical research.

In 2007, a meta-analysis was published comparing HoLEP to TURP (the current standard treatment). Follow-up of patients until at least 1 year showed similar improvements in International Prostate Symptom Score and maximal flow rate between the two techniques. Concerning the assessment of perioperative outcomes, HoLEP involves reduced catheter times (17.7–31 h versus 43.4–57.8 h) and hospital stays required compared with TURP (27.6–59.0 h vs 48.3–85.5 h). There were no recorded blood transfusions in any patients undergoing a HoLEP procedure.

Complications at 1 year were similar with a stricture rate of 2.6% for HoLEP and 4.4% for TURP [12]. Similar results to these have been published in further meta-analyses and also review articles on BPH surgery [13]. The assessment of durability requires a longer-term follow-up. HoLEP data have been published up to 7 years postprocedure, showing very low reoperation rates of 0–5%, which is lower than that quoted for TURP and open prostatectomy [14].

The literature published on HoLEP has shown it to be effective when compared with traditional techniques. This evidence has been used to justify its incorporation into current clinical guidelines. As standardization of patient care and treatment pathways become more important, physicians and patients rely on clinical guidelines from reputable organizations to guide patient management. HoLEP is currently the only laser therapy for the surgical treatment of BPH recommended by both the European Urology guidelines and the AUA guidelines. Level 1b evidence is also available for the use of HoLEP in the treatment of large prostate glands. This further confirms that HoLEP is now an established treatment for BPH and should be available for all patients considering BPH surgery

Learning curve

The learning curve has become a buzz word in the surgical literature as institutions, surgeons, researchers, and patients grapple with the definitions of competence and optimization of patient safety. Surgical audit has allowed identification of thresholds for procedures in which a surgeon is deemed competent. An absolute number is difficult to define though, as this is determined by the previous experience of the surgeon, the method of learning the technique, and how competence is defined. One of the usual criticisms of HoLEP has been the perceived difficulty of mastering the technique. Research has shown that, when properly mentored, approximately 20 HoLEP cases are required for competency and that this plateaus at around 50 cases [15]. This number is similar to, if not less than, many other routine operations performed by urologists [16]. In comparison with other "traditional" techniques, there are actually no adequate data on the learning curve for TURP, which is usually mastered as a urology resident and with assumed competence after a large number of cases [17]. Anecdotal evidence from centers that regularly perform HoLEP shows that residents pick up the technique as quickly as, if not more quickly than, those learning TURP. HoLEP is a procedure that requires mentoring and an appropriate number of cases for the surgeon to become competent. Being self-taught significantly prolongs the learning curve, and full proficiency may never be attained. For those starting the learning process, it is advisable to perform surgery initially only on patients with smaller prostate glands and to build up to larger glands, as these are technically more challenging As more and more residents come through programs specializing in laser management of BPH, this issue will become better understood.

Conclusion

The use of the holmium laser, and the HoLEP technique specifically, is now an established surgical treatment option for the management of BPH. The technique is reproducible and learnable, and shows an effectiveness comparable with traditional surgical options and with less morbidity.

Dos and don'ts

- Understand how the laser works and the properties of this unique wavelength, and conform to laser safety regulations.
- If introducing this technique, do have the appropriate equipment available including a morcellator, and undertake some form of proctorship or mentorship.
- When first starting out, do not try and perform the procedure on men with large prostates; work up to this, as it is more technically challenging.
- At all times during the procedure, be aware of appropriate anatomical landmarks to avoid inadvertent injury.
- Ensure that the initial incisions are made at the appropriate depth, as this allows the capsular plane between adenoma to be easily entered.
- When carrying out the lateral lobe enucleation, do not be too quick to commence the 12 o'clock incision but rather ensure that the plane from below has been adequately created up to or past 3 and 9 o'clock.
- Morcellation is a safe process if basic principles are followed: Ensure good vision with meticulous haemostasis, ensure the bladder is distended, maintain the morcellator in the correct midline position just inside the bladder neck, and visualize the mobility of the fragment being morcellated.
- When morcellating, the use of two inflow channels enables the bladder to remain distended to help avoid inadvertent bladder mucosal injury.
- Do be aware of the versatility of the holmium laser to treat not only BPH but also associated stones and strictures.

Bibliography

1 McVary KT, Roehrborn CG, Avins AL, Barry MJ, Bruskewitz RC, Donnell RF, *et al.* Update on AUA guideline on the management of benign prostatic hyperplasia. *J Urol.* 2011;185(5):1793–803.

2 *EAU guidelines, edition presented at the 25th EAU Annual Congress, Barcelona.* Arnhem, The Netherlands: EAU Guidelines Office; 2010.

3 Lowrance WT, Southwick A, Maschino AC, Sandhu JS. Contemporary practice patterns for endoscopic surgical management of benign prostatic hyperplasia among United States urologists. *J Urol.* 2013; 189(5):1811–6.

4 Gilling PJ, Cass CB, Malcolm AR, Fraundorfer MR. Combination holmium and Nd:YAG laser ablation of the prostate: initial clinical experience. *J Endourol.* 1995;9(2):151–3.

5 Mottet N, Anidjar M, Bourdon O. Randomized comparison of transurethral electroresection and holmium:YAG laser vaporization for symptomatic benign prostatic hyperplasia. *J Endourol.* 1999; 13:127–30.

6 Gilling PJ, Cass CB, Creswell MD, Fraundorfer MR. Holmium laser resection of the prostate: preliminary results of a new method for the treatment of benign prostatic hyperplasia. *Urology.* 1996;47:48–51.

7 Westenberg AM, Gilling PJ, Kennett KM, Frampton C, Fraundorfer MR Holmium laser resection of the prostate versus transurethral resection of the prostate: results of a randomized trial with 4-year minimum long-term follow-up. *J Urol.* 2004;172:616–9.

8 Tan AHH, Gilling PJ Holmium laser prostatectomy: current techniques. *Urology.* 2002;60:152–6.

9 Stewart GD1, Phipps S, Little B, Leveckis J, Stolzenburg JU, Tolley DA, *et al.* Description and vali-

dation of a modular training system for laparoscopic nephrectomy. *J Endourol.* 2012;26(11):1512–7.

10 Gerstein NS, Schulman PM, Gerstein WH, Petersen TR, Tawil I. Should more patients continue aspirin therapy perioperatively?: clinical impact of aspirin withdrawal syndrome. *Ann Surg.* 2012;255(5):811–9.

11 Tyson MD, Lerner LB. Safety of holmium laser enucleation of the prostate in anticoagulated patients. *J Endourol.* 2009;23(8):1343– 6.

12 Tan A, Liao C, Mo Z, Cao Y. Meta-analysis of holmium laser enucleation versus transurethral resection of the prostate for symptomatic prostatic obstruction. *Br J Surg.* 2007;94(10):1201–8.

13 Ahyai SA, Gilling P, Kaplan SA, Kuntz RM, Madersbacher S, Montorsi F, *et al.* Meta-analysis of functional outcomes and complications following transurethral procedures for lower urinary tract symptoms resulting from benign prostatic enlargement. *Eur Urol.* 2010;58(3):384–97.

14 Gilling PJ, Wilson LC, King CJ, Westenberg AM, Frampton CM, Fraundorfer MR. Long-term results of a randomized trial comparing holmium laser enucleation of the prostate and transurethral resection of the prostate: results at 7 years. *BJU Int.* 2012;109(3):408–11.

15 Shah HN, Mahajan AP, Sodha HS, Hegde S, Mohile PD, Bansal MB. Prospective evaluation of the learning curve for holmium laser enucleation of the prostate. *J Urol.* 2007;177(4):1468–74.

16 Kaul S, Shah N, Menon M. Learning curve using robotic surgery. *Curr Urol Rep.* 2006;7(2):125–9.

17 Schout BMA, Persoon MC, Martens EJ, Bemelmans BL, Scherpbier AJ, Hendrikx AJ. Analysis of pitfalls encountered by residents in transurethral procedures in master-apprentice type of training. *J Endourol.* 2010;24(4):621–8.

CHAPTER 16

Benign Prostatic Hyperplasia: GreenLight Laser Therapy

Alexis E. Te & Bilal Chughtai
Department of Urology, Weill Cornell Medical College, New York-Presbyterian Hospital, New York, NY, USA

Key points

- The 532 nm laser has a unique laser–tissue interaction that is suited to a transurethral aqueous procedure for a prostatectomy.
- The safety of the 532 nm laser prostatectomy has been studied in patients at high cardiopulmonary risk and has been demonstrated to have an excellent hemostatic profile.
- Laser prostatectomy performed with normal saline irrigation reduces dilutional hyponatremia, glycine-induced ammonia intoxication, and the direct toxic effect of glycine through its sealing zone of coagulative effect on tissue, which prevents fluid absorption.
- Studies evaluating GreenLight laser prostatectomy generally show positive outcomes with good efficacy, although the evidence base is not yet comparable with the extensive evidence-based data accumulated for transurethral resection of the prostate (TURP) over the years.
- Most studies on the 532 nm laser prostatectomy have been smaller cohorts with generally a short follow-up, which are not randomized and do not have a direct comparison against the gold standard of TURP.

532 nm wavelength laser

The high-power 532 nm laser system employs a high-powered green light visible wavelength utilizing laser systems also described as a potassium-titanyl-phosphate (KTP) laser, lithium triborate (LBO) laser, or GreenLight laser system, and the technique is often called photoselective vaporization of the prostate (PVP).

The original 532 nm high-power laser for PVP was a KTP-based laser system that contained a KTP crystal through which a 532 nm wavelength was generated. This had a different interaction with the prostate tissue when compared with its parent, Nd-YAG. The 532 nm wavelength is selectively absorbed by hemoglobin, which acts as an intracellular chromophore [1]. The 532 nm wavelength laser energy can be fully transmitted through aqueous irrigants into the cell, where it is absorbed by hemoglobin, which is then rapidly heated, leading to vaporization of prostate tissue. The short optical penetration that is associated with this wavelength confines its high-power laser energy to a superficial layer of prostatic tissue that is vaporized rapidly and hemostatically with only a 1–2 mm rim of coagulation. The thin coagulation zone arises as a result of the quasi-continuous emission characteristics of the 532 nm laser. Typically, continual irradiation of a single point causes heat to diffuse into deeper tissue layers, creating coagulation wherever there is enough convection thermal energy for protein denaturation but insufficient energy for vaporization.

60 W data

The first human trials with the 60 W KTP laser were conducted in a series of 10 patients described by Malek *et al.* in 1998 [2]. No patients suffered postoperative transurethral resection (TUR) syndrome or urinary retention; in fact, all patients were catheter-free within 24 h after the procedure. Patients experienced a significant improvement in Q_{max} (142%) by 24 h postoperatively.

Initial trials with the 60 W KTP laser were followed by a larger series of 55 patients in 2000 [3]. The 2-year experience with the higher-powered KTP laser again corroborated initial findings. Patients experienced statistically significant, enduring improvements in postoperative American Urological Association (AUA) symptom score (mean = 14, 82% improvement), Q_{max} (mean = 29.1 mL/s, 278% improvement), and postvoid residual (PVR; 27 mL, 75% improvement) with 2 years of follow-up, comparing favorably with published results for conventional transurethral resection of the prostate. The mean operative time was 44 min. All patients in the series were catheter-free 24 h after the procedure; none required recatheterization or experienced TUR syndrome. Hematuria was negligible despite the use of antiplatelet agents by many patients. These early results demonstrated level 4 evidence that prostatectomy with the prototype 60 W

KTP laser was as effective as conventional TURP and in fact demonstrated postoperative complications comparable with those of TURP and even other laser therapies, such as Ho:YAG.

80 W data

Despite the effectiveness of the 60 W KTP laser in prostatectomy, its less-than-ideal speed of vaporization inherently limited the size of prostate that could be resected. The next logical improvement therefore lay in increasing the laser power to speed up tissue ablation, and this led to the first clinically available 532 nm laser, which was a quasi-continuous 80 W KTP based laser. Early level 3 evidence led to its popular use.

Te *et al.* presented the first large, multicenter series on the use of an 80 W KTP laser in laser prostatectomy for 145 patients with long-term follow-up [4]. This early study represented the initial PVP experience with these centers, testing the ease of use. Significant and enduring improvements in AUA Symptom Index (AUA SI) scores, quality-of-life (QoL) scores, Q_{max}, and PVR were demonstrated up to 12 months postoperatively. Mean AUA symptom scores declined from 24 to 1.8 at 12 months; mean QoL scores improved from 4.3 to 0.4, Q_{max} from 7.7 to 22.8 mL/s, and PVR volume from 114.2 to 7.2 mL. The mean prostate volume, as determined by ultrasound, decreased from 54.6 to 34.4 mL. The mean operative time was 36 min, and no patient required a blood transfusion. More than 30% of patients were sent home without a catheter; those with postoperative catheters had them removed in a mean of 14 h. Reported morbidities were generally minor. Eight percent of patients experienced mild-to-moderate dysuria lasting more than 10 days, 8% had transient hematuria, and 3% had postoperative retention. Among the 56 men who were potent prior to the procedure, 27% experienced retrograde ejaculation, but none of them experienced impotence.

As a novel procedure, there are growing numbers of reports of long-term outcomes of 80 W KTP laser prostatectomy. Ruszat et al. published the largest series of 80 W KTP laser prostatectomies [5]. At a single center, 500 patients underwent PVP, including 45% taking oral anticoagulation. After 3 years, 26.2% of patients had a follow-up, and the mean AUA SI, PVR, and QoL were significantly improved compared with baseline. At 60 months, the retreatment rate was 6.8%, and the reoperation rate was 14.8%. Urethral and bladder neck strictures were observed in 4.4% and 3.6% of patients, comparable with the rate in TURP. Te et al. reported a 3-year multicenter long-term follow-up in 139 patients who underwent 80 W KTP laser prostatectomy. At 3 years, 33.8% of patients had a follow-up, and improvements in symptom relief and urinary flow rate endured [6]. The retreatment rate was 4.3%.

The 80 W KTP/532 nm laser was also studied on larger glands with good reported outcomes and an excellent safety profile. Sandhu et al. reported on large prostate volume resection with the 80 W KTP laser [7]. Sixty-four men with benign prostatic hyperplasia (BPH) who had prostates with volumes of at least 60 mL and who had failed medical therapy were included for vaporization with the 80 W KTP laser. The mean preoperative prostate volume was 101 mL with a mean operative time of 123 min. The International Prostate Symptom Score (IPSS) decreased from 18.4 to 6.7 at 12 months; Q_{max} increased from 7.9 mL/s to 18.9 mL/s, while PVR decreased from 189 mL to 109 mL. No transfusions were

required; nor was there any evidence of postoperative hyponatremia. All patients were discharged within 23 h. This was the first evidence that the 80 W KTP laser could be used as a safe and effective means with enduring results for large-volume prostatectomy.

Pfitzenmaier et al. conducted a comparative study between vaporization of prostates greater than or equal to 80 mL and those smaller than 80 mL. Thirty-nine of 173 patients had prostates ≥80 mL [8]. The authors found that PVP was safe and effective in prostates ≥80 mL, but the reoperation rate was higher. In another study, Rajbabu et al. assessed 54 consecutive patients with prostates >100 mL who underwent 80 W KTP laser prostatectomy [9]. Consistent with other published series, these studies further support the procedures safety, efficacy, and enduring improvements on IPSS and QoL.

The safety of the 80 W KTP laser prostatectomy has been studied in patients at high cardiopulmonary risk and has been demonstrated to be excellent due to the excellent hemostatic profile and perioperative hemodynamic stability of the procedure. Reich et al. performed an 80 W laser prostatectomy on 66 patients with an American Anesthesiology Score of 3 or greater [10]. Of these patients, 29 were being treated with ongoing oral anticoagulation or had a severe bleeding disorder. No major complications occurred during or following the procedure, and no blood transfusions were required. Two patients required reoperation within 12 months due to recurrent urinary retention. Mean improvements in IPSS (20.2 to 6.5) and peak flow (6.7 mL/s to 21.6 mL/s) endured at 12 months.

One specific safety application of the 80 W KTP laser was its use in anticoagulated patients at high risk for clinically significant bleeding. A series of 24 anticoagulated patients with BPH treated with laser prostatectomy using the 80 W KTP laser were studied [11]. Of these, eight were on warfarin, two on clopidogrel, and 14 on aspirin. Eight (33%) of these patients had a previous myocardial infarction, seven (29%) cerebrovascular disease, and seven (29%) peripheral vascular disease. No patients developed clinically significant hematuria postoperatively, and none developed clot retention. No transfusions were required, and there were no thromboembolic events. Follow-up revealed a decrease in IPSS from 18.7 to 9.5 as well as an increase in Q_{max} from 9.0 to 20.1 mL/s at 12 months. PVR decreased from 134 to 69 mL at 1 month but was not statistically significant beyond that time point. All patients underwent PVP safely without any adverse thromboembolic or bleeding events. Significantly, more energy and time were used for lasing per gland size in these patients.

The largest published series is a study by Chung et al. [12], who reported on outcomes and complications after PVP in a group of 162 high-risk men with a high degree of systemic anticoagulation who underwent photoselective vaporization of the prostate. The mean age was 72 years, mean baseline prostate volume 91 g, and mean prostate-specific antigen 4.1 ng/mL. Thirty-one patients (19%) were on warfarin, 101 (62%) were on acetylsalicylic acid, 19 (12%) were on clopidogrel, and 11 (7%) were on two or more anticoagulants. The median American Society of Anesthesiologists class was 3, and the mean Charlson comorbidity index was 5. The median operative time was 105 min, and the mean energy use was 280 ± 168 kJ. The immediate mean hematocrit decrease was 1.94%. One patient who received excessive intravenous fluids experienced heart failure. Complications within 30 days included urinary tract infection in four patients (2.5%) and delayed bleeding in six (4%). Three of these patients (50%) required blood transfusion, and one (17%)

required reoperation. In 2 years of follow-up, three patients (2%) required repeat PVP. No incontinence or urethral stricture developed. Significant improvements occurred in IPSS, Q_{max}, and PVR. This series supports the use of 532 nm PVP in patients at high risk on systemic anticoagulation, even those on two or more anticoagulation agents and with a large prostate requiring a longer operative time. Few complications developed, and significant enduring clinical improvement was seen in this high surgical risk cohort treated with PVP.

There is a growing body of level 2 to 3 evidence comparing 80 W KTP laser prostatectomy with TURP. Ruszat et al. conducted a study with 396 patients randomized to either 80 W laser prostatectomy or TURP [13]. Interim 24-month follow-up data found that the rates of intraoperative bleeding (3% vs 11%), blood transfusion (0 vs 5.5%), capsule perforations (0.4% vs 6.3%), and early postoperative clot retention (0.4% vs 3.9%) were significantly lower in the laser group. There were no significant differences in IPSS and PVR. After 12 months, the size reduction was greater in the TURP group (66% vs 44%), and the rate of repeat procedure was greater in the PVP group (6.9% vs 3.9%, not significant). Bouchier-Hayes et al. reported data on 120 patients randomized to undergo TURP or 80 W laser PVP [14]. At 12 months, improvements in IPSS and flow rates were demonstrated. Length of hospitalization, length of catheterization, and adverse events were lower in the laser group. In a nonrandomized study, Bachmann et al. studied 101 patients who had undergone either TURP or laser prostatectomy [15]. Perioperative morbidity and symptom improvement were similar between the groups at 6 months. Another randomized study has yielded divergent results. In this study, 76 patients with a prostate size of >70 mL were randomized to TURP and 80 W laser prostatectomy [16]. The procedure time was shorter for the TURP group, and the hospitalization stay and catheterization time were significantly shorter in the laser group. There was a significant difference in favor of TURP in terms of improvement in IPSS, PVR, and Q_{max} as well as volume reduction in the TURP group. In addition, the reoperation rate was higher in the laser group. An Australian study had similar results when comparing patients randomized to either 80 W laser prostatectomy or TURP [17]. Both groups showed a significant increase in mean urinary flow rate, improvement in IPSS scores, and no difference in sexual function with 1-year follow-up.

120 W

The 80 W KTP laser system evolved to a higher-power system capable of delivering 80–120 W to increase the vaporization efficiency. This laser emits the same 532 nm wavelength, with the same hemostastic properties as the 80 W KTP but utilizing a different crystal. The 532 nm 80 W KTP laser is created by passing a 1064 nm Nd:YAG laser beam through a KTP crystal. In contrast, the 120 W HPS 532 nm wavelength is created by passing an Nd:YAG laser beam through an LBO crystal. The 532 nm LBO-based system also has a beam that is better collimated than the KTP-based beam.

A study by Al-Ansari et al. randomized 120 patients with BPH to TURP or a 120 W 532 nm laser [18]. The baseline characteristics were comparable. The mean operative time was significantly shorter for TURP. Compared with preoperative values, there was a significant reduction in hemoglobin and serum sodium levels at the end of TURP only. In the PVP, no major intraoperative

complications were recorded, and none of the patients required a blood transfusion. Among TURP patients, 12 (20%) required transfusion, three (5%) developed TUR syndrome, and capsule perforation was observed in 10 patients. There was a dramatic improvement in Q_{max}, IPSS, and PVP compared with preoperative values, and the degree of improvement was comparable in both groups during the follow-up. Storage bladder symptoms were significantly higher in PVP. A redo procedure was required in one TURP patient and six PVP patients ($P < 0.05$). Two TURP patients and four PVP patients developed bladder neck contracture ($P > 0.05$) treated by bladder neck incision; none in either group experienced a urethral stricture or urinary incontinence.

Lukacs et al. compared PVP with TURP in a multicenter randomized controlled trial [19]. IPSS, Euro-QoL questionnaire, uroflowmetry, Danish Prostate Symptom Score Sexual Function Questionnaire, sexual satisfaction, and adverse events were collected at 1, 3, 6, and 12 months. A total of 139 patients were randomized equally. The median IPSS scores at the 12-month follow-up were 5 for TURP versus 6 for PVP. Noninferiority could not be demonstrated. The median length of stay was significantly shorter in the PVP group than in the TURP group, with a median of 1 versus 2.5 days, respectively ($P < 0.0001$). The uroflowmetry parameters and complications were comparable in both groups. Sexual outcomes were slightly better in the PVP group without reaching statistical significance.

Several trials comparing TURP and PVP have been analyzed by Thangasamy et al. in a meta-analysis to provide a systematic review and meta-analysis of level 1 evidence studies to determine the effectiveness of PVP versus TURP for surgical treatment of benign prostatic hyperplasia [20]. The outcomes reviewed included perioperative data, complications, and functional outcomes. Biomedical databases from 2002 to 2012 and AUA and European Association of Urology conference proceedings from 2007 to 2011 were searched. Trials were included if they were randomized controlled trials, had PVP as the intervention, and had TURP as control. The meta-analysis was performed using a random effects model. Nine trials were identified with 448 patients undergoing PVP (80 W in five trials and 120 W in four trials) and 441 undergoing TURP. The catheterization time and length of stay were shorter in the PVP group by 1.91 days ($P<0.00001$) and 2.13 days ($P<0.00001$), respectively. The operation time was shorter in the TURP group by 19.64 min ($P=0.0003$). Blood transfusion was significantly less likely in the PVP group ($P=0.003$). There were no significant differences between PVP and TURP when comparing other complications. Regarding functional outcomes, six studies found no difference between PVP and TURP, two favored TURP, and one favored PVP. In summary, the authors found that perioperative outcomes of catheterization time and length of hospital stay were shorter with PVP, whereas the operative time was longer with PVP. Postoperative complications of blood transfusion and clot retention were significantly less likely with PVP; no difference was noted in other complications. Overall, no difference was noted in intermediate-term functional outcomes.

180 W 532 nm laser

The most current advancement is the recent Food and Drug Administration approval of a 180 W-capable 532 nm LBO-based laser system with a feedback mechanism to control energy exiting the fiber (GreenLight XPS™) system and a new redesigned, water-cooled, high-power fiber (MoXy™ Fiber, American Medical Systems). The modifications in this system are innovative in that the safety and efficacy of this laser prostatectomy are increased. One key technology is a feedback mechanism that utilizes an infrared-based technology that monitors heat generated at the fiber tip. One aspect that predisposes a fiber to degradation resulting in less collimation, and deflection of the laser pathway, is heating at the tip of the fiber, which can be caused by contact with tissue or adherence of tissue to the tip acting as a heat sink.

This infrared-based feedback technology is an automatic safety system that detects overheating conditions that cause fiber damage or failure, and it briefly disables the beam to allow cooling and maintain a safe temperature zone. If excessive temperatures are reached, the laser emission is stopped momentarily.

Another new modification is applied to the coagulation power mode. The new 180 W-capable system delivers the lower-power coagulation mode laser light at intermittent pulses at a frequency. This intermittent laser pulse modality mimics the intermittent coagulation pattern of the delivery of power by electrocautery coagulation for hemostasis. However, the more important utility is the ability to better utilize this fiber for contact coagulation of arterial bleeders. With intermittent pulses, laser coagulation heat on tissue contact is limited by the intermittent pulsing and continuous flow of room-temperature irrigant over the tip.

Finally, to improve the rate of vaporization efficiency, the power of the 180 W-capable system has been increased. To allow utilization of the 180 W, and maintain the same power density characteristic of the 120 W system and its fiber, a new fiber design was necessary. This new fiber provides a wider tissue-vaporization effect with a more efficient vaporization due to its increased laser fiber diameter from 600 μm to 750 μm. Through this modification, the beam area has been increased by 50% with an increase in fiber diameter of only 0.15 mm. In addition, the end cap of the fiber has been redesigned to limit stray beams during the procedure. Most importantly, the cap is actively cooled with room-temperature saline, at a rate of 1 mL/s, which flows through the fiber and exits at the beam point. This cooling feature enables a fiber to exhibit only a minimal reduction in the amount of light delivered to tissue over the course of a long lasering procedure with the same fiber. These modifications reduce fiber divitrification, a process by which the glass at the tip of the fiber becomes opaque, which then leads to power degradation during the procedure. Additionally, the continuous aqueous flow, metal cap, and feedback feature limit the buildup of coagulated tissue on the tip of the fiber, thereby preventing fiber failure. With these features, one fiber may be all that is needed for large prostates.

Early level 4 evidence for the 180 W laser with the actively cooled fiber shows it to be extremely efficient in the hands of experience users, with equal efficacy and safety [21]. With the new aqueous cooled fibers and the 180 W laser system, up to 180 W of power can be utilized. However, at 120 W or above, the higher efficiency seems to be obtained at the expense of hemostasis. The increased power and efficiency highlight a concern that any misfiring within the bladder at settings such as 180 W could result in damage to the bladder or ureteral orifices, including bladder perforation etc.

(and so rapidly that it could escape the surgeon's attention).

Complications

All reported studies have noted markedly less morbidity associated with laser prostatectomy than with traditional surgical approaches. Bleeding is the main complication of traditional electrocautery TURP, often necessitating transfusion and causing associated problems such as clot retention, premature termination of the procedure, and inadequate relief of obstruction [22]. However, these are older data. Bleeding can also result in continuous catheter irrigation and complications such as stricture secondary to traction on the Foley catheter. Rarely, uncontrolled bleeding can even require open packing of the prostatic fossa. Poor visibility because of bleeding is also thought to be a cause of sphincteric damage and incontinence resulting from TURP. The incidence of hemorrhage requiring blood transfusion is 3.9% and increases twofold if the amount of resected tissue exceeds 45 mL or if the resection time is longer than 90 min. In contrast to transurethral electroresection, which cuts across the prostatic parenchyma and opens prostatic venous sinuses, laser prostatectomy seals blood vessels as it coagulates the transition zone and prevents both absorption of irrigating fluid and hemorrhage; the hemostasis associated with laser prostatectomy is thus superior, with even multiple studies of anticoagulated patients undergoing resection without any bleeding complications [11,23].

Irrigant fluid absorption during electrocautery TURP results in a 2% incidence of TURP syndrome because of dilutional hyponatremia, glycine-induced ammonia intoxication, or the direct toxic effect of glycine [22]. As with bleeding, fluid absorption increases with larger glands and longer resection times.

The incidence of urethral stricture after electrocautery TURP is 3.1%; if bladder neck contractures are included, this figure approaches 5% [22]. Stricture formation is thought to be secondary to trauma induced by the large size of the resectoscope as well as the use of a low-intensity, coagulating current, which penetrates deeper into tissue than cutting currents. Since laser procedures do not use electrical current, the cystoscopes utilized are smaller, the overall operative time is usually shorter, and the incidence of stricture is lower following laser procedures. The incidence of reoperation for residual obstructive tissue is difficult to determine, since most published series of laser prostatectomy have documented initial experiences with this technology. Our experience with strictures and bladder neck contracture has demonstrated that the incidence is higher in patients with bladder dysfunction or bladder diverticulum, or with long procedures utilizing larger-diameter scopes.

Postoperative infections may also occur after TURP. The incidence of urinary tract infection following TURP is 15.5% (median), while epididymitis occurs in 1.2% [22]. Urinary-tract infections have been reported in 1–20% of patients following laser prostatectomy and epididymitis in 5–7% of patients [24]. The treatment of such infections may be more problematic in laser prostatectomies secondary to the residual necrotic prostate tissue that remains *in situ* for several weeks after laser coagulation. When this occurs, the most common manifestation is subacute prostatitis, characterized by significant and persistent irritative voiding symptoms, with mild prostatic and/or epididymal tenderness on examination, persistent pyuria, and positive urine cultures [24,25].

Finally, retrograde ejaculation represents another potential side effect of electrocautery TURP, occurring in up to 90% of patients. Eighty-watt KTP laser data show that retrograde ejaculation also represents a potential problem in laser prostatectomy, with a 27% incidence of retrograde ejaculation [4]. Similarly, the incidence of impotence following electrocautery TURP ranges from 4% to 13% [22]. However, the overall incidence of impotence following all forms of laser prostatectomy is rare. While data are limited, available 80 W KTP data show no loss of potency in patients treated with laser prostatectomy.

Conclusion

Laser prostatectomy has proved to be a safe and efficacious surgical intervention to relieve symptomatic bladder outlet obstruction based on a large body of level 1 to 4 evidence.

Dos and don'ts

- Laser resection may begin with either the medial lobe or lateral lobes but should always be started proximally and continued distally, working away from the bladder neck and toward the verumontanum.
- The optimal distance from the tissue is close within one fiber cap in a noncontact technique.
- The prostate should be systematically swept so that there is no deep tissue penetration leading to undue postoperative irritative symptoms from coagulation necrosis.
- The risks of GreenLight treatment on active anticoagulation therapy should be clearly explained to the patient, as the risk of bleeding is always higher while on anticogulation medication than off it.

Overall morbidity contrasts favorably with standard surgical approaches. Moreover, laser technology is generally accessible to the practicing urologist. The transurethral endoscopic approach and operative techniques are not complex. These attributes have positioned laser prostatectomy as an accepted surgical treatment for BPH.

Bibliography

1 Kuntzman RS, Malek RS, Barrett DM, Bostwick DG. Potassium-titanyl-phosphate laser vaporization of the prostate: a comparative functional and pathologic study in canines. *Urology*. 1996;48(4):575–83.

2 Malek RS, Barrett DM, Kuntzman RS. High-power potassium-titanyl-phosphate (KTP/532) laser vaporization prostatectomy: 24 hours later. *Urology*. 1998;51(2):254–6.

3 Malek RS, Kuntzman RS, Barrett DM. High power potassium-titanyl-phosphate laser vaporization prostatectomy. *J Urol*. 2000;163(6):1730–3.

4 Te AE, Malloy TR, Stein BS, Ulchaker JC, Nseyo UO, Hai MA, *et al*. Photoselective vaporization of the prostate for the treatment of benign prostatic hyperplasia: 12-month results from the first United States multicenter prospective trial. *J Urol*. 2004;172(4 Pt 1):1404–8.

5 Ruszat R, Seitz M, Wyler SF, Abe C, Rieken M, Reich O, *et al*. GreenLight laser vaporization of the prostate: single-center experience and long-term results after 500 procedures. *Eur Urol*. 2008;54(4):893–901.

6 Te AE, Malloy TR, Stein BS, Ulchaker JC, Nseyo UO, Hai MA. Impact of prostate-specific antigen level and prostate volume as predictors of efficacy in photoselective vaporization prostatectomy: analysis and results of an ongoing prospective multicentre study at 3 years. *BJU Int*. 2006;97(6):1229–33.

7 Sandhu JS, Ng C, Vanderbrink BA, Egan C, Kaplan SA, Te AE. High-power potassium-titanyl-phosphate photoselective laser vaporization of prostate for treatment of benign prostatic hyperplasia in men with large prostates. *Urology*. 2004;64(6):1155–9.

8 Pfitzenmaier J, Gilfrich C, Pritsch M, Herrmann D, Buse S, Haferkamp A, *et al*. Vaporization of prostates of > or =80 mL using a potassium-titanyl-phosphate laser: midterm-results and comparison with prostates of <80 mL. *BJU Int*. 2008;102(3):322–7.

9 Rajbabu K, Chandrasekara SK, Barber NJ, Walsh K, Muir GH. Photoselective vaporization of the prostate with the potassium-titanyl-phosphate laser in men with prostates of >100 mL. *BJU Int*. 2007;100(3):593–8; discussion 8.

10 Reich O, Bachmann A, Siebels M, Hofstetter A, Stief CG, Sulser T. High power (80 W) potassium-titanyl-phosphate laser vaporization of the prostate in 66 high risk patients. *J Urol*. 2005;173(1):158–60.

11 Sandhu JS, Ng CK, Gonzalez RR, Kaplan SA, Te AE. Photoselective laser vaporization prostatectomy in men receiving anticoagulants. *J Endourol*. 2005;19(10):1196–8.

12 Chung DE, Wysock JS, Lee RK, Melamed SR, Kaplan SA, Te AE. Outcomes and complications after 532 nm laser prostatectomy in anticoagulated patients with benign prostatic hyperplasia. *J Urol*. 2011;186(3):977–81.

13 Ruszat R, Wyler SF, Seitz M, Lehmann K, Abe C, Bonkat G, *et al*. Comparison of potassium-titanyl-phosphate laser vaporization of the prostate and transurethral resection of the prostate: update of a prospective non-randomized two-centre study. *BJU Int*. 2008;102(10):1432–8; discussion 8–9.

14 Bouchier-Hayes DM, Anderson P, Van Appledorn S, Bugeja P, Costello AJ. KTP laser versus transurethral resection: early results of a randomized trial. *J Endourol*. 2006;20(8):580–5.

15 Bachmann A, Ruszat R, Wyler S, Reich O, Seifert HH, Muller A, *et al*. Photoselective vaporization of the prostate: the basel experience after 108 procedures. *Eur Urol*. 2005;47(6):798–804.

16 Horasanli K, Silay MS, Altay B, Tanriverdi O, Sarica K, Miroglu C. Photoselective potassium titanyl phosphate (KTP) laser vaporization versus transurethral resection of the prostate for prostates larger than 70 mL: a short-term prospective randomized trial. *Urology*. 2008;71(2):247–51.

17 Bouchier-Hayes DM, Van Appledorn S, Bugeja P, Crowe H, Challacombe B, Costello AJ. A randomized trial of photoselective vaporization of the prostate using the 80-W potassium-titanyl-phosphate laser versus transurethral prostatectomy, with a 1-year follow-up. *BJU Int*. 2010;105(7):964–9.

18 Al-Ansari A, Younes N, Sampige VP, Al-Rumaihi K, Ghafouri A, Gul T, *et al*. GreenLight HPS 120-W laser vaporization versus transurethral resection of the prostate for treatment of benign prostatic hyperplasia: a randomized clinical trial with midterm follow-up. *Eur Urol*. 2010;58(3):349–55.

19 Lukacs B, Loeffler J, Bruyere F, Blanchet P, Gelet A, Coloby P, *et al.* Photoselective vaporization of the prostate with GreenLight 120-W laser compared with monopolar transurethral resection of the prostate: a multicenter randomized controlled trial. *Eur Urol.* 2012;61(6):1165–73.

20 Thangasamy IA, Chalasani V, Bachmann A, Woo HH. Photoselective vaporisation of the prostate using 80-W and 120-W laser versus transurethral resection of the prostate for benign prostatic hyperplasia: a systematic review with meta-analysis from 2002 to 2012. *Eur Urol.* 2012;62(2):315–23.

21 Bachmann A, Muir GH, Collins EJ, Choi BB, Tabatabaei S, Reich OM, *et al.* 180-W XPS GreenLight laser therapy for benign prostate hyperplasia: early safety, efficacy, and perioperative outcome after 201 procedures. *Eur Urol.* 2012;61(3):600–7.

22 Mebust WK, Holtgrewe HL, Cockett AT, Peters PC. Transurethral prostatectomy: immediate and postoperative complications. A cooperative study of 13 participating institutions evaluating 3,885 patients. *J Urol.* 1989;141(2):243–7.

23 Kabalin JN, Gill HS. Urolase laser prostatectomy in patients on warfarin anticoagulation: a safe treatment alternative for bladder outlet obstruction. *Urology.* 1993;42(6):738–40.

24 McCullough DL, Roth RA, Babayan RK, Gordon JO, Reese JH, Crawford ED, *et al.* Transurethral ultrasound-guided laser-induced prostatectomy: National Human Cooperative Study results. *J Urol.* 1993;150(5 Pt 2):1607–11.

25 McCullough DL, Schulze H. Transurethral ultrasound guided laser induced prostatectomy (TULIP): U.S. Cooperative Study and University of Bochum results. *Prog Clin Biol Res.* 1994;386:529–33.

CHAPTER 17

Principles of Electrocautery-Based Techniques

Aaron M. Bernie & Richard Lee

Department of Urology, Weill Cornell Medical College, New York-Presbyterian Hospital, New York, NY, USA

Key points

- Electrosurgically based transurethral resection of the prostate (TURP) represents the gold standard in endoscopic treatment of symptomatic benign prostatic hyperplasia (BPH).
- Monopolar TURP (mTURP) has been used for a long period of time, which has allowed for large studies with extensive follow-up, thus confirming its efficacy and efficiency in both the short and long term.
- Commonly cited complications of mTURP include bleeding, transurethral resection (TUR) syndrome, and uretheral strictures.
- Transurethral electrovaporization involves a combination of fulguration, vaporization, and desiccation of tissue.
- Bipolar TURP (bTURP) is performed using a system where both electrodes are contained within the operative device, which not only allows for the use of isotonic saline but also decreases the risk of thermal burns.
- The goal of bTURP is to resect large amounts of prostatic tissue while decreasing the most common complications of mTURP, such as perioperative bleeding requiring transfusion and TUR syndrome.
- Comparative studies have shown that bTURP provides a reasonable and efficacious alternative for transurethral resection of the prostate when compared with the traditional modality of mTURP.

Overview

BPH represents one of the few conditions that virtually all men will experience to some degree secondary to an enlarging prostate as they age [1–3]. In fact, up to 90% of men who have received no intervention report symptoms of BPH by the age of 85 [4].

Surgical intervention can be divided into minimally invasive surgical therapies (needle ablation of the prostate and transuretheral microwave thermotherapy) as well as possible various transurethral resection, electrovaporization, vaporization, and enucleation procedures in addition to traditional open-surgery techniques, such as simple prostatectomy [5].

Electrosurgically based transurethral resection of the prostate (TURP) represents the gold standard in endoscopic treatment of symptomatic BPH. With the introduction of improved medical therapy combined with minimally invasive options, the number of TURPs performed in the United States has declined [6], but the procedure still remains

Male Lower Urinary Tract Symptoms and Benign Prostatic Hyperplasia, First Edition.
Edited by Steven A. Kaplan and Kevin T. McVary.
© 2014 John Wiley & Sons, Ltd. Published 2014 by John Wiley & Sons, Ltd.

the most effective treatment option after failure of conservative management and medical therapy.

Multiple electrosurgical transurethral options are available for treating BPH. These range from the classic monopolar TURP to the newer bipolar and laser technologies. In this chapter, we discuss both mTURP and bTURP, and provide a comparison of these two techniques.

Monopolar transurethral resection of the prostate

Monopolar transurethral resection of the prostate (mTURP) has been performed for almost 100 years for BPH in men with symptomatic lower urinary tract symptoms (LUTS) and bladder outlet obstruction (BOO) with proven long-term efficacy and improvement in symptoms [7,8]. Monopolar resection utilizes a high-frequency electrical current that is driven by an electrosurgical generator. Because the electrical current that is used to power most everyday tools can cause damage to the patient, the electrosurgical generator converts this energy to higher frequencies of 100,000 Hz and greater so that it can be safely used in the body. The electrical circuit in monopolar technology consists of the generator that is converting the energy, the resection loop through which the energy is conducted, and a return electrode, typically in the form of a grounding pad that is placed on the patient before surgery begins. The tissue that comes into contact with the resection loop receives the energy created by the generator and acts as a resistor through which the energy can pass, thus resulting in resection of tissue via cutting and coagulation [9].

Unlike many other modalities for treatment of BPH, mTURP has been used widely and extensively for a long period of time, which has allowed for large studies with extensive follow-up, thereby confirming its efficacy and efficiency in both the short and long term. The prototypical study for mTURP lies with the Veterans Affairs Cooperative Study Group on Transuretheral Resection of the Prostate study reported Wasson *et al.* In this trial, 556 men over the age of 54 with moderate symptoms of BPH were randomized to mTURP versus watchful waiting with an average follow-up of 2.8 years [10]. Surgery was associated with a better improvement in symptom score (–9.6 vs –5.5, $P < 0.001$), postvoid residual volume (PVR; –60 vs –41, $P = 0.015$), Q_{max} (6.3 vs 0.4, $P < 0.001$), and quality-of-life (QoL) scores from urinary bother (+29.6 vs 9.6, $P < 0.001$). Surgery was not associated with incontinence or impotence. Surgery was associated with a 52% reduction in treatment failure compared with watchful waiting. Twenty-four percent of the men assigned to watchful waiting underwent surgery within 3 years after the assignment.

While the rates of satisfaction and reoperation rate have shown good long-term results, the perioperative morbidity of mTURP has traditionally been an area of criticism and the driving force for the use of medical therapy and other surgical technologies for symptomatic BPH. Early perioperative mortality reports, from the mid 20th century, on mTURP were as high as 2.5% but have improved to below 0.5%, largely owing to the changes in available technology and perioperative medical care. Madersbacher *et al.* analyzed over 20,000 cases of men undergoing mTURP, and determined that 8 years after initial operation, 7.4% of men required another TURP due to a return of symptoms. They also found that the 90-day postsurgical mortality in this cohort was 0.7%; it must be considered that this finding is likely not as much due to operative intervention as it is to the fact that over 25% of these patients had at least one other medical comorbidity [11,12].

Complications rate with mTURP have also been relatively low. The most commonly cited complications of mTURP include bleeding, TUR syndrome, and uretheral strictures [13]. After 15 years of follow-up, Zwergel *et al.* showed that urethral strictures and bladder-neck contractures are seen in less than 3% of men undergoing mTURP, and that patients were still satisfied with the outcome of their procedure 15 years after it was performed [14].

One of the most well-known complications of mTURP is TUR syndrome, which is a complication that occurs due to the use of glycine as the irrigant solution in mTURP. TUR syndrome is a result of three different components: dilutional hyponatremia, fluid overload, and glycine toxicity [15]. TUR syndrome can be avoided by shortening the length of resection, taking care to monitor patients during and after the procedure, as well as using other solutions during mTURP such as glucose in a normal saline solution [16].

Other improvements in technology have also allowed for mTURP to be performed with improved morbidity. High-definition video-assistance cameras and continuous-flow resectoscopes allow surgeons to complete resections in shorter periods of time, decreasing the rates of TUR syndrome. One of the largest studies to date by Tasci *et al.* examined the outcomes of more than 3500 patients undergoing mTURP. Their experience showed that major complications such as perforation occurred in <1% of patients, and minor complications such as clot retention and recatheterization occurred at low rates as well, that is, 2.3% and 5.4%, respectively. With a follow-up of 7 years, patients

demonstrated an International Prostate Symptom Score (IPSS) improvement of 6.8 and a Q_{max} improvement of 19.5 mL/s [17].

Early experience with monopolar electrovaporization technology

Before widespread use of bipolar technology in transurethral resection of the prostate, early studies in electrovaporization of the prostate with a plasmakinetic system showed safety as well as efficacy when used in prostatic surgery [18–22]. Transurethral electrovaporization of the prostate (TEVP) involves the use of a high-energy cutting current to resect the prostate while decreasing bleeding and electrolyte and fluid absorption [20,23]. Specifically, electrovaporization involves a combination of fulguration as well as vaporization and desiccation of tissue; when the cutting current is applied, the tissue is quickly heated, which results in tissue explosion, that is, vaporization. This process is localized to the tissue in contact with the electrode, which greatly decreases damage to surrounding tissue [24].

An early study by Kaplan *et al.* followed 114 patients over an 18-month period after TEVP. These patients were evaluated at 1, 3, 6, 12, and 18 months postoperatively. Peri- and postoperative parameters were followed, including changes in serum electrolytes and hematocrit as well as operative time, postoperative catheterization time, American Urological Association (AUA) symptom score, peak flow, PVR, and complications. AUA symptom score (−11.3, $P < 0.01$) and peak urinary flow (Q_{max}, +9.6 mL/s, $P < 0.001$) at 18 months both improved compared with preoperative values. There was no significant difference in PVR at 12 months

(64.5 vs 33.6 mL, $P = 0.07$). None of the patients required postoperative transfusion or experienced TUR syndrome postoperatively. The mean catheterization was 10.4 h with a mean hospital stay of 0.9 days [21].

A follow-up study by Kaplan, *et al.* compared the results of electrovaporization with mTURP for the treatment of LUTS in a group of 64 men. Patients were evaluated at 1, 3, 6, and 12 months postoperatively. Improvement in symptom score was superior in the TEVP group compared with mTURP (12.8 vs 12.2, $P < 0.02$), although mTURP showed a better improvement in Q_{max} versus (11.3 mL/s vs 9.7 mL/s, $P < 0.03$). PVR was not statistically different between the two groups (43.6 mL for TEVP vs 34.2 mL for mTURP, $P = 0.11$). The overall operative time was shorter in the mTURP group [34.6 min vs 47.6 min in transurethral vaporization of the prostate (TUVP), $P < 0.01$], but the durations of catheterization and hospitalization were significantly shorter for the TUVP group (catheterization: 12.9 h vs 67.4 h, $P < 0.01$; hospitalization: 1.3 days vs 2.6 days, $P < 0.03$). There was a significantly larger decrease in sodium levels with the mTURP group (3.9 vs 1.4 mEq/L, $P < 0.03$) as well as more days of work lost (18.4 days vs 6.7 days, $P < 0.02$) [22]. These early studies showed promise for the use of transurethral electrovaporization of the prostate [25].

Bipolar transurethral resection of the prostate

The goal of bipolar transuretheral resection of the prostate (bTURP) has been to conceptually use the same mechanism of mTURP in resecting large amounts of prostatic tissue but to do so while decreasing the most common complications, such as perioperative bleeding requiring transfusion, TUR syndrome, and postoperative complications [26]. A variety of bTURP systems have been created and applied in clinical use, including systems by Olympus America Inc. (TURIS, Gyrus plasmakinetic system, ACMI; Center Valley, PA) and Karl Storz Industrial-America (El Segundo, CA) [27]. Figure 17.1 shows the basic differences between mTURP and bTURP, and Figures 17.2–17.4 show the standard bTURP resection apparatus and resection button.

Bipolar TURP is performed in similar fashion to mTURP but with a difference in the operative electrodes. In bTURP, both electrodes are contained within the operative device, which not only allows for the use of isotonic saline but also decreases the risk of thermal burns. In mTURP, one of the electrodes is in the instrument itself, and the other is typically on the exterior in the patient in the form of a grounding electrode. Because of the distance between electrodes in mTURP, a nonconductive solution such as glycine is necessary to ensure that the current does not dissipate; this is not necessary in bTURP, since the electrodes are close to one another [9,27]. This difference decreases the incidence of TUR syndrome in patients undergoing bTURP, as irrigant solutions such as isotonic saline may be used without fear of causing a short-circuit. The reduction in TUR syndrome also allows for a longer resection time and a decrease in one of the most feared complications of mTURP. Bipolar TURP is also able to utilize power more efficiently than mTURP, using approximately half of the electrical power that mTURP requires to cut through prostatic tissue, thus decreasing the risk of thermal burns [28,29].

A number of randomized controlled trials have been performed to compare bipolar versus monopolar transurethral resection

Traditional monopolar

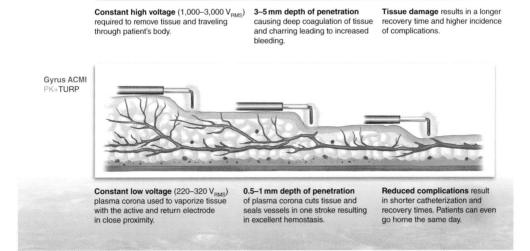

Constant high voltage (1,000–3,000 V$_{RMS}$) required to remove tissue and traveling through patient's body.

3–5 mm depth of penetration causing deep coagulation of tissue and charring leading to increased bleeding.

Tissue damage results in a longer recovery time and higher incidence of complications.

Gyrus ACMI PK+TURP

Constant low voltage (220–320 V$_{RMS}$) plasma corona used to vaporize tissue with the active and return electrode in close proximity.

0.5–1 mm depth of penetration of plasma corona cuts tissue and seals vessels in one stroke resulting in excellent hemostasis.

Reduced complications result in shorter catheterization and recovery times. Patients can even go home the same day.

Figure 17.1 Schematic diagram of traditional monopolar transurethral resection of the prostate (top) vs. bipolar transurethral resection of the prostate (bottom). Olympus. Reproduced with permission of Olympus America Inc.

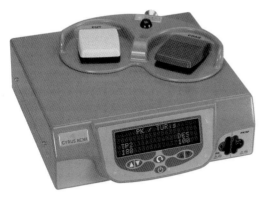

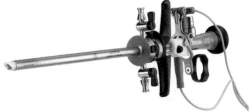

Figure 17.3 Olympus OES Pro Resectoscope apparatus with continuous flow sheath. Olympus. Reproduced with permission of Olympus America Inc.

Figure 17.2 Olympus PlasmaKinetic™ SuperPulse bipolar current generator with cut and coagulation foot pedal. Olympus. Reproduced with permission of Olympus America Inc.

(see Table 17.1). One of the largest studies with the longest duration of follow-up was reported in Erturhan *et al.*'s study, where 120 patients were randomized to either plasmakinetic bTURP or mTURP for treatment of symptomatic BPH. Catheterization time was shorter in the bTURP group (3 vs 4.5 days, $P < 0.001$) as were the time to discharge (3 vs 5 days, $P < 0.001$) and operative time (36 vs 57 min, $P < 0.001$). The improvement in Q_{max} was also better in the bTURP group (12.3 mL/s improvement vs 11.3 mL/s, $P < 0.001$).

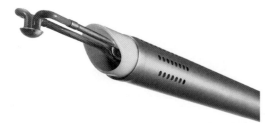

Figure 17.4 Olympus PlasmaButton™ vaporization electrode inside of continuous flow resectoscope sheath. Olympus. Reproduced with permission of Olympus America Inc.

The IPSS score improved similarly in both groups (20 points mTURP group vs 19 points bTURP group) after 12 months, as did both QoL scores (2 in both groups) and PVR (–110 mL for mTURP vs –99 mL for bTURP). Clot retention was significantly higher for patients undergoing mTURP (17 vs 2 paitents, $P = 0.0001$) as well as bleeding requiring transfusion (7 vs 1 patient, $P = 0.0001$) and severe dysuria (7 patients vs 2 patients, $P = 0.025$). Not all complications, however, were confined to the mTURP group. Interestingly, TUR syndrome was not significantly different between the two groups (2 vs 0 patients, $P = 0.15$). More urethral injuries (3 vs 0 patients, $P = 0.01$) and meatal strictures (3 vs 2 patients, $P = 0.025$) occurred in the bTURP group. Overall, this study suggests that while symptom improvements are similar using both technologies, several of the complications are seen at a reduced rate with bTURP [30]. This study, like many of the early studies, is limited by the relatively low number of patients and short duration of follow-up.

Another large randomized control trial reported by Michielsen *et al.* examined the use of bipolar TURis, that is, bipolar resection performed in saline versus mTURP [31]. They found that, in contrast to the above study, there was no difference in the rates of complications, specifically clot retention (6 vs

4, $P = 0.75$), blood transfusion (1 vs 4, $P = 0.21$), TUR syndrome (1 vs 0, $P = 1.0$), hospital stay (4.9 vs 5.1 days, $P = 0.591$), catheterization time (4.0 vs 4.5 days, $P = 0.2$), or urinary retention (5 vs 3, $P = 0.72$) in mTURP vs bTURP, respectively. The only difference seen between the groups was operative time, which was significantly shorter in the mTURP group (44 min vs 56 min, $P = 0.001$) at the cost of a larger decrease in serum sodium levels for mTURP patients (–2.23 vs –1.47; no P value given). The number needed to treat to avoid an episode of TUR syndrome from mTURP calculated in this study was 50 patients. There were no data regarding symptom score, Q_{max}, or PVR improvement in this study. This study did not have any long-term follow-up data, as the presented data were only collected during these patients' initial hospital stay (no mean follow-up reported). The authors concluded that bipolar TUR was safe and efficacious compared with mTURP, although the difference in postoperative complication rates was not clinically significant [31].

Yoon *et al.* reported on a study of 102 men undergoing mTURP ($N = 53$) versus bTURP ($N = 49$) [32]. Improvements in IPSS (11.7 bTURP vs 12.1 mTURP, $P > 0.05$) and Q_{max} (10.1 bTURP vs, 10.2 mTURP, $P > 0.05$) were no different between the two groups as was the rate of postoperative complications. The durations of both catheterization and hospitalization were significantly lower in the bTURP group (2.28 days vs 3.12 days, $P = 0.012$; 3.52 days vs 4.27 days, $P = 0.034$, respectively).

There are a number of other randomized control trials reporting on the outcomes of bipolar versus monopolar resection (see Table 17.1). The table includes the largest available trials, as well as those with the longest follow-up data. All of their results

Table 17.1 Studies comparing monopolar TURP (mTURP) with bipolar TURP (bTURP)

Authors	Trial size	Follow-up	Operative time	Catheterization time	TUR syndrome	Postop change in hemoglobin	Hospital stay	Change in Q_{max} (mL/s)	Change in postvoid residual
Xie et al. [39]	110 mTURP, 110 bTURP	60 months	60.01 min mTURP, 55.03 min bTURP (P = 0.033)	3.61 days mTURP, 2.70 days bTURP (P < 0.001)	2 patients mTURP, 0 patients bTURP (P = 0.477)	1.58 g/dL mTURP, 1.22 g/dL bTURP (P = 0.014)	5.19 days mTURP, 4.18 days bTURP (P < 0.001)	15.29 mL/s mTURP, 16.55 mL/s bTURP (P = 0.176)	81.91 mL mTURP, 82.79 bTURP (P = 0.176)
Chen et al. [40]	50 mTURP, 50 bTURP	24 months	60 min mTURP, 59 min bTURP (P = 0.82)	NA	0 patients mTURP, 0 patients bTURP	1.6 g/dL mTURP, 1.1 g/dL bTURP (P = 0.008)	NA	16.9 mL/s mTURP, 18.4 mL/s bTURP (P = 0.72)	NA
Michielsen et al. [31]	120 mTURP, 118 bTURP	18 months	44 min mTURP, 56 min bTURP (P < 0.001)	4.5 days mTURP, 4.0 days bTURP (P = 0.201)	1 patient mTURP, 0 patients bTURP (P = 1.00)	1.3 mg/dL mTURP, 1.4 mg/dL bTURP	5.1 days mTURP, 4.9 days bTURP (P = 0.591)	NA	NA
Yoon et al. [32]	53 mTURP, 49 bTURP	12 months	72.6 min mTURP, 74.2 min bTURP (P = 0.451)	3.12 days mTURP, 2.28 days bTURP (P = 0.012)	NA	0.62 g/dL mTURP, 0.67 g/dL bTURP (P = 0.278)	4.27 days mTURP, 3.52 days bTURP (P = 0.034)	10.2 mL/s mTURP, 10.1 bTURP (P = NS)	NA
Starkman and Santucci [38]	18 mTURP, 25 bTURP	18 months	NA	3.2 days mTURP, 1.8 days bTURP (P = 0.12)	NA	NA	2.1 days mTURP, 1.2 days bTURP (P = 0.11)	NA	NA
Autorino et al. [36]	35 mTURP, 35 bTURP	48 months	53 min mTURP, 49 min bTURP (P = 0.07)	NA	NA	1.0 g/dL mTURP, 0.8 bTURP g/dL (P = 0.09)	NA	15 mL/s mTURP, 12.7 bTURP (P = 0.44)	30 mL mTURP, 38 mL bTURP (P = 0.3)
Kong et al. [33]	51 mTURP, 51 bTURP	12 months	NS (no values given)	57.7 h mTURP, 37.2 h bTURP (P = 0.03)	NA	1.8 g/dL mTURP, 0.6 g/dL bTURP (P = 0.01)	2.6 days mTURP, 1.5 days bTURP (P = 0.02)	11.91 mL/s mTURP, 12.63 mL/s bTURP (P = NS)	81.63 mL mTURP, 82.79 mL bTURP
Ho et al. [41]	52 mTURP, 48 bTURP	12 months	58 min mTURP, 59 min bTURP (P = NS)	NA	2 patients mTURP, 0 patients bTURP (P < 0.05)	1.8 mg/dL mTURP, 1.2 mg/dL bTURP (P = NS)	NA	At 12 months, NS difference (no exact values given)	NA

Dos and don'ts

- mTURP, TEVP, and bTURP can all be used effectively in the surgical management of BPH.
- Both mTURP and bTURP are effective in the treatment of symptomatic BPH and BOO, so a definitive decision as to which is more effective for each individual treatment cannot be made.
- Several modalities exist for performance of bTURP.
- Symptomatic improvement occurs with all forms of electrosurgical management of BPH.
- Both monopolar and bipolar TURP have long-term follow-up studies that provide information about what can be expected several years after the procedure has been performed.

echo the studies cited, suggesting that bTURP is an effective and efficacious way to perform a resection of the prostate [33–36].

The advent of bipolar technology and its use in TURP have produced results comparable with that of mTURP but with decreased prevalence of TUR syndrome and potentially bleeding complications postoperatively in addition to potentially shorter resection times and durations of postoperative catheterization [8,37]. It has also been suggested that the use of bTURP decreases postoperative hospitalization stay, which can on average reduce the cost by over $1000 per patient per day [38]. While more long-term studies on efficacy of bTURP are necessary to confirm these early trends, it appears that bTURP provides a reasonable and efficacious alternative for transurethral resection of the prostate when compared with traditional modalities.

Bibliography

1 Djavan B, Nickel JC, de la Rosette J, Abrams P. The urologist view of BPH progression: results of an international survey. *Eur Urol.* 2002;41(5): 490–6.

2 Verhamme KM, Dieleman JP, Bleumink GS, van der Lei J, Sturkenboom MC, Artibani W, *et al.* Incidence and prevalence of lower urinary tract symptoms suggestive of benign prostatic hyperplasia in primary care – the Triumph project. *Eur Urol.* 2002;42(4):323–8.

3 Chute CG, Panser LA, Girman CJ, Oesterling JE, Guess HA, Jacobsen SJ, *et al.* The prevalence of prostatism: a population-based survey of urinary symptoms. *J Urol.* 1993;150(1):85–9.

4 Roberts RO, Jacobsen SJ, Jacobson DJ, Reilly WT, Talley NJ, Lieber MM. Natural history of prostatism: high American Urological Association Symptom scores among community-dwelling men and women with urinary incontinence. *Urology.* 1998, 51(2):213–9.

5 McVary KT, Roehrborn CG, Avins AL, Barry MJ, Bruskewitz RC, Donnell RF, *et al.* Update on AUA guideline on the management of benign prostatic hyperplasia. *J Urol.* 2011;185(5):1793–803.

6 Merrill RM, Hunter BD. The diminishing role of transurethral resection of the prostate. *Ann Surg Oncol.* 2010;17(5):1422–8.

7 Reich O, Gratzke C, Stief CG. Techniques and long-term results of surgical procedures for BPH. *Eur Urol.* 2006;49(6):970–8; discussion 978.

8 Mamoulakis C, Ubbink DT, de la Rosette JJ. Bipolar versus monopolar transurethral resection of the prostate: a systematic review and meta-analysis of randomized controlled trials. *Eur Urol.* 2009;56(5):798–809.

9 Issa MM. Technological advances in transurethral resection of the prostate: bipolar versus monopolar TURP. *J Endourol.* 2008;22(8):1587–95.

10 Wasson JH, Reda DJ, Bruskewitz RC, Elinson J, Keller AM, Henderson WG. A comparison of transurethral surgery with watchful waiting for moderate symptoms of benign prostatic hyperplasia. The Veterans Affairs Cooperative Study Group on Transurethral Resection of the Prostate. *N Engl J Med.* 1995;332(2):75–9.

11 Holtgrewe HL, Valk WL. Factors influencing the mortality and morbidity of transurethral prostatectomy: a study of 2,015 cases. *J Urol.* 1962;87: 450–9.

12 Madersbacher S, Lackner J, Brossner C, Rohlich M, Stancik I, Willinger M, *et al.* Reoperation, myocardial infarction and mortality after transurethral and open prostatectomy: a nation-wide, long-term analysis of 23,123 cases. *Eur Urol.* 2005; 47(4):499–504.

13 Ho HS, Cheng CW. Bipolar transurethral resection of prostate: a new reference standard? *Curr Opin Urol.* 2008;18(1):50–5.

14 Zwergel U, Wullich B, Lindenmeir U, Rohde V, Zwergel T. Long-term results following transurethral resection of the prostate. *Eur Urol.* 1998; 33(5):476–80.

15 Smith RD, Patel A. Transurethral resection of the prostate revisited and updated. *Curr Opin Urol.* 2011;21(1):36–41.

16 Yousef AA, Suliman GA, Elashry OM, Elsharaby MD, Elgamasy Ael N. A randomized comparison between three types of irrigating fluids during transurethral resection in benign prostatic hyperplasia. *BMC Anesthesiol.* 2010;10:7.

17 Tasci AI, Ilbey YO, Tugcu V, Cicekler O, Cevik C, Zoroglu F. Transurethral resection of the prostate with monopolar resectoscope: single-surgeon experience and long-term results of after 3589 procedures. *Urology.* 2011;78(5):1151–55.

18 Te AE, Santarosa R, Kaplan SA. Electrovaporization of the prostate: electrosurgical modification of standard transurethral resection in 93 patients with benign hyperplasia. *J Endourol.* 1997;11(1): 71–75.

19 Te AE, Kaplan SA. Transurethral electrovaporization of the prostate. *Mayo Clin Proc.* 1998;73(7): 691–5.

20 Kaplan SA, Te AE. Transurethral electrovaporization of the prostate: a novel method for treating men with benign prostatic hyperplasia. *Urology.* 1995;45(4):566–72.

21 Kaplan SA, Santarosa RP, Te AE. Transurethral electrovaporization of the prostate: one-year experience. *Urology.* 1996;48(6):876–81.

22 Kaplan SA, Laor E, Fatal M, Te AE. Transurethral resection of the prostate versus transurethral electrovaporization of the prostate: a blinded, prospective comparative study with 1-year followup. *J Urol.* 1998;159(2):454–58.

23 Hammadeh MY, Philp T. Transurethral electrovaporization of the prostate (TUVP) is effective, safe and durable. *Prostate Cancer Prostatic Dis.* 2003;6(2):121–6.

24 Cabelin MA, Te AE, Kaplan SA. Transurethral vaporization of the prostate: current techniques. *Curr Urol Rep.* 2000;1(2):116–23.

25 Patel A, Fuchs GJ, Gutierrez-Aceves J, Andrade-Perez F. Transurethral electrovaporization and vapour-resection of the prostate: an appraisal of possible electrosurgical alternatives to regular loop resection. *BJU Int.* 2000;85(2):202–10.

26 Ubee SS, Philip J, Nair M. Bipolar technology for transurethral prostatectomy. *Expert Rev Med Devices.* 2011;8(2):149–54.

27 Rassweiler J, Schulze M, Stock C, Teber D, De La Rosette J. Bipolar transurethral resection of the prostate – technical modifications and early clinical experience. *Minim Invasive Ther Allied Technol.* 2007;16(1):11–21.

28 Patel A, Adshead JM. First clinical experience with new transurethral bipolar prostate electrosurgery resection system: controlled tissue ablation (coblation technology). *J Endourol.* 2004;18(10):959–64.

29 Botto H, Lebret T, Barre P, Orsoni JL, Herve JM, Lugagne PM. Electrovaporization of the prostate with the Gyrus device. *J Endourol.* 2001, 15(3): 313–6.

30 Erturhan S, Erbagci A, Seckiner I, Yagci F, Ustun A. Plasmakinetic resection of the prostate versus standard transurethral resection of the prostate: a prospective randomized trial with 1-year follow-up. *Prostate Cancer Prostatic Dis.* 2007;10(1):97–100.

31 Michielsen DP, Debacker T, De Boe V, Van Lersberghe C, Kaufman L, Braeckman JG, *et al.* Bipolar transurethral resection in saline – an alternative surgical treatment for bladder outlet obstruction? *J Urol.* 2007;178(5):2035–9; discussion 2039.

32 Yoon CJ, Kim JY, Moon KH, Jung HC, Park TC. Transurethral resection of the prostate with a bipolar tissue management system compared to conventional monopolar resectoscope: one-year outcome. *Yonsei Med J.* 2006;47(5):715–20.

33 Kong CH, Ibrahim MF, Zainuddin ZM. A prospective, randomized clinical trial comparing bipolar plasma kinetic resection of the prostate versus conventional monopolar transurethral resection of the prostate in the treatment of benign prostatic hyperplasia. *Ann Saudi Med.* 2009, 29(6):429–32.

34 Seckiner I, Yesilli C, Akduman B, Altan K, Mungan NA. A prospective randomized study for comparing bipolar plasmakinetic resection of the prostate with standard TURP. *Urol Int.* 2006; 76(2):139–43.

35 de Sio M, Autorino R, Quarto G, Damiano R, Perdona S, di Lorenzo G, *et al.* Gyrus bipolar versus standard monopolar transurethral resection of the prostate: a randomized prospective trial. *Urology.* 2006;67(1):69–72.

36 Autorino R, Damiano R, Di Lorenzo G, Quarto G, Perdona S, D'Armiento M, *et al.* Four-year outcome of a prospective randomised trial comparing bipolar plasmakinetic and monopolar transurethral resection of the prostate. *Eur Urol.* 2009; 55(4):922–29.

37 Fagerstrom T, Nyman CR, Hahn RG. Complications and clinical outcome 18 months after bipolar and monopolar transurethral resection of the prostate. *J Endourol.* 2011;25(6):1043–1049.

38 Starkman JS, Santucci RA. Comparison of bipolar transurethral resection of the prostate with standard transurethral prostatectomy: shorter stay, earlier catheter removal and fewer complications. *BJU Int.* 2005;95(1):69–71.

39 Xie CY, Zhu GB, Wang XH, Liu XB. Five-year follow-up results of a randomized controlled trial comparing bipolar plasmakinetic and monopolar transurethral resection of the prostate. *Yonsei Med J* 2012;53(4):734–41.

40 Chen Q, Zhang L, Fan QL, Zhou J, Peng YB, Wang Z. Bipolar transurethral resection in saline versus traditional monopolar resection of the prostate: results of a randomized trial with a 2-year follow-up. *BJU Int.* 2010;106(9):1339–43.

41 Ho HS, Yip SK, Lim KB, Fook S, Foo KT, Cheng CW. A prospective randomized study comparing monopolar and bipolar transurethral resection of prostate using transurethral resection in saline (TURIS) system. *Eur Urol.* 2007;52(2):517–22.

Index

Male Lower Urinary Tract Symptoms and Benign Prostatic Hyperplasia, First Edition.
Edited by Steven A. Kaplan and Kevin T. McVary.
© 2014 John Wiley & Sons, Ltd. Published 2014 by John Wiley & Sons, Ltd.